THE CLINICAL CARDIAC ELECTROPHYSIOLOGY HANDBOOK

Jason G. Andrade, MD

Matthew T. Bennett, MD
Marc W. Deyell, MD, MSc
Nathaniel Hawkins, MD
Andrew D. Krahn, MD
Laurent Macle, MD
Stanley Nattel, MD

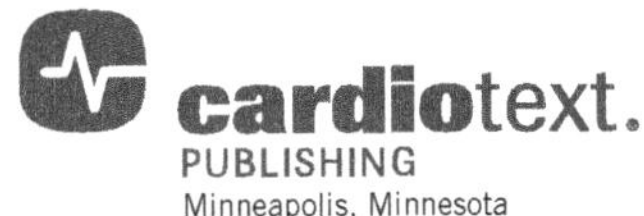

Minneapolis, Minnesota

Cardiotext Publishing, LLC
3405 W. 44th Street
Minneapolis, Minnesota 55410
USA

www.cardiotextpublishing.com

Any updates to this book may be found at:
www.cardiotextpublishing.com/clinical-cardiac-electrophysiology-handbook

Comments, inquiries, and requests for bulk sales can be directed to the publisher at: info@cardiotextpublishing.com.

This book is intended for educational purposes and to further general scientific and medical knowledge, research, and understanding of the conditions and associated treatments discussed herein. This book is not intended to serve as and should not be relied upon as recommending or promoting any specific diagnosis or method of treatment for a particular condition or a particular patient. It is the reader's responsibility to determine the proper steps for diagnosis and the proper course of treatment for any condition or patient, including suitable and appropriate tests, medications, or medical devices to be used for or in conjunction with any diagnosis or treatment.

Due to ongoing research, discoveries, modifications to medicines, equipment and devices, and changes in government regulations, the information contained in this book may not reflect the latest standards, developments, guidelines, regulations, products, or devices in the field. Readers are responsible for keeping up to date with the latest developments and are urged to review the latest instructions and warnings for any medicine, equipment, or medical device. Readers should consult with a specialist or contact the vendor of any medicine or medical device where appropriate.

Except for the publisher's website associated with this work, the publisher is not affiliated with and does not sponsor or endorse any websites, organizations, or other sources of information referred to herein.

The publisher and the author specifically disclaim any damage, liability, or loss incurred, directly or indirectly, from the use or application of any of the contents of this book.

Unless otherwise stated, all figures and tables in this book are used courtesy of the authors.

Library of Congress Control Number: 2015956425

ISBN: 978-1-942909-00-2

Printed in The United States of America
2 3 4 5 6 7 8 9 20 19 18 17

We are extremely grateful to our colleagues and technical staff at the Montreal Heart Institute and Vancouver General Hospital, without whom this book would not have been possible.

For Becky, Amélie, and Noah

CONTENTS

ABOUT THE AUTHORS

Jason G. Andrade, MD
Montreal Heart Institute
Université de Montréal, Montreal, Canada
University of British Columbia, Vancouver, Canada

Contributors

Matthew T. Bennett, MD
University of British Columbia, Vancouver, Canada

Marc W. Deyell, MD, MSc
University of British Columbia, Vancouver, Canada

Nathaniel Hawkins, MD
University of British Columbia, Vancouver, Canada

Andrew D. Krahn, MD
University of British Columbia, Vancouver, Canada

Laurent Macle, MD
Montreal Heart Institute
Université de Montréal, Montreal, Canada

Stanley Nattel, MD
Montreal Heart Institute
Université de Montréal, Montreal, Canada

PREFACE

The clinical science of interventional cardiac electrophysiology is a rapidly evolving area. In the early days, it was referred to as "His bundle electrophysiology," because about the only procedure available was to record the electrical potential arising in the common bundle of His with a catheter electrode and use the results to localize/quantify conduction abnormalities to identify patients needing pacemakers. But a lot has changed since then: Programmed stimulation produced a revolution in the 1970s, followed in the 1980s by ablation and more advanced recording methods (beginning with the recording of potentials from accessory pathways). Progress advanced to include sophisticated invasive and noninvasive mapping systems and complex access and intervention approaches. Implantable devices were introduced as simple right ventricular pacemakers implanted by surgeons, developing over time into implantable defibrillators, and from there to highly sophisticated units capable of complex data recording and acquisition, high levels of programmability and interrogation capacity, complex antitachycardia pacing algorithms combined with intelligent defibrillation maneuvers, and even leadless devices. Basic science advances have revolutionized our understanding of arrhythmia mechanisms and created exciting new therapeutic possibilities. Large, randomized clinical trials have provided solid bases for clinical decision-making.

One consequence of these formidable developments has been the challenging mass of information that needs to be mastered in order to understand and apply clinical cardiac electrophysiology interventions. This volume of knowledge is particularly daunting to trainees and paramedical personnel, who perform vital functions requiring high-level skills but who lack the extensive training, knowledge base, and experience of established clinical electrophysiologists.

This was the reason to create *The Clinical Cardiac Electrophysiology Handbook*: to offer in a succinct presentation all the *practical* information needed to understand the subtleties of a wide range of cardiac electrophysiology problems and approaches. Our focus is on the "how to," with the goal of providing key knowledge about approaches to identify, diagnose, and manage a broad range of cardiac rhythm disorders. However, the user will also find a lot of information on the "why"—the underlying fundamental and clinical science basis for clinical electrophysiology decision-making.

We took the approach that our book should look like what you might expect to find if a brilliant clinical electrophysiology fellow had transcribed notes about all that he or she was taught and was able to obtain from the literature, including all the most important information without any filler in between. It is intended to be a quick source for information in the EP lab or on the wards, as well as a guide to learning—offering the ability to quickly review the essential components prior to a case or to rapidly reinforce new notions and practices encountered during a case.

Overall, we hope users will find that *The Clinical Cardiac Electrophysiology Handbook* constitutes a valuable new tool, occupying an important niche that was largely empty prior to its completion and offering readers a key contribution to the learning material in this area.

—Stanley Nattel, MD

ABBREVIATIONS

A	atrial
AAD	antiarrhythmic drug
ABG	arterial blood gasses
ACI	average complex interval
ACLS	advanced cardiac life support
ACT	activated clotting time
AD	autosomal dominant
AEAT	automatic ectopic atrial tachycardia
AERP	atrial effective refractory period
AF	atrial fibrillation
AFL	atrial flutter
AMVL	anterior mitral valve leaflet
AP	accessory pathway
APD	action potential duration
APERP	accessory pathway effective refractory period
ARP	atrial refractory period
ARVC	arrhythmogenic right ventricular cardiomyopathy
AS	aortic stenosis
ASA	apirin
ASD	atrial septal defect
ASH	asymmetric septal hypertrophy
AT	atrial tachycardia
ATP	anti-tachycardia pacing
AV	atrioventricular
AVBCL	atrioventricular block cycle length
AVD	atrioventricular delay
AVN	atrioventricular node

AVNERP	atrioventricular node effective refractory period
AVNRT	atrioventricular nodal reentrant tachycardia
AVRT	atrioventricular reciprocating tachycardia
BB	β-blocker (beta-blocker)
BBB	bundle branch block
BC	blood culture
BCL	basic cycle length
BBR-VT	bundle branch reentrant-venous tachycardia
BNP	brain natriuretic peptide
BSA	body surface area
CAD	coronary arterial disease
CBC	complete blood count
CCB	calcium-channel blockers
CCS-SAF	Canadian Cardiovascular Society (CCS) Severity of Atrial Fibrillation (SAF)
CFAE	complex fractionated atrial electrogram
CHF	congestive heart failure
CIED	cardiac implantable electronic devices
CL	cycle length
CMC	circular mapping catheter
CMR	cardiovascular magnetic resonance
CO	cardiac output
COPD	Chronic obstructive pulmonary disease
cPPI	corrected post-pacing interval
CPVT	catecholaminergic polymorphic ventricular tachycardia
Cr	creatinine
CRT	Cardiac Resynchronization Therapy
CS	coronary sinus
CSNRT	corrected sinus node recovery time
CTI	cavotricuspid isthmus
DAD	delayed afterdepolarization
DAP	decremental atrial pacing
DCCV	direct-current cardioversion
DCM	dilated cardiomyopathy
dCS	distal coronary sinus
DFT	defibrillator threshold testing

DI diabetes insipidus
DSM dynamic substrate mapping
DVT deep vein thrombosis

EAD early afterdepolarization
EAM electroanatomic mapping
EAT atrial ectopic (unifocal) tachycardia
EC extracellular
ECG electrocardiogram
EDV end diastolic volume
EF ejection fraction
eGFR estimated glomerular filtration rate
EGM electrogram
EHRA European Heart Rhythm Association
EP electrophysiology
EPS electrophysiology study
ERAT early recurrence of atrial tachyarrhythmias
ERI elective replacement indicator
ERP effective refractory period
ESC European Society of Cardiology
ESV end systolic volume

FAT focal atrial tachyarrthmia
FPERP Fast Pathway Effective Refractory Period
fQRS filtered QRS
FRP functional refractory period

GA general anesthesia

HB His Bundle
HBE His bundle EGM
HCM hypertrophic cardiomyopathy
HF heart failure
HPS His-Purkinje system
HRA high right atrial/high right atrium
H-RB-LB His-right bundle-left bundle
HR heart rate
HRT heart rate turbulence

HRV	heart rate variability
HTLS	high thoracic left sympathectomy
HTN	hypertension
IART	intraatrial reentrant tachycardia
IC	intracellular
ICD	implantable cardioverter-defibrillator
ICE	intracardiac echocardiography
ICH	intracranial hemorrhage
ICL	Interval Confidence Level
IHR	intrinsic heart rate
ILR	insertable loop recorder
INR	International normalized ratio
IST	inappropriate sinus tachycardia
IV	intravenous, intravenously
IVCD	intraventricular conduction delay
JET	junctional ectopic tachycardia
JT	junctional tachycardia
JVP	jugular venous pressure
LAA	left atrial appendage
LAC	local activation time
LACA	left atrial circumferential ablation
LAD	left anterior descending (artery)
LAO	left anterior oblique
LAS	low-amplitude signal
LAT	local activation time
LAVD	long arteriovenous delay
LB	left bundle
LBB	left bundle branch
LBBB	left bundle branch block
LCSD	left cardiac sympathetic denervation
LCX	left circumflex artery
LDAC	left-dominant arrhythmogenic cardiomyopathy
LGE	late gadolinium enhancement
LIPV	left inferior pulmonary vein
LLSB	left lower sternal border
LOC	loss of consciousness

LQT	long QT
LQTS	long QT syndrome
LRL	lower rate limit
LSPV	left superior pulmonary vein
LV	left ventricle, left ventricular
LVEF	left ventricle ejection fraction
LVH	left ventricular hypertrophy
LVOT	left ventricular outflow tract
LVSD	left ventricle systolic dysfunction
MAAC	Multi-Array Ablation Catheter
MAD	mean absolute deviation
MAP	mean arterial pressure
MASC	Multi-Array Septal Catheter
MAT	multifocal atrial tachyarrhythmia
MDMA	3,4-methylenedioxy-methamphetamine
MDP	mid-diastolic potential
MEA	multi-electrode array
MI	myocardial infarction
MIBG	meta-iodobenzylguanidine
MRAT	macroreentrant atrial tachycardia
MRI	magnetic resonance imaging
MRSA	Methicillin-resistant *Staphylococcus aureus*
MS	mitral stenosis
ms	millisecond
MV	mitral valve
MVA	mitral valve area
MVC	mitral valve closure
MVP	mitral valve prolapse
NAFAT	non-automatic focal atrial tachycardia
NCT	narrow-complex tachycardia
NCX	Na^+/Ca^{2+} exchange
ND-CCB	non-dihydropyridine calcium-channel blocker
NIDCM	non-ischemic dilated cardiomyopathy
NPV	negative predictive value
NSR	normal sinus rhythm
NSTEMI	non-ST segment-elevation MI
NSVT	non-sustained ventricular tachycardia

OAC	oral anticoagulant
ORT	orthodromic reentrant tachycardia
OS	ostium
P1	late diastolic Purkinje potential
P2	pre-systolic Purkinje potential
PA	pulmonary artery
PAC	premature atrial contraction
PAVPB	post-atrial ventricular blanking period
pCS	proximal coronary sinus
PE	pulmonary embolism
PEA	pulseless electrical activity
PEI	pre-excitement index
PET	positron emission tomography
PFO	patent foramen ovale
PIP	pill-in-the-pocket
PLAX	parasternal long axis
PMT	pacemaker-mediated tachycardia
PMVT	polymorphic ventricular tachycardia
POTS	postural orthostatic tachycardia syndrome
PPI	post-pacing interval
PPI – TCL	post-pacing interval – tachycardia cycle length
PPV	positive pressure ventilation
PS	pulmonary stenosis
PSAX	parasternal short-axis
PSNS	parasympathetic nervous system
PSVT	paroxysmal supraventricular tachycardia
PV	pulmonary vein
PVABP	post-ventricular atrial blanking period (a.k.a., far-field blanking)
PVAC	Pulmonary Vein Ablation Catheter
PVARP	post-ventricular atrial refractory period
PVC	premature ventricular contraction
PVD	peripheral vascular disease
PVI	pulmonary vein isolation
PVP	pulmonary vein potentials
QOL	quality of life
QTc	corrected QT interval

RA	right atrial, right atrium
RAO	right anterior oblique
RB	right bundle
RBB	right bundle branch
RBBB	right bundle branch block
RCA	right coronary artery
RCM	restrictive cardiomyopathy
RF	radiofrequency
RIPV	right inferior pulmonary vein
RR	relative risk
RRP	relative refractory period
RRR	relative risk reduction
RSPV	right superior pulmonary vein
RV	right ventricle, right ventricular
RVa	right ventricular apex
RVEDV	right ventricular end-diastolic volume
RVEF	right ventricular ejection fraction
RVH	right ventricular hypertrophy
RVOT	right ventricular outflow tract
SA	sinoatrial
SACT	sinoatrial conduction time
SAECG	signal averaged ECG
SAM	systolic anterior motion
SAVD	short arteriovenous delay
SCD	sudden cardiac death
SCI	shortest complex interval
SEM	systolic ejection murmurs
SN	sinus node
SND	sinus node dysfunction
SNRT	sinus node reentrant tachycardia / sinus node recovery time
SNS	sympathetic nervous system
SPERRI	shortest pre-excited RR interval
SR	sustained release
SSRIs	selective serotonin reuptake inhibitors
ST	sinus tachycardia
Staph	*Staphylococcus*
STEMI	ST segment elevation MI

SVC	superior vena cava
SVT	supraventricular tachycardia
TARP	total atrial refractory period
TCA	tricyclic antidepressant
TCL	tachycardia cycle length
TEE	transesophageal echocardiography
TFC	thoracic fluid content
TIA	transient ischemic attack
TRT	total recovery time
TSH	thyroid stimulating hormone
TTE	transthoracic echocardiogram
TV	tricuspid valve
TVA	tricuspid valve annuloplasty
TVAC	tip versatile ablation catheter
TWA	T-wave alternans
URL	upper rate limit (pacemaker)
V	ventrical
VA	ventriculoatrial
VBP	ventricular blanking period
VERP	ventricular refractory period
VF	ventricular fibrillation
VPB	ventricular premature beat
VRP	ventricular refractory period
VSD	ventricular septal defect
VT	ventricular tachycardia
VUS	variants of unknown significance
WBC	white blood cell
WCL	Wenckebach cycle length
WCT	wide-complex tachycardia
WMA	wall motion abnormality
WPW	Wolff-Parkinson-White syndrome

CHAPTER

1

Fundamentals

THE CARDIAC ACTION POTENTIAL

Myocardial tissue contains 5 main properties that integrate the electrical and mechanical activity.

- **Automaticity**: The ability of a cell/tissue to initiate an impulse or stimulus. In the absence of external stimulation, the pacemaker cells spontaneously depolarize. This property generates sinus rhythm at a rate appropriate to the body's needs.
- **Excitability**: The ability of a cell/tissue to respond to an impulse or stimulus. Myocardial cells respond to the impulse generated by the pacemaker cells of the cardiac conduction system through depolarization and repolarization.
- **Conductivity**: The ability of a cell or tissue to transmit impulses to other areas. While conductivity is much more efficient in the conduction system, the cells in the conduction system and the myocardium also have this property.
- **Refractoriness**: The property that governs the time following excitation until the tissue can be re-excited. This property prevents tissue from being re-excited too soon after the previous excitation, thereby protecting against dangerously rapid rates and reentrant arrhythmias.
- **Contractility**: The ability of a cell or tissue to respond to electrical stimulation with mechanical action.

The "Fast-Channel" Cardiac Action Potential

Characteristic of action potentials found in the atrial and ventricular myocardium, as well as the rapidly conducting His-Purkinje system—consisting of the bundle of His, right and left bundle branches, fascicular Purkinje cells, and endocardial Purkinje-cell conduction system.

These action potentials have a true resting potential, a rapid depolarization phase, and a prolonged plateau phase.

The Clinical Cardiac Electrophysiology Handbook © 2016 Jason Andrade.
Cardiotext Publishing, ISBN: 978-1-942909-00-2.

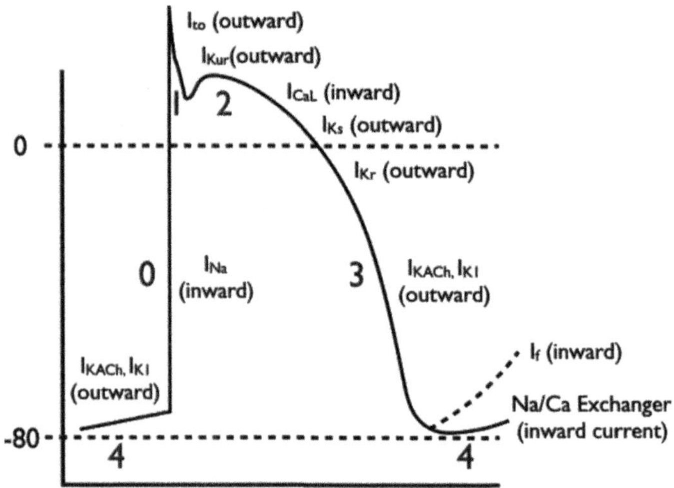

Depolarization

When the cardiac muscle cell is stimulated, the cell undergoes an electrical event called depolarization.

- **Phase 0: Rapid depolarization phase ("upstroke")**
  - With stimulation, the fast sodium (Na) channels are activated, resulting in a rapid increase in sodium membrane conductance (G_{Na}) and/or rapid influx of sodium ions (I_{Na}) into the cell.
  - The entry of positively charged sodium ions produces a rapid change in the electrical charge of the interior of the cell, providing the energy for rapid impulse propagation (conduction velocity of ~1 m/s).

Repolarization

Almost immediately after depolarization, the inactivation of the fast sodium channels arrests Na^+ movement into the cell, allowing the cell to initiate the restoration of its (inactive) resting state.

- **Phase 1: Early repolarization**
  The early repolarization phase starts with the opening of rapid, outward potassium current (I_{to}). This currents result in rapid repolarization to about 0 mV (with time-dependent inactivation).
- **Phase 2: "Plateau" phase**
  A "stable" membrane potential is observed resulting from a balance of the inward movement of calcium through L-type calcium channels ($I_{Ca,L}$) and the outward movement of K^+ through the delayed rectifier (rapid and slow components: I_{Kr} and I_{Ks}) and the inward rectifier (I_{K1}) potassium channels. The sodium–calcium exchange current ($I_{Na/Ca}$) and the sodium–potassium pump current ($I_{Na/K}$) also play minor roles in the maintenance of the current, and major roles in the maintenance of physiological intracellular sodium, potassium, and calcium concentrations.
- **Phase 3: Rapid repolarization at the conclusion of the plateau phase**
  Initially, the net negative change in membrane potential is driven by the inactivation of L-type Ca channels. The rapid delayed rectifier K^+ channel (I_{Kr}) and inwardly rectifying K^+ current (I_{K1}) activate, causing a more rapid net outward current, causing the cell to repolarize to baseline. This phase governs refractoriness

by controlling action potential duration (APD). I_{Na} is inactivated at voltages positive to –60 mV, so following the phase 0 upstroke, the cell cannot be reactivated until it returns to –60 mV during phase 3. The APD to –60 mV determines the "effective refractory period" (ERP) of fast-channel tissue.

- **Phase 4: Resting phase**
  The resting phase constitutes a steady, stable, polarized membrane (~–90 mV in working myocardial cells). When membrane potential is restored to baseline, the delayed rectifier K^+ channels close. Voltage-regulated inward rectifiers (I_{K1}) remain open, regulating resting membrane potential.

Ventricular Action Potential

Compared to the atrium, the ventricular action potential has a:

- Longer duration
- Higher phase 2 (absent I_{Kur})
- Shorter phase 3, with faster repolarization

Action Potential of the His-Purkinje System

Compared to the myocardium, the action potential of the **His-Purkinje system** displays the following differences:

- More prominent early (phase 1) repolarization
- Longer plateau phase (phase 2)
- Automaticity: Spontaneous, phase 4 depolarization

The "Slow-Channel" Cardiac Action Potential

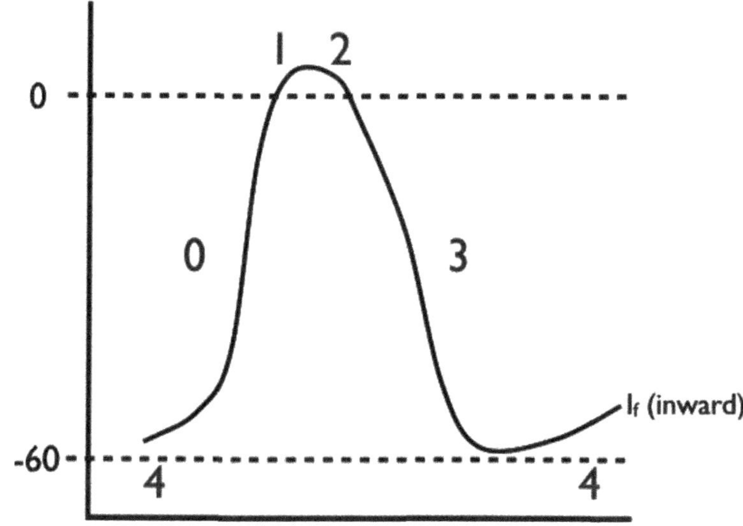

Characteristic of action potentials found in the sinoatrial (SA) and atrioventricular (AV) nodes. The key features of these action potentials are the property of automaticity, as well as the fact that the depolarization phase is slower, and with a shorter APD than "fast-channel" action potentials.

- **Phase 0: Rapid depolarization phase ("upstroke")**
  This phase is slower (conduction velocity of ~0.02 to 0.05 m/s) due to a smaller inward current that governs activation (generated by $I_{Ca,L}$, rather than I_{Na}).
- **Phase 1: Early repolarization phase**
  Early repolarization is not perceptible in slow-channel tissue, because I_{to} is small and partially inactivated by the relatively positive resting potential.
- **Phase 2: "Plateau" phase**
  In principle, this phase is similar to that of fast-channel tissue, except that because of the small phase 0 current, the transitions from phase 0 to phase 1 and subsequently to phase 2 are much less defined.
- **Phase 3: Rapid repolarization at the conclusion of the plateau phase**
  This phase has similar ionic mechanisms to fast-channel phase 3. Because $I_{Ca,L}$ is smaller and recovers much more slowly than I_{Na}, the main factor determining ERP in slow-channel tissue is slow, time-dependent recovery of $I_{Ca,L}$. Therefore, unlike fast-channel tissue, APD is not the main determinant of ERP and changes in APD have relatively little effect on ERP. The time-dependent recovery of $I_{Ca,L}$ results in reduced current at fast rates, greatly limiting the maximum follow frequency of the AVN. This is an important protective property that prevents excessively rapid ventricular rates during very rapid supraventricular tachyarrhythmias like atrial flutter (AFL) and atrial fibrillation (AF).
- **Phase 4: "Resting" phase**
  Automaticity results from the combination of: (1) spontaneous diastolic depolarization due to phase 4 I_f (a poorly selective, inward current carried mainly by Na and activating upon repolarization), activation of T-type Ca^{2+} current ($I_{Ca,T}$), and inactivation of delayed rectifier K^+ currents; and (2) the maximum negative "resting" potential ("maximum diastolic potential" or MDP) being closer to the depolarization threshold (–50 to –60 mV vs. –80 mV for fast-channel potentials). As a result, the SA node acts as the predominent cardiac pacemaker, with the AVN acting as the primary backup "escape" if the SA node fails.

ARRHYTHMIA MECHANISMS

General Classification of Arrhythmia Mechanisms

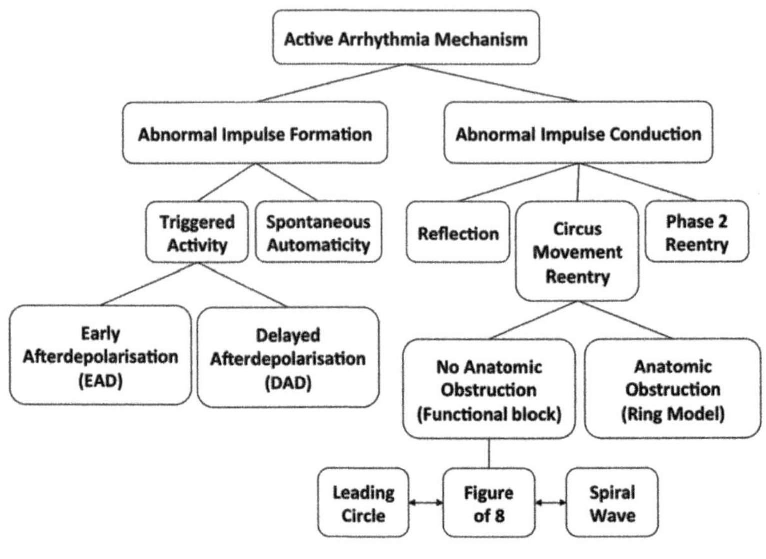

Table 1.1 Characteristics of Arrhythmia Mechanisms

		Focal		
	Macroreentry	Microreentry	Triggered Activity	Automaticity
Initiation by programmed stimulation	Yes	Yes	Yes	No
Termination by programmed stimulation	Yes (Abrupt)	Yes	Yes (Gradual)	No (Transient suppression)
Resetting	Yes	Yes	Yes	Yes
Entrainment	Yes	Yes	No	No
Site specificity of entrainment	Yes	Yes	No	No
Overdrive suppression	No	No	Yes	Yes
Overdrive acceleration	Yes	Yes	Yes	No
Adenosine sensitivity	No	No	Yes (Terminates)	No (Transient suppression)
Catecholamine sensitivity	Maybe	Maybe	Yes	Yes
Activation recorded throughout the cycle	100%	100% (50% local EGM)	<50%	<50%
Size	>2 atrial segments	≤2 atrial segments	1 atrial segment	1 atrial segment
Ablation target	Bidirectional block across critical isthmus	Origin		

Altered Impulse Formation

Automaticity

The ability of a cell to depolarize itself to threshold and spontaneously generate an action potential.

- Driven by spontaneous, phase 4 depolarization in the absence of external stimulation.
- May be influenced by neurohormonal (sympathetic and parasympathetic) input.
- While all cardiac tissues can initiate depolarization, only certain cell or tissue types routinely possess this pacemaker function (in ascending order of importance):
  - Sinus node
  - Specialized atrial cells, such as the AVN
  - Bundle of His
  - Right and left bundle branches
  - Fascicular Purkinje cells
  - Ventricular endocardial Purkinje conduction system
- **Abnormal automaticity** (accelerated phase 4 upslope) can lead to extrasystoles or sustained tachyarrhythmias.
  - Most often these arrhythmias are due to metabolic causes:
    - Acute ischemia or hypoxia
    - Myocardial stretch
    - Electrolyte abnormalities (hypoxemia, hypokalemia, hypomagnesemia, acid-base disorders)
    - High sympathetic tone
  - **Arrhythmias arising from abnormal automaticity**
    - May exhibit a rate increase at onset ("warm-up") or a rate decrease at termination ("cool-down").
    - They generally cannot be induced by pacing, and therefore are not amenable to provocative electrophysiology (EP) testing.

Triggered Activity

Refers to a situation where heart tissue is stimulated once, but the stimulus results in the production of more than one conducted beat.

- Arrhythmias can have features characteristic for automaticity and reentry.
  - **Automaticity:** A new action potential can be generated by the leakage of positive ions into the cell.
    - The arrhythmia displays typical warm-up and cool-down and may respond to calcium- or sodium-channel blockers.
  - **Reentry** can be induced by premature beats and programmed pacing.
    - In contrast to typical reentry, the induction of triggered activity may require the introduction of a pause into the pacing sequence ("pause-dependent" arrhythmias).

- The two most common forms of triggered activity are:
  - **Early afterdepolarization (EAD)**, which occurs **before** complete cellular repolarization.
    - EADs result from the reactivation of $I_{Ca,L}$ and/or spontaneous Ca^{2+} release from the sarcoplasmic reticulum (SR).
    - Plateau EAD occurs during phase 2.
    - Late EADs occur during phase 3 and are caused by reactivation of I_{Na} or spontaneous Ca^{2+} release from the SR.
  - **Delayed afterdepolarization (DAD)** occurs **after** complete repolarization of the cell during phase 4 of the action potential.
    - DAD is caused by intracellular Ca^{2+} overload or RyR2 dysfunction, with spontaneous release of Ca^{2+} from the SR resulting in a depolarizing current via Na^{+}/Ca^{2+} exchange (NCX) current. When extruding excess Ca^{2+} from inside the cell, NCX-mediated efflux of 1 calcium ion in exchange for 3 sodium ions results in membrane depolarization during the diastolic interval.

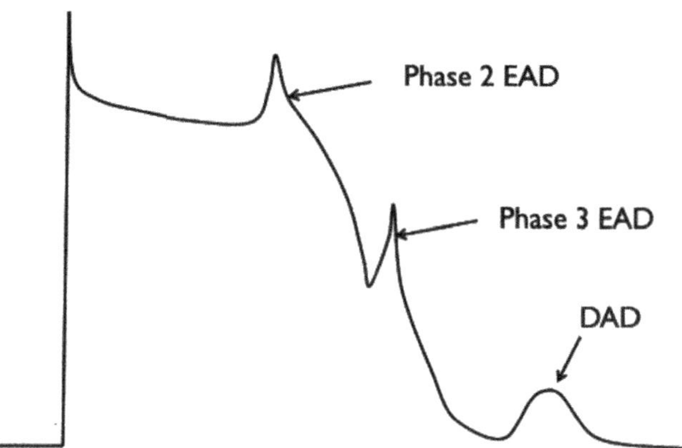

Altered Impulse Conduction

Reentry

Inhomogeneous conduction results in reentry of an impulse into an area that was just depolarized and has since repolarized.

- Requires 2 discrete parallel conducting "pathways" that:
  - Connect proximally and distally
  - Are separated by a barrier
    - Anatomic: Valve, vessel, scar
    - Functional: A central core that is either continuously depolarized by centripetal waves (leading circle) or excitable, but not excited (spiral wave)
  - Contain different electrophysiologic properties
    - One of the pathways must have a refractory period substantially longer than the refractory period of the other ("fast" β pathway), and the pathway with the shorter refractory period must conduct electrical impulses more slowly than the other pathway ("slow" α pathway).

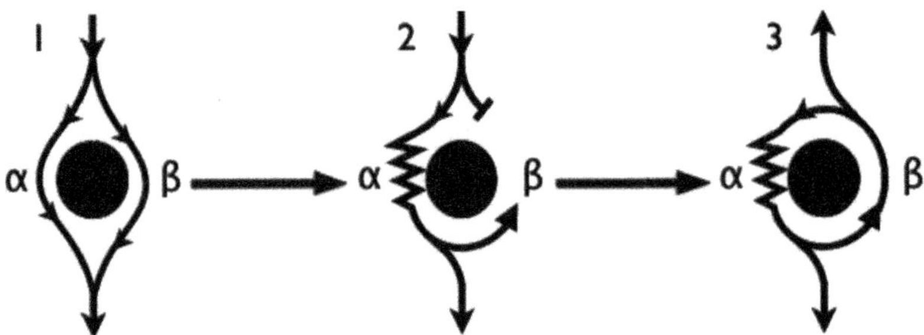

- **Mechanism of reentry** (anatomical)
  - In sinus rhythm, the wavefront depolarizes both pathways simultaneously (**Panel 1**).
  - An event (i.e., atrial or ventricular extrasystole) exposes the presence of the pathways due to their differing conduction velocity and recovery.
    - Premature impulse enters the circuit when the β (fast) pathway is refractory and at a time when the α (slow) pathway has recovered and is able to accept the impulse (**Panel 2**).
    - While the α pathway slowly conducts the impulse, the β pathway has the chance to recover.
    - By the time the impulse reaches the distal end of the α pathway, the β pathway has recovered and is able to conduct retrograde back up to the atria (echo beat: **Panel 3**).
    - If the α (slow) pathway has recovered, then the impulse can reenter the α (slow) pathway and initiate a circular impulse movement arrhythmia.
  - Note: There is no single point of origin of activation.
    - Reentrant activation can be recorded throughout the entire cycle length (CL); a point of earliest activity does not exist.
    - Atrial myocardium surrounding the circuit is activated from various parts of the circuit.

Terminology of Reentry

- **Cycle length**: Time required for depolarization to complete the circuit and return to its spatial origin
- **Wavelength**: The minimum path length that can support reentry
  - Wavelength is the product of the **conduction velocity** and the **refractory period** (the shortest coupling interval that captures the reentrant circuit).
- **Temporal excitable gap**: The time interval during the CL when the circuit may be "excited"
  - The temporal excitable gap is the difference between the CL and the refractory period.
- **Spatial excitable gap**: The spatial distance within the circuit that is excitable
  - The spatial excitable gap is the difference between the total circuit distance and the wavelength.

Classification of Reentry

- **Microreentry**: A reentry circuit too small to be seen on the surface electrocardiogram (ECG) (e.g., atrioventricular nodal reentry tachycardia [AVNRT])
- **Macroreentry**: A reentry circuit large enough to be seen on the surface ECG (e.g., AFL)

ENTRAINMENT

Demonstration of entrainment is proof that an arrhythmia is due to a reentrant circuit with an excitable gap between the tail of one wavefront and the head of the next.

- A reentrant tachycardia may be reset by premature extrastimuli.
- If a train of pacing stimuli is delivered with a pacing CL shorter than the tachycardia cycle length (TCL), the tachycardia may be continuously reset with each successive pacing stimulus.
    - Continuous resetting is called entrainment.
    - Entrainment is present when at least two consecutive stimuli are conducted orthodromically through the circuit with the same conduction time.

Criteria of Entrainment

- There is constant fusion at a pacing rate and the last beat is entrained but not fused.
    - Pattern of activation represents a combination of pacing and tachycardia.
    - When pacing is terminated, the last paced beat is early (entrained) but propagates around the circuit (activation pattern similar to spontaneous arrhythmia).
- There is progressive fusion as the pacing rate increases:
    - At a pacing CL just short of the tachycardia, there is minimal invasion of the circuit and activation mainly resembles the spontaneous tachycardia (fusion).
    - With progressive shortening of the pacing CL, the circuit is invaded to a greater extent, leading to an alteration in activation closer to that of pacing.
- Tachycardia interruption is accompanied by a block to a recording site, followed by activation at the same site from a different direction.
- There is demonstration of a change in conduction time and electrogram (EGM) morphology at one recording site when pacing from another site at 2 different constant pacing rates, each of which is faster than the spontaneous rate of tachycardia but fails to interrupt it.

Uses of Entrainment

- Proves the arrhythmia mechanism is reentry
    - Note: Entrainment does not prove that the pacing site is within the circuit, because if the excitable gap is large, then entrainment can be achieved by pacing at a large distance from the circuit.
- Indicates the location is part of the reentrant circuit
- May also indicate a good site for ablation (i.e., concealed fusion with latency and good post-pacing interval [PPI])

Entrainment and Specific Arrhythmias

- AFL
    - Entrainment of the cavotricuspid isthmus (CTI) is important to show it is part of the circuit.
- Supraventricular tachycardia (SVT)
    - Ventricular entrainment is useful to distinguish atrial tachycardia (AT) (a VAAV response) from AVNRT/atrioventricular reciprocating tachycardia (AVRT) (a VAV response).
    - His synchronous VPBs may reset AVRT but not AVNRT.

- Ventricular tachycardia (VT)
  - Entrainment mapping is used to complement activation mapping, substrate mapping, and pace mapping.
  - The diastolic pathway is a target for ablation and may be identified by concealed entrainment with latency and a PPI-TCL of <30 ms.

RESETTING

The Physiologic Basis of Entrainment

- During sustained arrhythmia, a premature impulse may enter the excitable gap of the circuit before dividing into two wavefronts:
  - Antidromic/retrograde wavefront (opposite in direction to the reentrant tachycardia), which collides with the preceding tachycardia wavefront
  - Anterograde/orthodromic wavefront, which conducts through the reentrant circuit and exits at an earlier time (compared to the next expected beat of the tachycardia)
- Resetting is defined as:
  - The advancement of the tachycardia by at least 20 ms
  - The return tachycardia has the same activation/morphology and CL
  - The premature impulse should find the excitable gap and invade the reentrant circuit

Post-pacing Interval (PPI)

- The return CL as measured from the last stimulus to the return EGM in the pacing electrode
- Represents the time taken for the impulse to travel from the pacing site to the tachycardia circuit, around the circuit, and back to the pacing site
  - An in-circuit response is defined as a PPI of less than 30 ms.
- Note:
  - The range of coupling intervals from onset of resetting to arrhythmia termination reflects the duration of the excitable gap.
  - Resetting response may be characterized by plotting the return CL against the coupling intervals.
    - Flat, increasing (increasing return cycles with decreasing coupling intervals), or mixed flat and increasing curves are typical for reentrant tachycardia.
    - Flat or decreasing curves may be seen with triggered activity.
    - Flat response may be seen with automatic tachycardia.
  - Pacing from different sites may affect the resetting response in a reentrant tachycardia.
    - Site specificity of resetting is not a feature of automaticity or triggered activity.

FUSION

Two wavefronts of activation (one from the pacing stimulus and one from the exit of the reentrant circuit) occur at the same time, resulting in a QRS morphology, P-wave morphology, or activation sequence that is an intermediate of the two wavefronts (fully paced and reentrant tachycardia).

- Manifest fusion (or fusion that is evident on ECG) requires:
  - There is a significant degree of dissimilarity between the paced rhythm and the reentrant tachycardia.
  - A significant proportion of the myocardium is activated by both wavefronts (i.e., enough to alter the ECG).
  - A pacing CL is short enough to reset the tachycardia.
- **Local fusion** is the resetting of the tachycardia. The local EGM within the circuit is unchanged in morphology, and there is no apparent ECG fusion.
- **Concealed fusion** occurs when the pacing site is within the circuit (or a bystander), resulting in orthodromic conduction within the circuit before exiting the normal site (hence P/QRS morphology is unchanged).

LEFT-SIDED ACCESS: TRANSAORTIC AND TRANSSEPTAL APPROACH

Table 1.2 Transaortic (Retrograde) vs. Transseptal (Anterograde) Approaches

	Benefit	Drawback
Transaortic	Avoids risks of transseptal puncture Easier access to left posteroseptal space	**Unstable** in anterolateral or lateral region Risk of coronary artery or aortic valve damage
Transseptal	Easier catheter manipulation Pre-shaped sheaths permit stable mapping and ablation Easier access to anterolateral or lateral space	Difficult to access left posteroseptal space

Transaortic (Retrograde) Approach

- **Complications**
  - Aortic or aortic valve damage
  - Coronary artery injury, myocardial infarction
  - Embolism (aortic atheroma): Stroke, peripheral embolization
- **Contraindications**
  - Significant peripheral vascular disease
  - Significant aortic valve disease or replacement surgery
- **Procedure**
  - The catheter is advanced to the aortic valve in right anterior oblique (RAO) projection.
  - Catheter is tightly curved in the posterior direction and prolapsed through the aortic valve.
  - Once the left ventricle (LV) is entered, the "J" curve of the catheter is rotated counterclockwise to turn the tip posteriorly toward the mitral annulus.
  - The curve should then be opened to engage the sub-annular area.
  - The ideal positioning is achieved through:
    - Slight catheter movements in the annulus-engaged position
    - Repeated advancement, flexion, torque, and then reengagement

Transseptal (Anterograde) Approach

- **Complications**
  - Pericardial effusion or tamponade
  - Aortic root or pulmonary artery puncture
  - Right atrial (RA) or left atrial (LA) wall needle puncture
  - Pleuritic chest pain
  - Embolism: Stroke, myocardial infarction, peripheral embolization
  - Persistent atrial septal defect
    - Potential for right to left shunting associated with stroke and migraine
  - Transient ST segment elevation in the inferior ECG leads with or without chest pain (0.6% of cases):
    - Due to (1) coronary air embolism or (2) vagal response (mechanical disruption of the autonomic network by the transseptal apparatus)
- **Anatomy**
  - The true interatrial septum is relatively small
    - Makes up only a small part of the medial RA wall
  - Anatomic relations of the interatrial septum (clockwise)
    - Superior: Superior vena cava (SVC)
    - Antero-superior: Aortic root (non-coronary sinus)
    - Anterior: Triangle of Koch and septal tricuspid annulus
    - Antero-inferior: Coronary sinus (CS) ostium
    - Inferior: Inferior vena cava
    - Postero-superior: Pulmonary artery (PA)

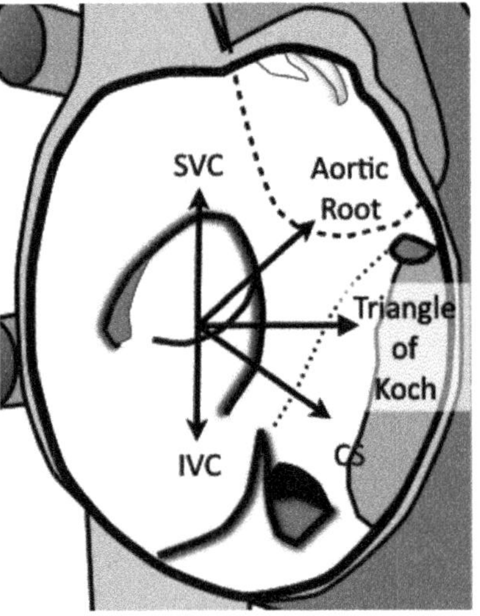

- **Equipment**
  - Needle (standard length 71 cm): BRK-1, BRK-0, or BRK-2 mechanical needle, radiofrequency (RF) needle
  - Sheath (standard sheath length 63 cm, dilator length 67 cm): SL0 or SL1
  - Pressure line: To monitor LA pressure (vs. aortic or pulmonary artery pressure)
- **Procedure**
  - Aortic anatomic reference markers are placed according to operator preference.
    - **Direct reference**: Retrograde placement of a pigtail catheter in the aortic root
    - **Indirect reference**: The bundle of His typically lies adjacent to the aortic root
  - Transseptal sheath and dilator are advanced over a 135-cm 0.032–0.035 J-tipped wire placed into the SVC.
  - The guidewire is removed and the apparatus' lumen is aspirated and flushed with heparinized saline.
  - The transseptal needle is then introduced under fluoroscopic guidance (to avoid SVC injury).
  - After removal of the stylet the transseptal needle is aspirated and attached to a pressure transducer.

- The entire transseptal apparatus (needle-sheath-dilator) is then fixed together.
  - The needle held in the fingers of the right hand
  - The sheath and dilator assembly held with the left hand
- With fluoroscopy in the left anterior oblique (LAO) projection (30°), the transseptal assembly is rotated clockwise (posteromedial to approximately ~4–5 o'clock) and withdrawn smoothly from the SVC to the RA.
- While continuously observing the catheter under fluoroscopy, two distinct "jumps" should be noted:
  - The first will be the catheter falling into the RA from the SVC.
  - The second is seen as the catheter falls from the muscular intra-atrial septum into the fossa ovalis.
- In the fossa ovalis, the transseptal apparatus should be gently advanced.
  - If the apparatus is in the correct position, it will catch the lip of the fossa.
  - If the needle does not catch the lip of the fossa ovalis and slides back into the superior RA, then the whole assembly should be rotated slightly clockwise or counterclockwise and withdrawn from SVC to RA again.
- As the transseptal apparatus abuts the interatrial septum, the pressure tracing should demonstrate a transition from RA pressure to progressive damping.
- **Confirmation of position should be done in the LAO and RAO projections.**

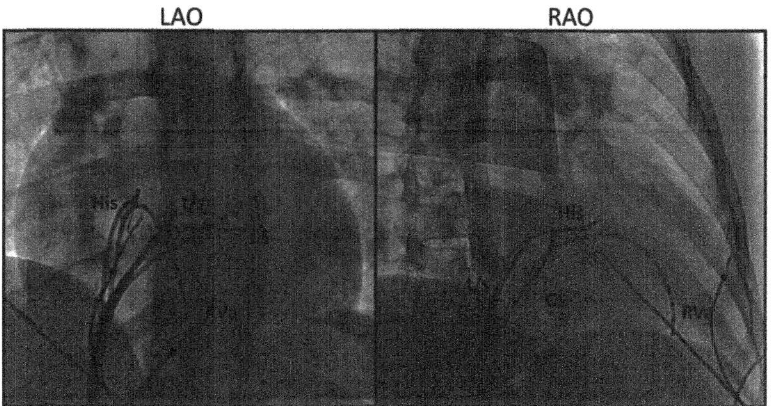

- LAO:
  - The apparatus should lie:
    - Superior to the proximal CS
    - Inferior and rightward of aortic marker
- RAO:
  - The apparatus should lie:
    - Parallel to the CS
    - Posterior to the CS and aortic marker

- Once position is confirmed, transseptal puncture should be performed in the LAO projection.
  - With the transseptal sheath and dilator fixed by the operator's left hand, the needle should be advanced out of the sheath by the operator's right hand.
  - A pop may be felt as the needle passes through the fossa into the left atrium (LA).
- Before advancing the dilator or sheath across, it is critical to be sure the needle is in the LA.
  - **Pressure tracing**: Should demonstrate LA pressure.
    - Note: An atrial pressure tracing may be seen with a pericardial puncture.

- **Arterial blood**: Bright red blood should be freely withdrawn from the transseptal needle.
  - Note: Arterial blood may be withdrawn from the aorta but the pressure tracing differs, pericardial puncture should not have any return, and if the needle is in the RA or PA the blood will be darker.
- **Contrast injection**: Contrast injection into the LA may delineate LA anatomy and confirm placement.
  - Note: Contrast should flow inferiorly from the LA to the LV; suspect aortic puncture with superior flow.
- **Echocardiographic visualization**
  - Direct visualization of the sheath in the fossa and subsequently the LA. Saline flushing via the sheath results in LA bubbles.

- If there is any doubt about transseptal position, then the needle should be withdrawn and the process restarted.
- Once position is confirmed, the needle is fixed in position with the right hand and the dilator and sheath are advanced slightly into the LA with the left hand.
  - The give as the dilator crosses the septum is felt and observed on fluoroscopy.
- The needle and dilator are then fixed in position with the right hand and the sheath advanced into the LA with the left hand.
  - If a pressure transducer has been attached throughout, then LA pressure should be seen when both the dilator and sheath are advanced.
  - Loss of LA pressure suggests either that the apparatus is against the back wall of the LA or that it has prolapsed back into the RA.
- Finally, the dilator and needle are gently withdrawn.
  - The transseptal sheath is then aspirated via the side arm (to ensure no air bubbles) and then connected to a continuously flushing pressure line.

- **Dealing with the difficult transseptal**
  - **Anterior fossa**
    - A fossa located closer to 3 o'clock rather than 4–5 o'clock confers a higher risk of aortic perforation.
    - Access may be safely facilitated by echocardiographic guidance.
  - **Tough septum**
    - Due to puncture of the muscular septum or a fibrosed septum (e.g., from previous transseptal previous punctures).
    - Access may be facilitated by RF or two-part Endrys needle.
  - **Sheath slides up and down the septum freely**
    - Access may be facilitated by positioning the sheath 0.5 cm below the usual anatomic reference. Once in place, the needle can be advanced out of the sheath and the entire apparatus gently advanced.
    - With the needle out, it should catch the septum and puncture; however, if it slides freely, then abandon the puncture and proceed with echocardiographic guidance.
  - **Sheath does not reach the fossa**
    - With RA dilatation, the standard curve on the transseptal needle may not reach the fossa.
    - Access may be facilitated by sharper curves (e.g., BRK-2 needle or manually increasing the curve).

- **Management of transseptal sheaths**
  - Sheaths should be continuously/intermittently irrigated with heparinized saline while in place.
  - Catheters should be advanced and withdrawn slowly so as to not entrain air.
  - After a catheter is removed, blood should be aspirated to ensure that no air remains in the apparatus.

INTRACARDIAC ELECTROGRAM (EGM)

- This is the recording of localized electrical activity within the heart, determined by the voltage difference between two electrodes (anode and cathode).
- This signal undergoes filtering and gain modification.
  - **High band pass filtering**: Attenuates frequencies lower than the cut-off
    - Used to eliminate low-frequency oscillations due to respiration or catheter movements, repolarization artifact, and far-field signals (the high-frequency content attenuates more rapidly with increasing distance from the site of origin thus leaving only the low-frequency component)
    - **General settings**: 30–40 Hz (0.5 Hz for unipolar EGMs)
  - **Low band pass filtering**: Attenuates frequencies higher than the cut-off
    - Used to eliminate environmental or electrical noise
    - If filter settings are too high: Lose signal components to filtering.
    - If filter settings are too low: Lose signal components to noise.
    - **General settings**: 250 Hz to 400–500 Hz
  - **Notch filter**
    - Attenuates signals around 50–60 Hz (attenuates noise due to alternating current [AC])
    - Use may result in loss of signal components to filtering.
    - Recording can be **unipolar** or **bipolar**.

Table 1.3 Differences Between Unipolar and Bipolar Electrograms (EGMs)

Unipolar EGM	Bipolar EGM
• Morphology is important (QS vs. RS)	• Timing is important (morphology less useful)
• Affected by far-field signals	• Represents local electrical activity
• Useful for activation mapping	• Widespread use in EP
• Less useful for mapping scar tissue	• Able to map small fractioned EGMs in scar

Unipolar EGM

- **Recording**: EGM represents current flow between the intracardiac electrode (anode) and the dispersive electrode on the patient's back (cathode).
- **Morphology**: The unipolar EGM can be used to determine direction of wavefront propagation or source location.
  - **Maximum negative QS deflection** observed with the electrode positioned at the source
  - **Equiphasic (RS) to positive deflection** as the electrode moves away from source

- **Local activation time (LAT)**
  - With a recording electrode at a fixed location:
    - **Slow (shallow) positive deflection** as the wavefront approaches the electrode
    - **Steep negative (–dV/dt) deflection** as the wavefront passes the electrode tip
    - **Shallow negative deflection** as the wavefront moves away from the electrode
  - **Maximum negative slope (dV/dt)** coincides with maximum sodium channel conductance (i.e., the local arrival of the activation wavefront).
- **Advantages**
  - Gives more precise measure of local activation timing
  - Gives information about the directionality (unfiltered)
- **Disadvantages**
  - Poor signal to noise ratio; far-field signals may obscure local potentials
    - Hard to separate out small amplitude local EGMs (i.e., scar tissue)
  - Inability to record an undisturbed EGM around pacing
    - Effectively impossible to do entrainment mapping

Bipolar EGM

- **Recording**: EGM represents current flow between adjacent intracardiac catheter electrodes.
  - Distal electrode acts as the cathode, and the proximal electrode is the anode.
- **Morphology**
  - EGM acts as a summation of the potentials from each of the two electrodes at a given point of time (i.e., a sum of the two unipolar EGMs).
  - The initial peak of the bipolar signal ("intrinsic deflection") corresponds to depolarization beneath the electrodes.
- **LAT**:
  - **Healthy tissue**: Onset of the first rapid deflection
    - Initial peak of a filtered (30–300/500 Hz) signal
    - Absolute maximum EGM amplitude
  - **Diseased tissue**: Harder to determine (choose the bipolar signal that coincides with the unipolar monophasic QS EGM).
    - **Fractionated potentials**: Choose local timing at the earliest activation.
    - **Double potentials**: Choose local timing at the larger of the two EGMs.
- **Advantages**
  - Improved signal to noise ratio facilitates identification of high-frequency components (e.g., local signal in scar).
- **Disadvantages**
  - Morphology does not give information about directionality.
  - It is not possible to simultaneously pace and record from the same pair of electrodes.
    - Need to pace from 1 and 3 while recording from 2 and 4

Classification and Interpretation of EGMs

- **Low amplitude**
  - Definition: Amplitude <1.5 mV
  - Interpretation: Area of fibrosis/scar; poor catheter contact; far-field signal
- **Fractionated**
  - Definition: Prolonged (>70 ms), low-amplitude potentials with multiple peaks/troughs
  - Interpretation: Peri-infarct or slow conduction zone; catheter movement; arborized connections
- **Split**
  - Definition: Two components of the potential separated by an isoelectric interval (>60 ms)
  - Interpretation: Local conduction block (anatomic/functional) or slow conduction zone
- **Late component**
  - Definition: Potential occurring at the end of the surface QRS
  - Interpretation: Delayed activation; local conduction block (anatomic/functional) or slow conduction
- **Continuous**
  - Definition: Potential that runs throughout the cardiac cycle with no diastolic isoelectric interval
  - Interpretation: Slow conduction zone; artifact; electromagnetic interference
    - Note: Continuous activation during the diastolic period represents slow/fractionated conduction in diseased myocardium (may not be an essential area of the circuit).
- **Mid-diastolic**
  - Definition: Discrete potential that occurs in mid-diastole with isoelectric intervals on either side
    - Usually occurs approximately 10–100 ms before the major ventricular deflection
  - Interpretation: Represents activation of the diastolic pathway (zone of slow conduction)
- **Low frequency**
  - Definition: Small-amplitude potential with shallow slope (low dV/dt)
  - Interpretation: Far-field signal; artifact
- **Monophasic**
  - Definition: Pattern seen with injury current
  - Interpretation: Too much contact pressure; injury to tissue locally

3D CARDIAC MAPPING

General Principles

- When to use 3D mapping:
  - Sustained focal atrial or ventricular arrhythmias
  - Macroreentry in the context of previous cardiac surgery/atrial scar
  - AT after AF ablation
  - Endocardial and epicardial ablation of scar-mediated VT
  - Substrate mapping for ablation of unmappable (unstable) VT
  - Desire to perform multiple chamber mapping and non-contact mapping (i.e., multiple tachycardia)
- **Limitations of 3D mapping**
  - Sequential site mapping can be time consuming (usually at least 30–40 points need to be obtained to define the arrhythmia mechanism and circuit).
  - Mapping of non-sustained or poorly tolerated tachycardia is very difficult.
  - A change in TCL or morphology requires a new map of the chamber.
- **Electroanatomical data can be shown as:**
  - **LAT map**: The timing of each individual recorded signal relative to a chosen reference is allocated a specific color (earliest red, latest purple).
    - The activation sequence and path of arrhythmia are displayed in 3D.
  - **Propagation map**: Animated version of the LAT map demonstrating the spread of wavefront propagation as a movie.
  - **Isochronal map**: Similar to LAT, but each color represents a specific duration (i.e., 5 ms) so that conduction velocity is better appreciated.
  - **Voltage map**: Recorded signal amplitudes are allocated colors and the scale is manually adjusted to highlight abnormal myocardium.
    - **Dynamic substrate map**: A voltage map generated from the multi-site array. Using a single cardiac cycle, the array defines areas of scar based on a percentage of peak maximal unipolar voltage.
  - **Complex Fractionated Atrial Electrogram (CFAE) map**:
    - **CARTO-Interval Confidence Level (ICL)**: The number of intervals identified between consecutive complexes identified as CFAE over a specified duration (i.e., 2.5 seconds). The more repetitions observed (higher ICL), the more confident the categorization of CFAE.
    - **CARTO-Shortest Complex Interval (SCI)** or **Average Complex Interval (ACI)**: The shortest or average interval between consecutive CFAE complexes (in ms) observed over a specified duration (i.e., 2.5 seconds). The shorter the interval, the more confident the categorization of CFAE.
    - **NAVx - Fractionation Index**: The mean or standard deviation of local peak-to-peak EGM CL intervals over a specified duration (i.e., 1–8 seconds). The shorter the mean CL the more rapid and fractionated the EGM.

3D Electroanatomic Mapping (EAM) Systems

CARTO (Biosense Webster, Diamond Bar, CA)

- Ultra-low-magnetic fields generated by three coils mounted under the examination table are used to localize a special ablation catheter that contains a magnetic sensor at the distal catheter electrode. The three-dimensional position and orientation of the catheter can be determined (pitch, roll, yaw) relative to an external reference electrode placed on the patient's back (ideally in close proximity to the chamber of interest).

Ensite NavX (St. Jude Medical, St. Paul, MN)

- A transthoracic electrical field is generated by three pairs of cutaneous electrodes that are positioned to form orthogonal axes of *x* (left to right), *y* (neck to left leg), *z* (anterior to posterior).
- A 5.6 kHz low-level current is delivered alternatively between these pairs of patches, with catheter location determined by measuring the local voltage gradient along each axis (*x*, *y*, and *z*) with respect to a reference electrode.
- Note:
  - A stable reference catheter is essential (e.g., CS, aortic, or active fixation catheter).
  - Respiratory compensation corrects for changes in thoracic impedance during the procedure.
  - A field scaling algorithm may be applied to geometry construction to correct for impedance non-linearity that can distort the anatomical shape of the chamber.

Non-Contact Mapping

- The multi-electrode array (MEA) is a 64-electrode mesh designed to provide global, simultaneous electrical mapping of any cardiac chamber, allowing the entire arrhythmia circuit to be mapped in a single heartbeat.

Image Integration

Image integration involves the computational combination of two representations of the same cardiac chamber that are created by two separate modalities.

- There are three fundamental processes involved in image integration:
  - **Image acquisition**: Anatomic imaging by computed tomography, magnetic resonance imaging, intracardiac echocardiography, or rotational angiography
  - **Segmentation**: The isolation of an image of a cardiac chamber from neighboring structures
    - The process involves selecting the level of interest followed by adjustment of the blood pool density to highlight the chamber of interest. Thereafter, the chamber can be segmented from the surrounding structures with manual adjusting of the inaccuracies.
  - **Registration**: The alignment and incorporation of the segmented chamber within the electroanatomic mapping system (EAM)
- Pitfalls of image integration
  - Volume status may alter chamber size (perform acquisition as close to the procedure as possible).
  - Registration can be affected by movement artifact.
  - Tenting of the atrial roof or anterior wall may distort the EAM.
  - Rotational error can occur in the sagittal plane if only pulmonary vein (PV) ostia are used as landmarks.

ARRHYTHMIA MAPPING

Contact (Activation) Mapping

Assessment of the timing and directionality of intracardiac impulses in relation to a fixed reference.

- Useful for:
  - Hemodynamically stable tachycardia
  - Can be utilized for frequent extrasystoles

Process

- **Define the electrical reference**: The stable and consistent signal from which all interpretations of timing are based
  - Best: The onset of the earliest surface P wave (AT) or surface QRS complex (VT)
  - Surrogate: A stable intracardiac EGM indexed to the surface onset
- **Define the window of interest** (diagnostic landmarking): Used to determine local EGM timing relative to the reference (i.e., early vs. late)
  - **Window onset**: Should precede surface ECG tachycardia onset (~33%–50% of CL)
    - Note: If mapping during pacing, then employ 10 ms blanking after the pacing spike.
  - **Window duration**: Should cover >90% of the total tachycardia cycle
- **Mapping**
  - Use the surface 12-lead ECG to get a rough idea about the region of interest.
  - Confirm with simultaneous intracardiac mapping (e.g., high right atrium [HRA], CS, His, RV apex [RVa]).
  - Finally, utilize the roving catheter to compare local activation timing to the reference.
- **Signal acquisition**
  - Bipolar EGMs
    - **Healthy tissue: LAT** = onset of the first rapid deflection
      - Alternatives: Initial peak of a filtered (30–300/500 Hz) signal, or the absolute maximum EGM amplitude
    - **Diseased tissue: LAT** = harder to determine (choose the bipolar signal that coincides with the unipolar monophasic QS EGM).
      - **Fractionated potentials**: Choose local timing at the earliest activation.
      - **Double potentials**: Choose local timing at the larger of the two EGMs.
  - **Unipolar EGMs: LAT** = maximum negative slope (dV/dt)
    - Coincides with maximum sodium channel conductance
    - Should have a monophasic QS morphology
- **Data resolution**
  - ≥50–100 points are usually required to accurately define arrhythmia mechanisms.
  - ≥10–20 points should be focused on the area of interest.

Interpretation

- **Focal tachycardia**
  - The pattern of activation is centrifugal, arising from a discrete site.
  - Usually only 50% of the TCL can be mapped within the chamber.
  - **Goals**: Identify the site of arrhythmia origin.
- **Reentrant tachycardia**
  - The pattern of activation is circumferential with "early-meets-late" activation.
  - Usually >90% of the TCL can be mapped within the chamber.
  - **Goals**: Identify the critical isthmus.

Non-Contact Activation Mapping

The MEA is designed to provide global, simultaneous electrical mapping of any cardiac chamber. Theoretically requires only one beat to determine the activation pattern; however, in practice multiple beats must be analyzed to ensure consistent data.

- Useful for:
  - Hemodynamically unstable tachycardia
  - Rarely observed phenomena such as extrasystoles (PACs or VPBs) or nonsustained tachycardia

Process

- The MEA is advanced over a 0.035" guidewire to the cardiac chamber of interest.
- Anticoagulation is required: Target an ACT >250 (right-sided procedures) or >300 (left-sided procedures).
- **Geometry**
  - Conventional catheter is used to define the chamber geometry relative to the MEA.
  - A low-level current is passed at 5.68 kHz from the roving catheter to two ring electrodes of the MEA to allow determination of its location.
- **Settings**
  - **Low pass filter (25–300 Hz)**: Used to eliminate environmental noise
  - **High pass filter (0.1–32 Hz)**: Used to eliminate repolarization artifact and far-field (epicardium or adjacent chamber)
    - Start at 2Hz: Preserves low-amplitude depolarization/zones of slow conduction
    - Drop to 0.5–1 Hz if looking for areas with slow conduction/diastolic potentials
- **Defining the tachycardia mechanism and activation using isopotential mapping**
  - Intracavitary unipolar signals are acquired by the MEA, amplified, and processed using inverse mathematics to reconstruct 3360 "virtual" unipolar EGMs on the geometry.
  - Activation sequence should then be reviewed in slow playback (i.e., 1:50) over several beats.
    - Regions with differences in activation or timing (>40 ms) suggest conduction block.
  - Consider displaying EGMs at fast sweep speed (i.e., 400 mm/s).
    - The earliest QS complex denotes the earliest site of activation.
    - An initial R wave may suggest activation from a neighboring site or chamber.
  - Once an area of potential ablation has been identified, it should be confirmed using a contact mapping catheter.

Limitations

- Non-contact activation mapping is less suitable for larger chambers because the accuracy is compromised if the endocardium is >40 mm from the MEA.
- Low amplitude signals may not be detected (e.g., fractionation, diastolic potentials).
- Inadvertent endocardial or ablation catheter contact may cause data saturation or artifact.
- Isopotential maps are dependent on manual adjustment of filter settings and voltage thresholds.
- Chamber surface interpolations create a "false space."

Entrainment Mapping

- Demonstration of entrainment
  - Confirms the mechanism as reentry
  - Localizes the reentrant circuit to a specific chamber (or site)
  - Localizes the critical components of the reentrant circuit that sustain tachycardia (i.e., the isthmus of slow conduction or diastolic pathway)

Process

- Pacing during tachycardia at rates 20–30 ms faster than the TCL captures the chamber of interest and accelerates the tachycardia to the pacing rate.

Key Questions to Determine If the Pacing Site Is in a Critical Area of the Circuit

- Is there concealed entrainment or manifest fusion?
  - Concealed entrainment occurs when the paced morphology (QRS or P) and intracardiac activation are identical to the tachycardia.
  - Concealed entrainment indicates that the pacing is being performed within the inner part of the tachycardia circuit (i.e., the diastolic pathway [zone of slow conduction] or at a bystander zone).
  - Concealed entrainment differs from fusion where the paced morphology and intracardiac activation patterns are not identical to that of the clinical tachycardia.
    - Fusion may be due to pacing outside the circuit (outer loop, adjacent area, or bystander), bidirectional conduction, or multiple exit sites.
- What is the post-pacing interval (and PPI – TCL timing)?
  - The PPI is the time from the last entrained stimulus to the next local non-stimulated depolarization measured at the pacing site
  - **PPI variability**
    - Inconsistent PPIs (PPI variability > 30 ms): Focal atrial tachyarrthmia (FAT)
    - Consistent PPIs (PPI variability < 10 ms): Reentry (micro or macro)
  - **PPI timing (PPI – TCL)**
    - If the site is within the circuit, the PPI should be equal to the time it takes for the impulse to complete the circuit (PPI – TCL ≤ 20 ms).
      - Concealed entrainment with PPI = TCL: **In-circuit response**
    - If the site is a bystander, then the PPI is greater than the tachycardia cycle length.
      - Entrainment with fusion and PPI > TCL: **Out-of-circuit response**
      - Concealed entrainment with PPI > TCL: **Bystander location**
    - Note: Rapid pacing can result in decrement in the zone of slow conduction (a.k.a., rate-dependent PPI lengthening).
- What are the stimulation and activation times?
  - The activation time (time from local EGM to subsequent QRS; EGM-QRS) should equal (<25 ms) the stimulus time (time from paced EGM to subsequent QRS; Stim-QRS) if pacing is being performed within the circuit.
  - The location within the circuit can be estimated by Stim-QRS/TCL.
    - <30% = exit; 30%–50% = central; 50%–70% = proximal; >70% = inner loop

- If the site is a bystander, the stimulus time will exceed the activation time.

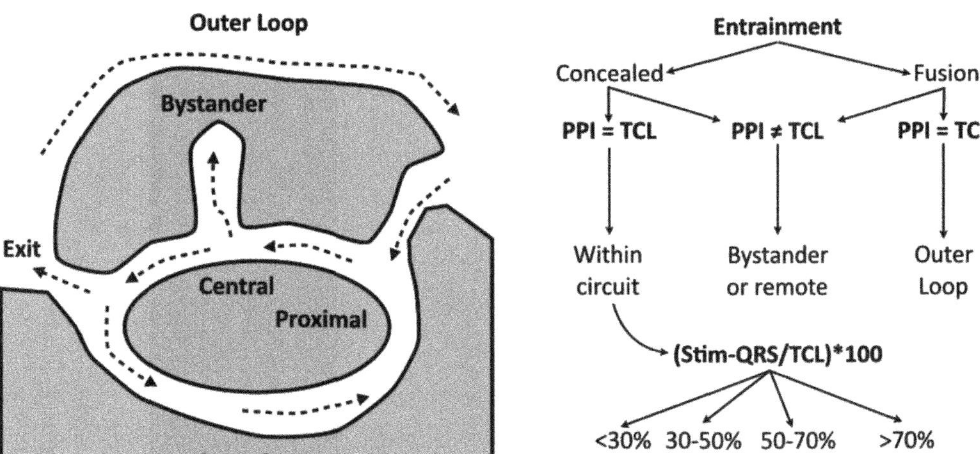

Substrate Mapping

Substrate mapping is based on the principle that areas of dense scar and zones of slow conduction can be differentiated from areas of normal healthy tissue.

- **Useful for scar-related tachycardia** (i.e., ischemic VT, incisional AT) that are not hemodynamically tolerated, non-inducible, or non-sustained at the time of ablation

Voltage Mapping in the Ventricle (Contact)

- **Dense scar**
  - Bipolar EGM < 0.5 mV
- **Border zone scar**
  - **Endocardial right ventricle (RV)**
    - Bipolar 0.5 mV to 1.5 mV
    - Unipolar 0.5 mV to 5.5 mV (free wall)
  - **Endocardial LV**
    - Bipolar 0.5 mV to 1.5–2.0 mV
    - Unipolar 0.7 mV to 8.3 mV (alternatively, may represent the endocardial manifestation of epicardial or mid-myocardial scar – a.k.a., "ghosting")
  - **Epicardial**: 0.5 mV to 1.0 mV
- **Normal tissue**
  - Bipolar > 1.5 mV

Voltage Mapping in the Atria (Contact)

- Bipolar amplitude:
  - >1.0 is considered normal
  - <0.5 mV is probably abnormal
  - <0.05–0.1 mV is likely scar
- As the approach is less well validated, the map should include electrically silent areas, double potentials, and fractionation in order to delineate potential reentry circuits.

Non-contact Substrate Mapping

- **Dynamic substrate mapping (DSM) algorithm**:
  - Uses a percentage of the peak negative chamber voltage
- Absolute cut-offs are not used because MEA reconstructed voltages can be affected by differences in chamber size and mass.
  - **Sinus rhythm**: Peak negative voltage <34% with DSM correlates with ventricular scar.
  - **Ventricular pacing**: Peak negative voltage <20% with DSM correlates with ventricular scar.
- High-low pass filter settings: 2–150 Hz

Pace Mapping

Pace mapping is based on the principle that pacing near the site of origin of the tachycardia, and at a similar CL, will result in similar myocardial activation similar to the tachycardia.

- Useful for any type of arrhythmia:
  - Works best for focal arrhythmias (especially idiopathic VT) where the ECG configuration is determined by the sequence of myocardial activation.
  - For reentry, the pace map will generally reflect the exit site.
- Usually used to confirm an activation map:
  - 12-lead ECG obtained during arrhythmia is compared to a 12-lead ECG obtained during pacing at the TCL (or coupling interval).
  - If in tachycardia, pace at 20–40 ms faster than TCL.

Interpretation

- **Matching**
  - Pace maps with identical or near-identical activation in all 12 leads suggest the site of origin.
  - **Subjective match**: Matching in ≥10 leads is considered adequate
  - **Objective match** (automated software): CORR (correlation coefficient) is more widely used; however, the MAD score (mean absolute deviation) is more sensitive to differences in waveform amplitude.
    - MAD ranges from 0% (identical) to 100% (completely different).
    - Score of <12% has 93% sensitivity and 75% specificity for successful ablation site.
    - Score of >12%–15% has 100% negative predictive value for successful ablation site, suggesting there is no utility to ablating at this location.
- **Stim-QRS during pace mapping**
  - Pacing in normal myocardium is associated with a Stim-QRS of <20–40 ms.
    - A Stim-QRS >40 ms is associated with a zone of slow conduction or a protected isthmus.
  - Stim-QRS can be used to map a protected isthmus in sinus rhythm and within ongoing VT.
    - The Stim-QRS should progressively lengthen as the pacing site moves along the isthmus from exit to entrance (see the Entrainment section).

Limitations

- **Imprecise**
  - Subjectively excellent (12/12) pace maps may be achieved over a large area (up to 1 cm^2).
  - Yet small differences (notching, amplitude change) can be seen over short distances (~5 mm).
- **False negatives** (the pace map QRS does not resemble VT despite pacing within the isthmus)
  - **Bidirectional conduction**: The exit in sinus is opposite to VT or is a fusion of multiple exits.
  - **Functional barrier exists only in tachycardia**: As an example, for VT, the QRS morphology in sinus may be completely different despite pacing being performed within the critical isthmus.
  - **Capture of other local tissue contaminates pacing in isthmus**.

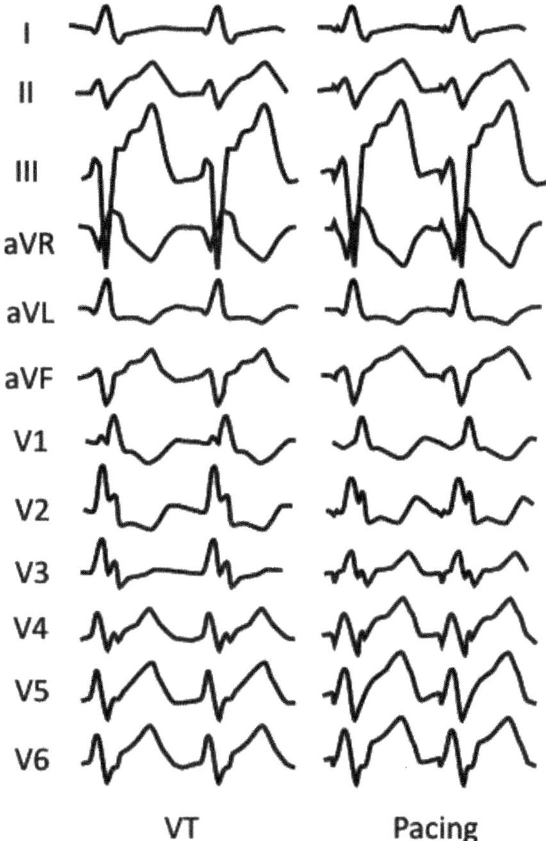

ABLATION ENERGY

Radiofrequency (RF) Energy

- The most commonly used ablation energy
- Compared to direct current (DC) ablation, RF ablation offers the advantages of:
  - Lessened discomfort during energy delivery
  - Absent skeletal- and cardiac-muscle stimulation
  - Relatively discrete ablation lesions with absent barotrauma
  - The potential for the premature termination of ablation to avoid impending complications
- **Mechanism of action**
  - AC is delivered between the catheter tip and the dispersive electrode.
  - This electromagnetic energy is converted to thermal energy as the RF current passes from the low-resistance catheter through high-resistance tissue (**resistive heating**).
    - The **heat** generated locally at the tip-tissue interface is then dispersed into surrounding tissue (**conductive heating** with subsequent thermal injury).

Table 1.4 Determinants of Ablation Lesion Size with RF

Factor	Effect on Lesion Size
Power	Directly proportional
Electrode temperature	Directly proportional
Energy delivery duration	Exponential: ~50% of the lesion is created within the first 5–10 seconds of ablation
Contact force	Directly proportional
Blood flow	May reduce lesion size if it acts as a heat sink
Electrode size	Directly proportional: Convective cooling due to greater surface area (electrode circumference and length) enables greater power delivery
Catheter irrigation	Irrigation by circulating fluid within the electrode (closed loop) or through small openings in the ablation electrode cools the electrode, allowing greater power delivery and deeper lesion creation

Cryothermal Energy

- **Mechanism of action**
  - **Freezing effect**: Progressive hypothermia results in:
    - Slowing of cellular metabolism: Ion pumps lose transport capability
    - Formation of ice crystals: First in the extracellular (EC) space (at tissue temperature below –15°C), then in the intracellular (IC) space (at tissue temperature below –40°C). The ice results in the EC space becoming hypertonic relative to the cell precipitating an osmotic gradient. Movement of water from the IC space results in cell shrinkage and precipitates a diffusion gradient (movement of H+ out of the cell). The increased IC solute concentration and acidic IC pH results in cellular dysfunction and death.
  - **Thawing and tissue healing**
    - Passive tissue rewarming induces cellular damage through: (1) recrystallization and coalescence of IC and EC ice, which intensifies the osmotic damage, and (2) restoration of microcirculatory function associated with a hyperemic vascular injury.
    - Concurrent to thawing is reactive inflammation, followed by repair and replacement fibrosis. The result is a mature lesion, with a well-circumscribed central dense fibrosis.

Table 1.5 Potential Benefits of Cryoenergy

Advantages	Clinical Implications
Reversibility of suppression of conduction tissue	"Safety mapping" has lower risk of inadvertent AV block "Efficacy mapping" predicts successful ablation site
Adhesion to cardiac tissue	Reduced risk of damage to adjacent structures Allows programmed stimulation during ablation
Well demarcated homogeneous lesions	Less pro-arrhythmogenic
Preservation of ultrastructural integrity	Reduced risk of thrombus/embolism Reduced risk of perforation, PV stenosis
Reduced patient discomfort during the procedure	More comfortable Less sedation

CHAPTER

2

Electrophysiology Study and Maneuvers

THE ELECTROPHYSIOLOGY STUDY

Indications

- Evaluation of sinus node function in patients in whom sinus node dysfunction is suspected (but not confirmed) as the cause of symptoms
- Evaluation of symptomatic patients in whom His-Purkinje block is suspected as a cause of symptoms
- Evaluation of narrow QRS complex tachyarrhythmias
  - Patients with frequent or poorly tolerated episodes who do not adequately respond to drug therapy
  - Patients who prefer catheter ablation to pharmacological therapy
- Evaluation of patients with wide QRS tachycardia in whom the diagnosis is unclear after clinical analysis, and for whom the correct diagnosis is essential for patient care
- Assessment of patients with Wolff-Parkinson-White syndrome
  - Patients being evaluated for catheter ablation or surgical ablation of an accessory pathway (AP)
  - Patients with ventricular pre-excitation with unexplained syncope or who have survived cardiac arrest
- Investigation of unexplained syncope, including suspected structural heart disease and syncope that remains unexplained after evaluation
- Assessment of patients surviving cardiac arrest without evidence of acute myocardial infarction (MI) or >48 h after the acute phase
- Assessment of patients with palpitations and inappropriately rapid pulse in whom the cause is not documented

Complications

- The incidence and type of complication depends on the procedure being performed (see Table 2.1).
  - Atrial tachycardia (AT) or atrial flutter has a complication rate of about 4%–5%.

- Ablation of the atrioventricular (AV) junction has a complication rate of about 2%–3%.
- Modification of the AV junction for atrioventricular nodal reentrant tachycardia (AVNRT) has a complication rate of about 3%–4%.
- Ablation of an AP has a complication rate of about 2%–4%.
- Ablation of ventricular tachycardia (VT) has a complication rate of about 5%–8%.

Table 2.1 Complications Associated with Various Diagnostic and Therapeutic Procedures

Complication	Diagnostic	Ablation
Death	<0.1%	0.3%
Access site complication	0.2%	0.6%
Embolism (systemic or cerebral)	<0.1%	0.2%–0.5%
Myocardial ischemia or infarction	<0.1%	0.1%–0.2%
AV block necessitating pacemaker	<0.1%	0.5%–2.0%
Pericardial effusion	<0.1%	0.3%–2.0%
Tamponade	<0.1%	0.2%–0.7%
Pericarditis/chest pain	<0.1%	<1.0%
Venous thrombosis	0.5%–1%	0.5%–1%
Major bleeding	<0.1%	0.2%–0.7%
Pacemaker lead dislodgment	<1%	<1%
Pneumothorax	0.1%	0.1%
Total	1%	3%

STANDARD CATHETER PLACEMENT

High Right Atrium

- Catheters used include Josephson or Cournand shape.
  - Quadripolar catheters are used for simultaneous stimulation and recording.
- Preferred position is high posterolateral wall at the junction of the superior vena cava (SVC) as this site approximates the sinoatrial (SA) node exit site.
  - Right atrial appendage (anterior) may be used if it is difficult to place.
  - Technique: In the anteroposterior projection, advance the catheter to the HRA and torque catheter posteriorly.
- While recording, keep in mind:
  - The EGM corresponds to the depolarization wavefront arriving at the atrial cells of the superior RA.
  - The timing of the EGM is close to the onset of the P wave on the surface ECG.

Right Ventricle

- Catheters used include Josephson or Cournand shape.
    - Catheters are quadripolar for simultaneous stimulation and recording, or bipolar (capture inferred from ECG).
- Preferred position is in the right ventricular apex (RVa).
    - Right ventriclar outflow tract (RVOT) is used in difficult cases or if dual-site pacing is required.
    - Technique: In anteroposterior or RAO projection, advance catheter to RVa.
- While recording, keep in mind:
    - EGM corresponds to the depolarization of the RV after the signal has exited the His-Purkinje.
    - Timing of the EGM is close to the onset of the QRS on the surface ECG.

His Bundle Catheter

- Catheters used include CRD2, Josephson, or Cournand shape.
- Usual location is approximately 1–2 o'clock on the Tricuspid valve (TV) in LAO projection where there is a large His EGM.
    - Technique: Position the catheter across the anterior-superior TV in antero-posterior or RAO projection, then gently withdraw the catheter with clockwise torque to assure septal contact.
- While recording, keep in mind:
    - Atrial EGM corresponds to depolarization of the cells located in the low RA near the atrioventricular node (AVN).
    - His EGM corresponds to depolarization of the proximal His-Purkinje after the EGM exits the AVN.
    - Ventricular EGM corresponds to the depolarization of the ventricular cells adjacent to the node.
        - The timing of the EGM is close to the surface QRS onset as the septum is one of the first areas activated.
- Caveats
    - An inadequate atrial EGM results in:
        - Underestimation of the HV interval due to the recording of a right bundle potential
        - Misinterpretation of the position of the AVN and aortic root

Coronary Sinus

- Multipolar catheter (8–10 electrodes) is utilized to record the LA activation sequence.
- Positioning depends on which approach is used.
    - Inferior approach
        - The catheter is positioned across the TV and deflected inferiorly. It is then withdrawn with clockwise torque until equal atrial and ventricular EGMs are recorded. Once the coronary sinus (CS) ostium is engaged, release the deflection while continuing to apply clockwise torque to allow the tip to turn superiorly and follow the course of the vein.

- Superior approach
  - Position the catheter across the TV and withdraw towards the IVC while applying clockwise torque until equal atrial and ventricular EGMs are recorded.
- Difficulties in positioning the catheter may include:
  - Failure to cannulate the CS ostium
  - Failure to advance catheter distally in the CS due to a distal valve
  - Recurrent catheter dislodgement; consider using a support sheath (SR0 or SL2) or switching to a superior approach

- While recording, keep in mind:
  - Atrial EGM corresponds to the depolarization of the LA cells adjacent to the mitral annulus.
    - As depolarization progresses from the sinoatrial node (SA Node) the activation pattern in the CS will be proximal to distal.
  - Ventricular EGM corresponds to the depolarization of the LV cells adjacent to the mitral annulus.
  - Caveats
    - Partial introduction with the distal poles at the mid-CS position and the proximal poles outside the ostium can result in misclassification of midline activation as eccentric.

MEASUREMENT OF BASIC CONDUCTION INTERVALS

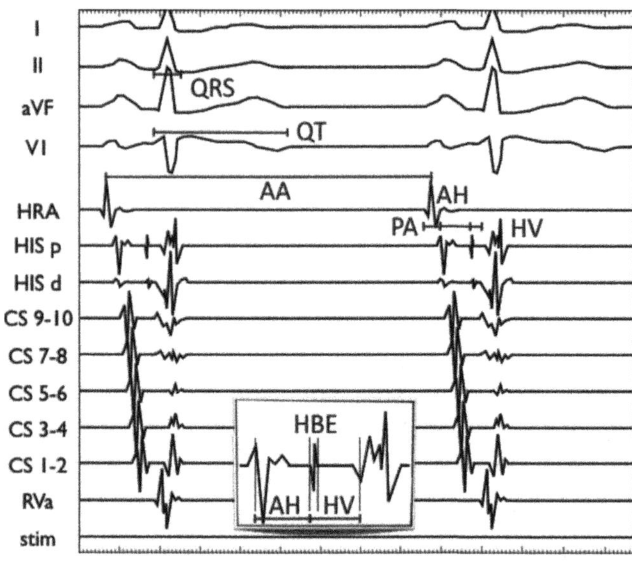

Conduction Intervals

PA: 25–55 ms
AH: 55–125 ms
HBE: <30 ms
HV: 35–55 ms

Sinus Node Function

Maximum SNRT: ≤1.5 sec
CSNRT: <550 ms
Maximum TRT: ≤5 sec
SACT: 50–115 ms

Refractory Periods

Atrial ERP: 180–330 ms
AV Nodal ERP: 250–400 ms (anterograde)
AV Nodal FRP: 330–550 ms
Ventricular ERP: 180–290 ms

Cycle Length

- Cycle length (CL) is the length of time between each successive heartbeat as measured in milliseconds.

PA Interval (normal: 25–55 ms)

- PA interval is an estimation of intra-atrial conduction.
  - It represents the time for activation to travel from the SA node region to the AVN region.
  - The PA interval is measured from the earliest atrial activation in any channel (surface P wave or earliest atrial EGM) to the rapid deflection of the atrial EGM on the His bundle catheter.

AH Interval (normal: 55–125 ms)

- AH interval is an estimation of AVN conduction time.
  - It represents the time for the impulse to travel from the low RA through the AVN to the His bundle.
  - The AH interval is measured on the His bundle catheter between the earliest rapid atrial deflection (low RA depolarization) and the beginning of the His EGM.
  - It can vary by up to 20 ms due to autonomic tone.

His Bundle EGM (HBE) Duration (normal: <30 ms)

- HBE is the time needed for activation of the His bundle.
  - The HBE duration is measured from the beginning to the end of the HBE.
  - Minor delay may cause a notching of the HBE, with significant delay causing a split HBE.

HV Interval (normal: 35–55 ms)

- The HV interval is the time needed for conduction from the His bundle through the His-Purkinje system to the ventricular myocardium.
  - It is measured from the onset of the HBE to the earliest ventricular activation (surface QRS or V EGM).

PR Interval

- The PR interval is the summation of the PA interval, the AH interval, and the HV interval.

QRS Duration (normal: <120 ms)

- The QRS duration is the time needed for ventricular activation to occur.

QT Interval (normal: <440 ms in men or <460 ms in women)

- The QT interval is the time needed for ventricular activation and repolarization to occur.

REFRACTORY PERIODS

- After cardiac depolarization, the period of time during which it cannot be depolarized again is termed the **refractory period** (usually from phase 0 to late phase 3 of the cell's action potential).
- With progressively shorter coupling intervals, three characteristic refractory periods are observed.

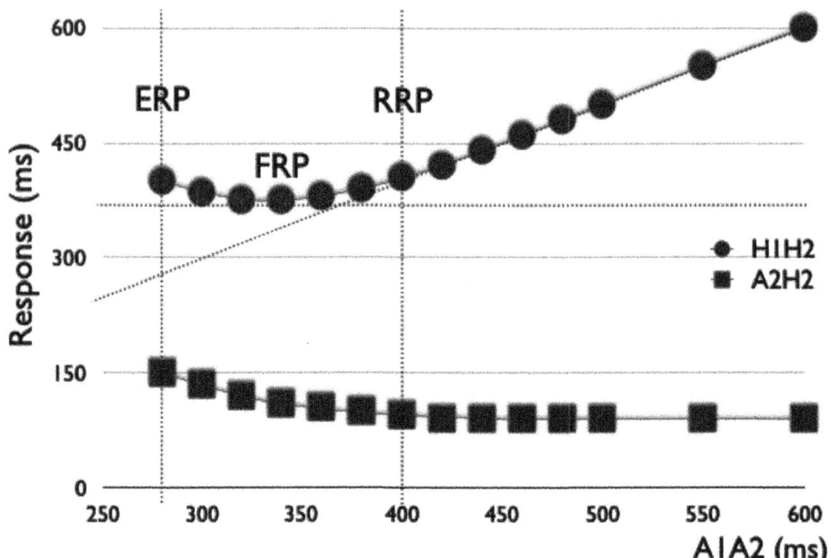

Relative Refractory Period (RRP): "Change"

- As the input coupling interval is steadily decreased, there is initially a steady relationship between the "input" (e.g., S1S2) and the solicited tissue response, or "output" (e.g., H1H2 or A2H2).
- With progressively shorter coupling intervals, the tissue response changes, whereby shorter output coupling intervals are still induced; however, the magnitude of effect is lessened.
- This point where the output interval begins to differ from the input is defined as the RRP.
- RRP is also known as the point at which latency or decremental conduction begins (i.e. if the impulse was delivered any later it would conduct normally).
  - **Decremental conduction**: Progressively shorter coupling results in slower conduction velocity.
    - Decremental conduction is seen with tissues dependent on "slow" inward calcium current for depolarization (e.g., AVN).
    - **Purkinje fibers** are dependent on "fast" sodium channels resulting in nearly no decrement.
    - **Myocardium** (atrial and ventricular) has minimal decremental properties.
  - **Latency** is the delay between the extrastimulus and the EGM generated by the tissue.
    - Latency is observed when the short-coupled extrastimulus impinges on the refractory period of the adjacent myocardium.

Functional Refractory Period (FRP): "Best"

- As the "input" coupling interval is progressively decreased, there is a change in the tissue response such that the "optimal" conduction interval is reached (i.e., shortest output coupling interval).
  - Functionally, this is a quantitative measure of tissue output (conduction velocity and refractoriness).
    - It defines the lower limit of the output that the tissue/structure can produce.

Effective Refractory Period (ERP): "Loss"

- Thereafter, shorter input coupling intervals result in a progressive "worsening" in tissue output down to the ERP.
- ERP is defined as the longest coupling interval for which an impulse fails to propagate through tissue (i.e., if the impulse were delivered any later, it would conduct).
  - ERP occurs during the last third of phase 3 of the AP.

Assessment of Refractory Periods

Incremental Pacing

- Pacing is initiated at a rate slightly faster than the patient's spontaneous rhythm.
  - Pacing CL is decreased step-wise to the point of block or to a minimum cycle of 200–300 ms.
- Determine the following:
  - The Wenckebach CL (WCL), which is the time when 1:1 conduction ceases.
  - The presence/absence of retrograde atrial activation.
  - The retrograde atrial activation sequence (concentric vs. eccentric).
  - The site of block (AH or HV).

Decremental Conduction as a Result of Incremental Atrial Pacing

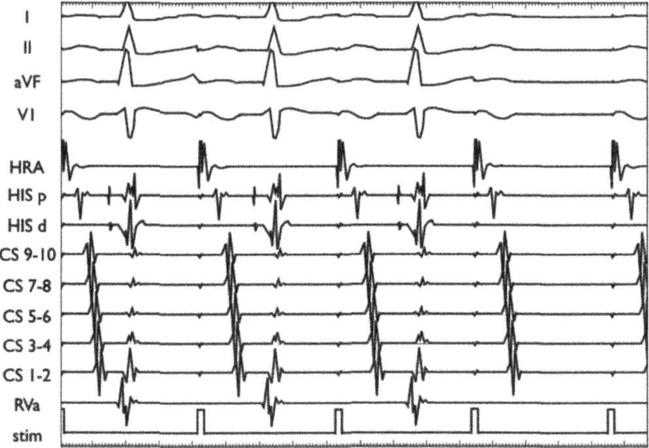

As the pacing CL is progressively decreased in the atria, the conduction decrements in the AVN before eventually blocking (second-to-last beat).

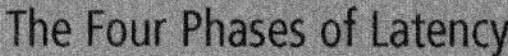

The Four Phases of Latency

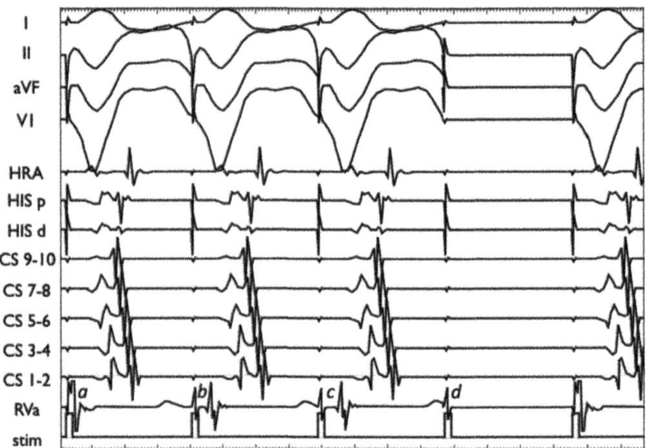

During ventricular pacing, there is no initial latency (a. V1V2 = S1S2). A delay is observed between the pacing stimulus (S) and the elicited EGM (V) as the paced beat (or extrastimulus) starts to impinge on the refractory period of the ventricular myocardium (b. Onset of latency: V1V2 > S1S2). Thereafter, a more marked latency is seen (c. V1V2 >> S1S2), followed by tissue refractoriness (d. No V2).

Extrastimulus

- Technique for inducing and assessing extrastimuli is as follows:
  - A series of impulses at fixed CL (8-beat S1) is followed by the introduction of one or more extrastimuli at a fixed coupling interval (S2, S3, etc.)
  - Typically, start with an 8-beat drive train (S1) at 600 ms with S2 at 580 ms.
  - The coupling interval (S2) is reduced by 10–20 ms to 200 ms or refractoriness.
  - Additional extrastimuli (S3, S4, etc.) can be introduced depending on the study protocol.
  - Note: As shorter S1 CLs decrease, the refractory period in most tissue (except the AVN) the refractory period must be measured over at least 2 basic CLs.
    - Usually repeated with an S1 of 400 ms (depending on the basal rate)
- Interpretation includes making the following assessments:
  - Anterograde refractory periods
    - **AVN effective refractory period** (AVNERP: Normal 250–400 ms)
    - **Atrial effective refractory period** (AERP: Normal 180–330 ms)
  - Retrograde refractory periods
    - VA refractory period (retrograde AVNERP or VAERP)
    - Ventricular refractory period (VERP: Normal 180–290 ms)

Decremental AV Conduction Using the Extrastimulus Technique

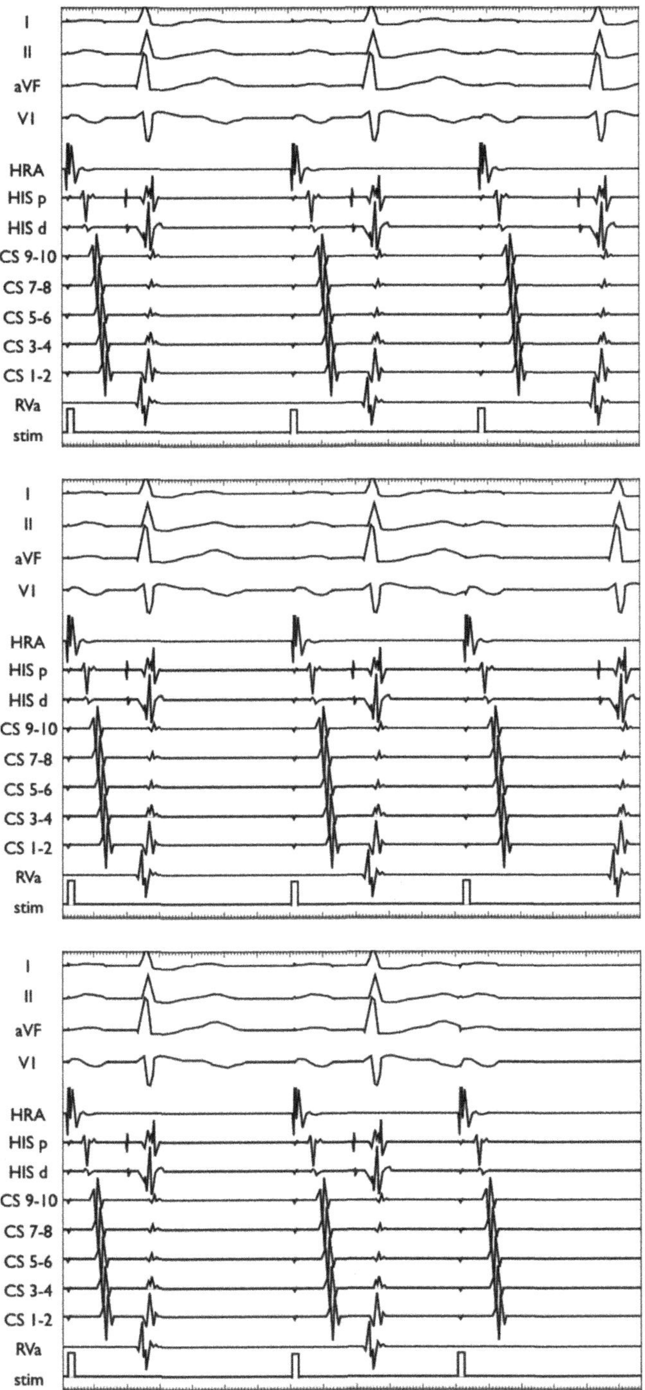

Using a stable drive train (S1), an extrastimulus (S2) is introduced at progressively shorter coupling intervals. AV conduction initially decrements in the AVN, resulting in AH prolongation. As the coupling interval is shortened, there is finally AV block at the level of the AVN (i.e., conduction block without His depolarization).

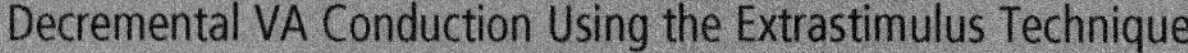

Decremental VA Conduction Using the Extrastimulus Technique

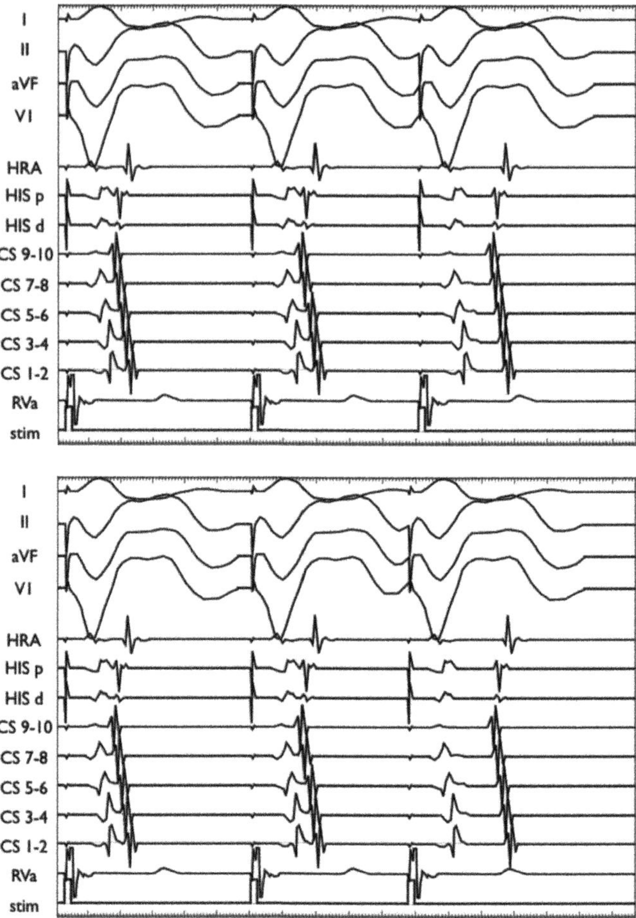

Using a stable drive train (S1), an extrastimulus (S2) is introduced at progressively shorter coupling intervals. The VA conduction demonstrates decremental conduction through the AVN as manifested by progressive VA prolongation with shorter S1S2 coupling intervals.

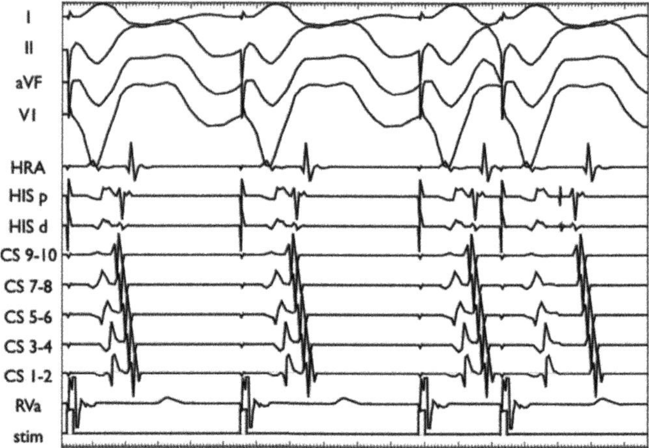

In contrast to the top two panels, the conduction delay in this panel occurs in the His-Purkinje system rather than the AVN (as demonstrated by the delay in the V2H2 interval).

Conduction Curves

- Technique includes assessment of the anterograde and retrograde conduction curves.
  - Anterograde conduction curve
    - Low atrial A1A2 interval (i.e., on His catheter) vs. output interval (H1H2)
    - Low atrial A1A2 interval (i.e., on His catheter) vs. low atrial A2H2 interval
  - Retrograde conduction curve
    - Low atrial V1V2 interval (i.e., on His catheter) vs. output interval (A1A2)
    - Low atrial V1V2 interval (i.e., on His catheter) vs. low atrial V2A2 interval
- Interpretation of normal anterograde conduction curve:

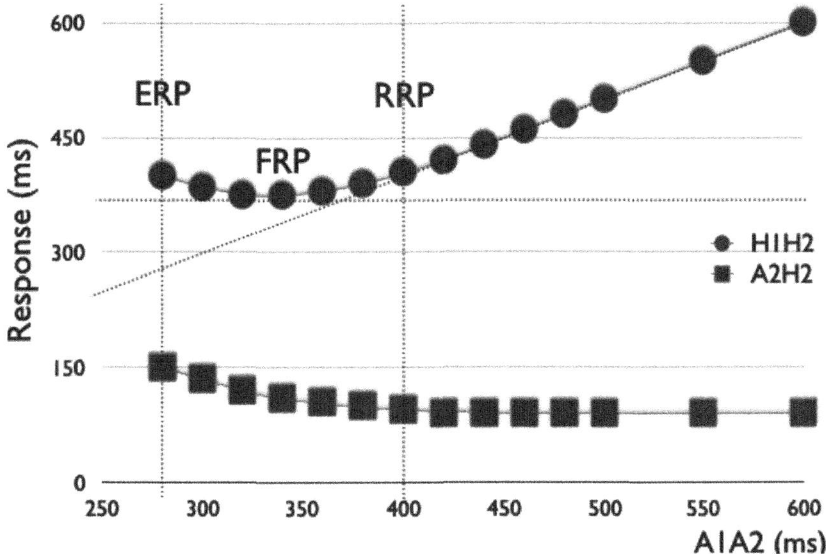

  - As the S1S2 coupling interval is decreased, there is initially a steady relationship with H1H2 and A2H2.
  - This is followed by:
    - Decremental AVN conduction, in which a gradual lengthening in the H1H2 and A2H2 intervals is observed with decreasing A1A2
    - Normal HV interval without decremental response, in which there is an increase in A1A2 with decreasing S1S2 at short coupling intervals due to the emergence of intra-atrial conduction delay
- Interpretation of discontinuous anterograde conduction curves:

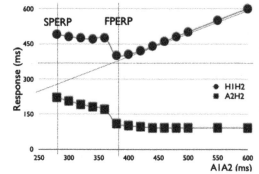

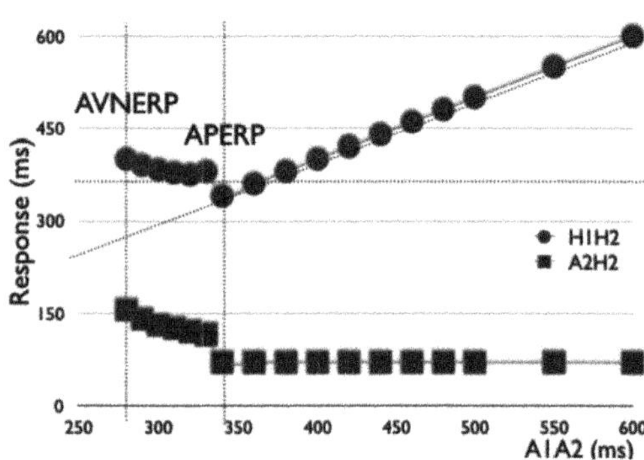

The initial portion of the curve represents decremental conduction through the fast pathway. When the refractory period is reached, conduction blocks in the fast pathway (FPERP) and "jumps" to the slow pathway (defined by a ≥50 ms increase in the A2H2 or H1H2 interval with a 10 ms decrease in the S1S2 coupling interval), where it remains decremental until the slow pathway ERP (SPERP). Note: An AH jump without echo beat may be seen in 30% of normal controls.

The initial portion represents non-decremental conduction through the AP. When the refractory period is reached, conduction blocks in the AP (APERP) and "jumps" to the AVN, where it becomes decremental until the AVNERP is reached. Note: There may be decremental AH conduction via the AVN with non-decremental AV conduction via the AP resulting in progressively more negative HV interval/more manifest pre-excitation.

Difficulties in Determining Refractory Periods

- Refractory periods are dependent on autonomic tone.
  - Sympathetic tone increases conduction velocity and decreases refractory periods.
  - Parasympathetic tone decreases conduction velocity and increases refractory periods.
- Accurate estimation of retrograde AVNERP
  - During ventricular stimulation, the AVN receives its input via the bundle of His.
  - By definition, the retrograde AVNERP is the longest H1H2 that fails to conduct across the node and back to the atria.
  - In the situation where the retrograde His is buried in the ventricular EGM, it is better to refer to the retrograde AVNERP as the retrograde ERP of the VA conduction system.
- Conduction of the AVN may continue to atrial tissue refractoriness due to:
  - The AVNERP being less than the atrial ERP (AERP)
  - Sufficient delay in the atrial tissue such that the coupling interval of the impulse arriving at the node remains above the AVNERP
- "Gap" phenomenon:
  - Conduction of an impulse may be blocked at a certain S1S2 interval, then reappear as the S1S2 interval is lowered further before finally disappearing at an even lower S1S2.

- This occurs when an impulse is conducted over 2 structures with differing ERPs in sequence.
  - At S1S2, there is block in the second structure (e.g., the His-Purkinje system or AVN).
  - At shorter S1S2, there is conduction delay (e.g., latency) in the first structure (e.g., the AVN or atrial myocardium) resulting in slowed conduction, thus allowing the impulse to reach the second structure (e.g., the His-Purkinje system or AVN) with an increased coupling interval (i.e., at a point when it has recovered).
  - At an even shorter S1S2, there is conduction block in the first structure.
- Conventionally, conduction is assumed to cease when the block first disappears.

- Arrhythmia induction:
  - As the risk of arrhythmias increases as the extrastimulus coupling interval falls, extrastimulus testing around AVNERP may be hampered by induction of supraventricular arrhythmias.

ANTEROGRADE CONDUCTION

Incremental Atrial Pacing

- Performed from the HRA or proximal CS (preferred), or distal CS (for potential left lateral AP)
- Determine the following:
  - Presence/absence of pre-excitation
  - The reterograde WCL:
    - WCL is defined as CL where 1:1 anterograde conduction ceases (normal 350–450 ms).
    - The location of the AV block should be noted (AH or HV).

Extrastimulus Testing

- Should be performed at 2 drive train CLs (typically 600 ms and 400 ms)
- Determine the following:
  - Anterograde conduction curve (see above)
  - Refractory periods:
    - AVNERP (normal 250–400 ms)
    - AERP (normal 180–330 ms)
      - Note: If AERP is reached before AVNERP, the use of a drive train with a shorter CL may decrease the AERP and increase the AVNERP.
      - Double extrastimuli (S2S3) may be required if too much intra-atrial conduction delay is observed at short coupling intervals.

Interpretation

- Normal findings are:
  - As the S1S2 coupling interval is decreased, there is initially a steady relationship with H1H2 and A2H2.
  - This is followed by decremental conduction in the AVN, leading to a gradual lengthening in the H1H2 and A2H2 intervals.

- Abnormal results include:
  - Discontinuous conduction curves (see above)
  - Echo beats
    - Extrastimulus is conducted down the anterior limb (e.g., slow pathway) and then back up the retrograde limb (e.g., fast pathway).
    - Presence of echo beats confirms tachycardia substrate.
    - Must be differentiated from **intra-atrial reentry**.
      - True nodal echoes have midline caudo-cranial activation (His before HRA).
      - VA timing of echoes should be consistent over many coupling intervals.

AV Nodal Echo Beat

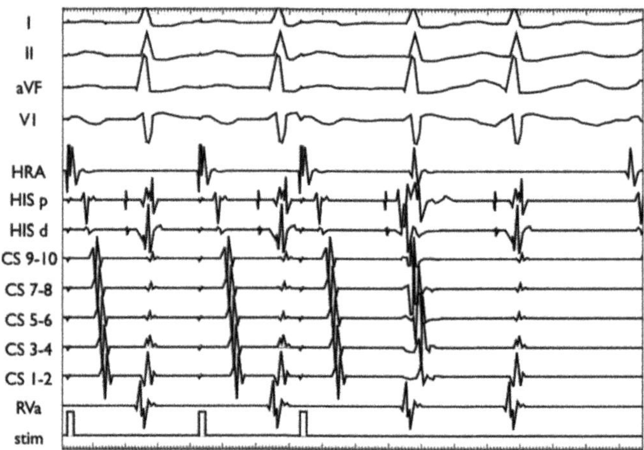

Using a stable drive train (S1), an extrastimulus (S2) is introduced and conducts anterogradely down the slow pathway and then back up the fast pathway. In this example, the impulse conducts back down the slow pathway, resulting in an echo beat before blocking retrogradely in the fast pathway.

RETROGRADE CONDUCTION

- Retrograde conduction is generally not as efficient as anterograde conduction.
  - Retrograde block occurs at longer CLs.
  - Normally, block occurs first in the His-Purkinje system.
  - Block can be hard to see, as His spike is buried in V.

Incremental Ventricular Pacing

- Assess
  - The presence (or absence) of retrograde atrial activation
  - The retrograde atrial activation sequence (concentric vs. eccentric)
  - The retrograde (VA) conduction time
  - The retrograde VA WCL
    - WCL is defined as CL where 1:1 retrograde conduction ceases.

Extrastimulus

- Should be performed at 2 drive train CLs (typically 600 ms and 400 ms)
- Assess
  - The retrograde conduction curve (see above)
  - Refractory periods:
    - VA conduction block (retro AVNERP)
    - **Ventricular myocardium ERP** (normal 180–290 ms)

Interpretation

- Normal findings are:
  - Absent VA conduction despite pharmacologic provocation

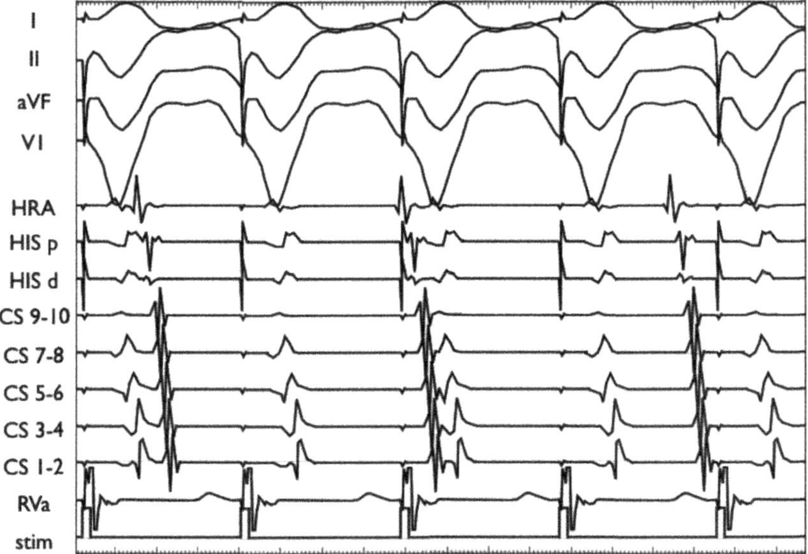

  - Concentric atrial activation (midline)

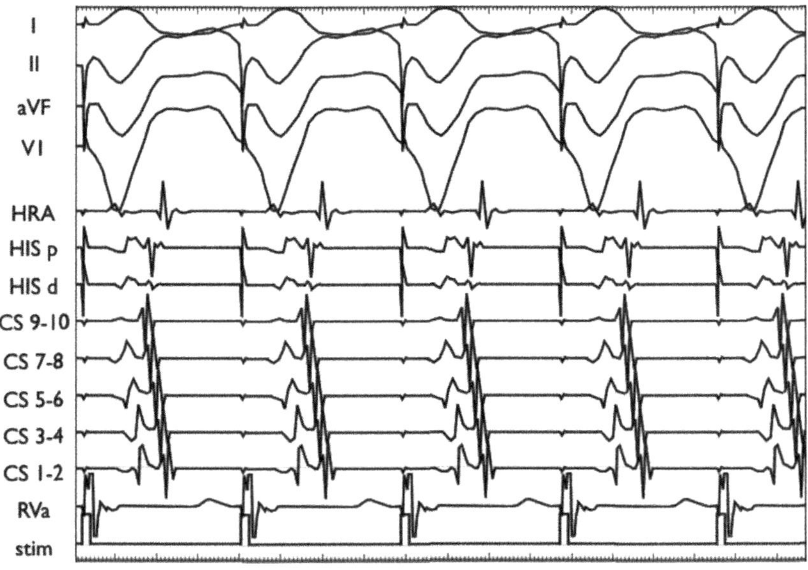

        - Decremental VA conduction
            - V2A2 > V1A1 with progressive increase in V2A2 with decreasing V1V2
    - Abnormal results include:
        - Eccentric atrial activation (right and left free wall APs)
        - Non-decremental VA conduction
        - VA jump due to:
            - Dual AVN physiology with a jump from the retrograde fast pathway to the slow pathway
            - Septal AP with a jump from AP to AVN conduction (AVNERP < APERP)
    - Ventricular extra beats post-extrastimulus due to:
        - Bundle branch reentry
            - Retrograde right bundle branch block (RBBB) allows S2 to cross the septum and conduct retrograde via the left bundle and then anterograde down the right bundle, which has recovered conduction.
        - Ventricular echo
            - Retrograde conduction up one limb blocks (typically the anterior limb, e.g., the slow pathway), allowing unopposed retrograde conduction up the retrograde limb (e.g., fast pathway) to return anterograde down the anterior limb (e.g., slow pathway).
        - Repetitive ventricular response
            - QRS morphology mimics the paced beats with RVa EGM at the onset of the QRS.

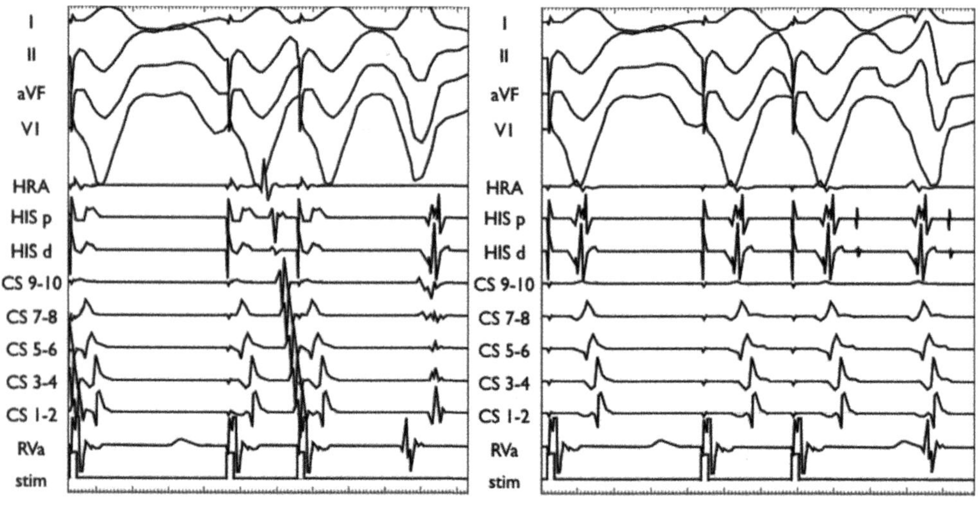

Repetitive Ventricular Response **Bundle Branch Reentry**

Difficulties in Interpreting Retrograde Curve

- AVN fusion and retrograde latency.
  - Retrograde atrial activation via the AVN can mask retrograde AP conduction.
  - Latent retrograde AP conduction can be unmasked by delaying the retrograde nodal activation relative to the AP (i.e., shifting atrial activation from midline to eccentric) via:
    - Retrograde extrastimuli
    - Pacing at shorter CLs
    - Pacing in the LV for left-sided APs (i.e., pacing closer to the AP insertion site)
    - IV adenosine to transiently block retrograde AVN conduction
- AVN and septal AP have similar retrograde conduction times.
  - No VA jump or change in midline activation as conduction switches between the AP and AVN
  - Pathway may be unmasked by:
    - Failure of IV adenosine to induce VA block
    - Parahisian pacing
    - Inducible supraventricular tachycardia (SVT) with advancement of atrial activation with His-synchronous ventricular premature beat (VPB)
- Retrograde AVN conduction is exclusively via fast pathway followed by VA block.
  - The presence of an AP may be refuted by:
    - VA block with IV adenosine administration
    - Parahisian pacing
    - Inducible SVT *without* advancement of atrial activation with His-synchronous VPB

ARRHYTHMIA INDUCTION

Importance of Arrhythmia Induction

- The mode of initiation may give clues to the mechanism of arrhythmia.
- Induction represents confirmation of the clinical arrhythmia.
- Induction permits assessment of hemodynamic consequences of the arrhythmia.
- Inducing the arrhythmia offers a baseline for comparison to post-treatment endpoint.
  - Also aids in assessment of methods to terminate arrhythmias

Techniques for Inducing Arrhythmia

- Burst or decremental pacing
  - Decremental pacing to refractoriness
  - Burst pacing at short CLs (near the refractory period) from multiple sites
- Programmed extrastimulus
  - Pacing with 1–3 extrastimuli from multiple sites (atrial: HRA and CS; ventricle: base and RVOT)
- Pharmacologic adjuncts, such as:
  - Isoproterenol 1–4 mcg/min IV infusion
  - Adrenaline 0.01–0.1 mcg/kg/min IV infusion
  - Atropine 500 mcg–1 mg IV bolus
  - Adenosine 6–18 mg IV bolus (most useful for AF induction)

Observations in Tachycardia

- After induction, the following key observations should be recorded:
  - Comparison to clinical tachycardia
  - Mode of initiation and termination
  - AV relationship during tachycardia
  - VA time and atrial activation sequence
  - Other observations

Atrial Tachycardia Initiation

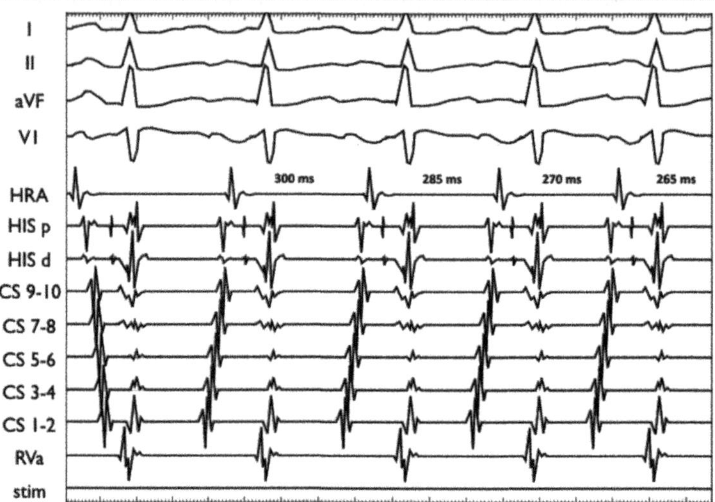

Arrhythmia onset is preceded by an atrial extrasystole (different P-wave morphology and atrial activation) when compared to the preceding sinus beat. Thereafter, an AT is initiated. Note the demonstration of a warm-up phenomenon — i.e., a gradual increase in tachycardia rate at arrhythmia onset.

AVNRT Initiation

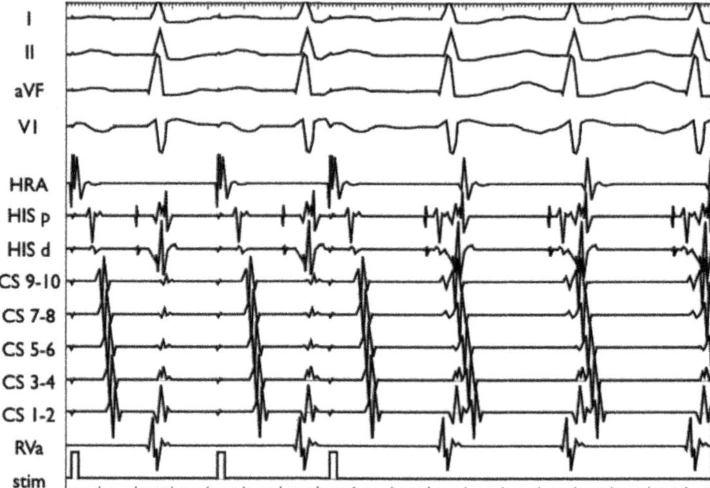

Atrial extrastimulus technique: Pacing in the HRA during the drive train demonstrates AVN conduction via the fast pathway. With an extrastimulus, there is block in the fast pathway resulting in a "jump" to the slow pathway. This impulse simultaneously conducts down to the ventricle and returns to the atria via the now-recovered fast pathway to complete the circuit.

Antidromic AV Reentrant Tachycardia Initiation

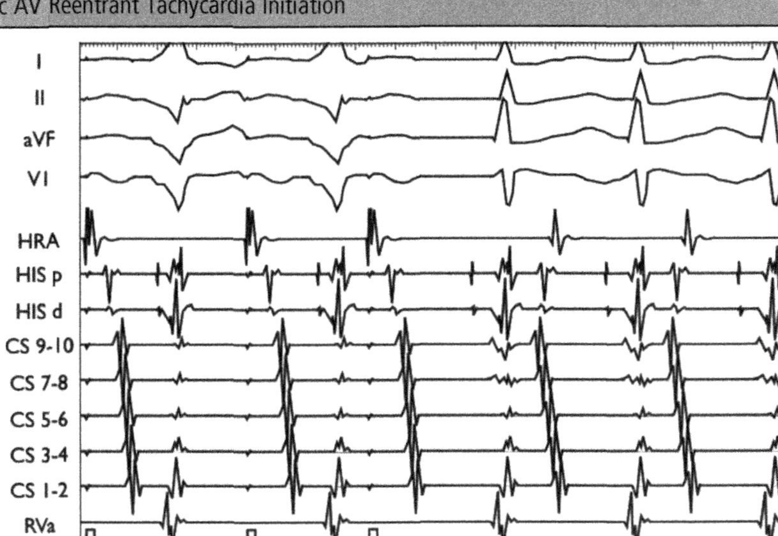

Atrial extrastimulus technique: Pacing in the HRA during the drive train demonstrates near-maximal pre-excitation from a posteroseptal AP. With an extrastimulus, there is block in the AP, resulting in anterograde conduction exclusively across the AVN. This impulse conducts down to the ventricle and returns to the atria via the now-recovered AP to complete the circuit (earliest A on the proximal CS).

PROGRAMMED VENTRICULAR STIMULATION

Background

- Sudden cardiac death is most commonly due to ventricular arrhythmias (VT, VF).
  - The most common mechanism of VT is reentry, which often occurs around scar (i.e., previous MI).
  - Less common mechanisms include triggered activity and automaticity.
- Ventricular stimulation is indicated:
  - For evaluation of unexplained syncope in patients at risk of SCD
  - To study and characterize the VT in order to aid in ablation

Principles

- The technique employs increasingly aggressive programmed stimulation using multiple extrastimuli.
  - Sensitivity is increased through:
    - The use of an increasing number of extrastimuli
    - Drive trains at multiple CLs
    - Multi-site ventricular pacing (typically RVa and RVOT)
    - Incremental pacing (i.e., burst pacing)
    - Isoproterenol infusion
  - Specificity is reduced by:
    - High stimulation outputs (more than twice the diastolic threshold)
    - Extrastimuli with coupling intervals <200 ms
    - The use of >3 extrastimuli

Procedure

- Start with an 8-beat drive train at 600 ms (S1), then a single extrastimulus (S2).
  - The S2 coupling interval is gradually reduced by 10 ms to 200 ms or ventricular refractoriness.
  - With S2 held at ERP, a second extrastimulus (S3) is introduced at ERP + 50 ms.
  - The S3 coupling interval is gradually reduced by 10 ms to 200 ms or ventricular refractoriness.
  - At S3 ventricular refractoriness, scan diastole by gradually reducing S2 by 10 ms until S3 captures again.
  - Repeat with progressively lower S3 and S2 until 200 ms or ventricular refractoriness.
- If no VT is induced, the process is repeated:
  - First, in the RVa at a 400 ms drive train
  - Second, in the RVOT at 600 ms and 400 ms
  - Third, with a third extrastimulus (S4) at both 600 ms and 400 ms in both the RVa and RVOT
- If VT is still not induced, consider:
  - Repeating the procedure with a isoproterenol infusion (or other agents: Adrenaline, atropine)
  - Incremental (burst) pacing
  - Long-short stimulus sequence (i.e., S1 train followed by long S2 and short-coupled S3)

Interpretation

- Initiation of sustained monomorphic VT is considered a positive test.
  - Intracardiac EGMs should demonstrate dissociation of atrial/His EGMs from ventricular EGMs.

Monomorphic Ventricular Tachycardia Initiation

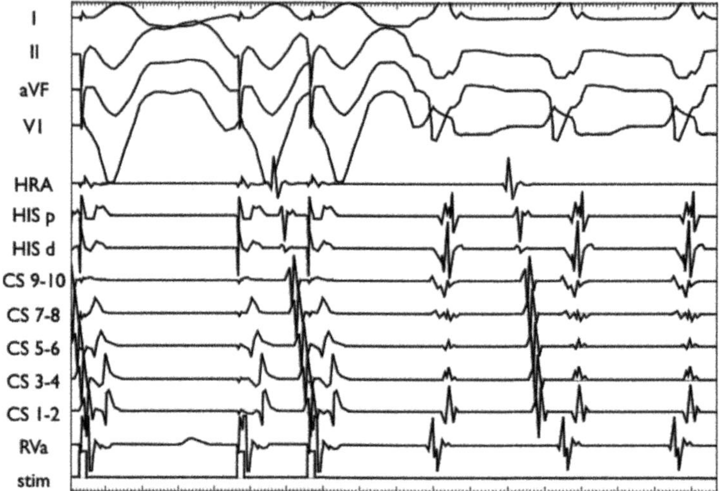

Pacing in the RV during the drive train does not demonstrate any evidence of VA conduction. With an extrastimulus, there is induction of a monomorphic VT. Note the AV dissociation.

- Confirmation with a 12-lead ECG should be obtained (compare to clinical VT if possible).
- Initiation of VF or non-sustained polymorphic VT is considered a non-specific result, but must be interpreted in the context of the reason for the test.
  - Better specificity if induced with >3 extrastimuli or late-coupled extrastimuli

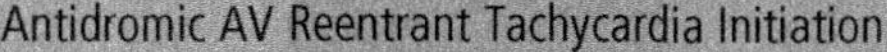

Antidromic AV Reentrant Tachycardia Initiation

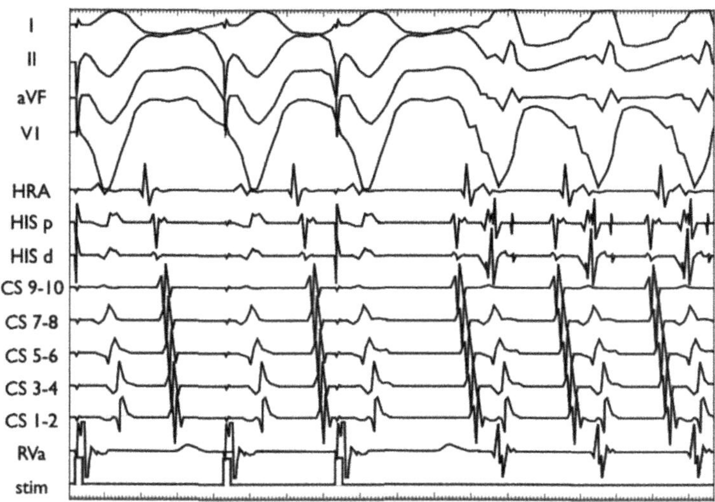

Pacing in the RV during the drive train demonstrates earliest atrial activation in the HRA, suggesting conduction across a right lateral AP. With an extrastimulus, there is block in the AP, resulting in retrograde conduction across the AVN (concentric atrial activation with earliest A on the His and PCS). This impulse conducts down to the ventricle via the now-recovered AP and returns to the atria via the His-Purkinje system (note the retrograde His deflection) to complete the circuit.

OBSERVATIONS IN TACHYCARDIA: ATRIAL ACTIVATION SEQUENCE

Normal Anterograde Activation

- The impulse starts from the sinus node and spreads in a radial fashion to the RA and LA, and inferiorly to the AVN (HRA → His bundle atrial EGM → proximal CS → distal CS).
- At the AVN, the impulse is delayed to allow for mechanical atrial emptying.
- The impulse then travels from the His-Purkinje system to the ventricles and is activated in a typical fashion from the Interventricular septum → Apices of RV and LV → Ventricular free walls → Basal ventricles, with the posterobasal LV activated last (latest V activation in the mid- to distal CS).

Normal Retrograde Activation

- The impulse moves through ventricular myocardium to the Purkinje fibers → Midline (His bundle atrial EGM) → Proximal to distal CS → HRA.

- Note: Assessment of atrial activation requires proper CS catheter positioning.
  - If the position is too proximal, a false chevron pattern with midline activation will be observed due to the mid CS bipoles being positioned over the CS ostium and thus activating early.
  - If the position is too distal, there will be a reverse chevron pattern with the distal and proximal CS being activated before the mid-CS due to anterior and posterior septal activation.

Interpretation

- Interpretation of the atrial activation sequence is most useful if performed during tachycardia, although information can be obtained during ventricular pacing in the presence of an AP.
- **Concentric (midline) atrial activation**
  - Earliest atrial activation is in the septum (**His A-EGM**), followed by the low LA (**CS** from proximal to distal), then the sinus node region (**HRA**; ~30 ms after His A-EGM).
  - Seen with: AVNRT, anteroseptal AP, slowly conducting AP, poorly conducting AP, atriofascicular AP

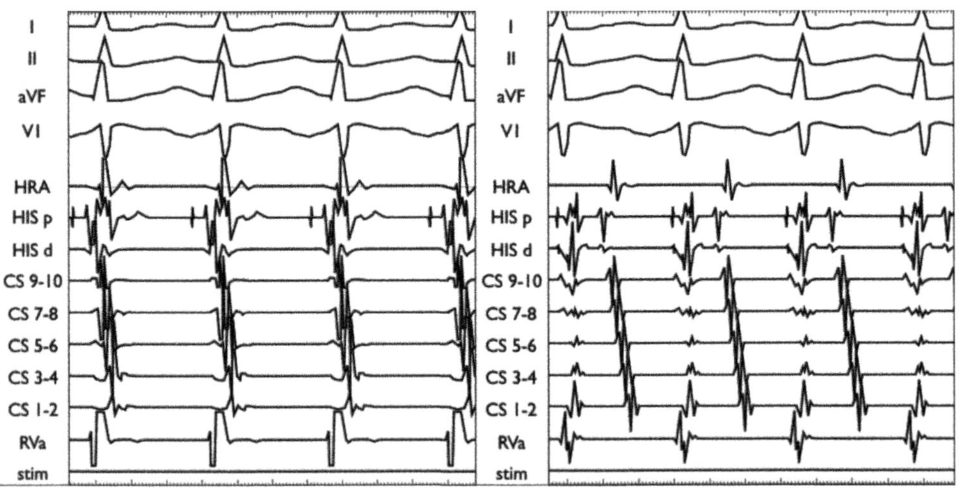

Typical AVNRT

Midline activation with a short VA time
Earliest activation on the His (anterior fast pathway exit)

Anteroseptal AP

Midline activation with a long VA time
Proximal CS and HRA timing is nearly simultaneous

- **Eccentric atrial activation**

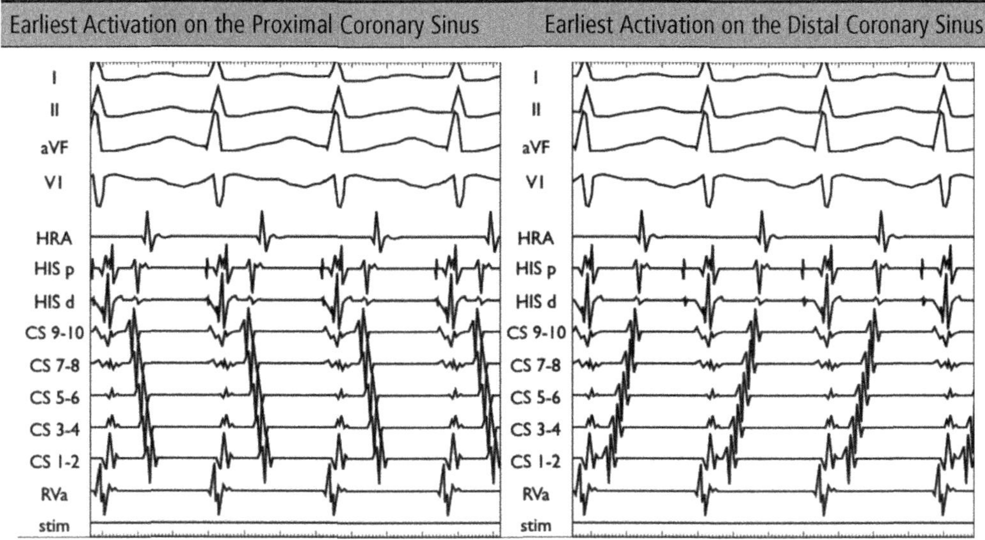

Activation: pCS → HBE → dCS → HRA
Due to:
- Retrograde AVN activation (AVNRT)
- Posteroseptal AP (AVRT)

Activation: dCS → pCS → HBE → HRA
Due to:
- Left lateral AP (AVRT)
- Left-sided AT

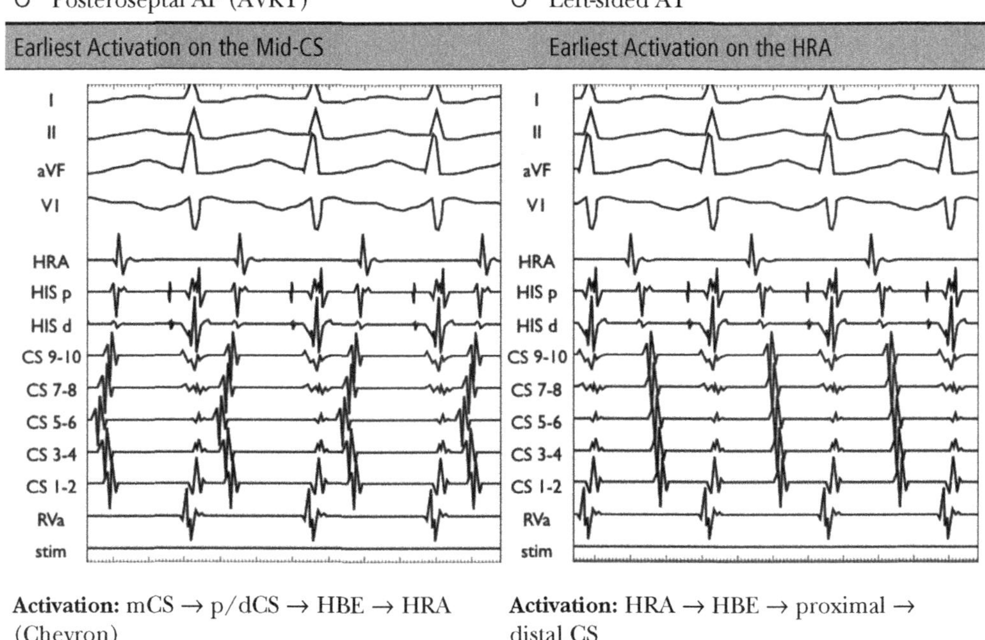

Activation: mCS → p/dCS → HBE → HRA (Chevron)
Due to:
- Left posterior AP (AVRT)
- Left-sided AVN connection (AVNRT)

Activation: HRA → HBE → proximal → distal CS
Due to:
- Right lateral AP (AVRT)
- Right-sided AT

Ventricular Entrainment from RV Overdrive Pacing

Atrial Activation Sequence

- Methodology
  - Pace the ventricle at a CL 10–40 ms (usually 20 ms) faster than the tachycardia cycle length (TCL).
  - Once the atria are entrained at the pacing rate, the pacing is stopped.
  - The atrial activation sequence during pacing is assessed and compared to tachycardia.
- Interpretation
  - Identical atrial activation sequences (e.g., pacing = tachycardia) may be due to:
    - AVNRT (slow pathway/fast pathway)
    - Atrioventricular reentrant tachycardia (AVRT; orthodromic reentrant tachycardia [ORT] via anteroseptal AP)
    - Failure to entrain may be secondary to:
      - Tachycardia termination during RV pacing (re-induce tachycardia and the repeat maneuver)
      - VA block at CL greater than TCL (in this case, the maneuver is not diagnostically useful)
    - Note: An identical activation sequence essentially excludes an AT.
  - Different atrial activation sequences (e.g., pacing ≠ tachycardia) may be due to:
    - AT
    - Concealed or bystander APs
    - Multiple APs
    - Note: AVRT (ORT via anteroseptal AP) remains possible in the circumstance where the pacing CL is less than the retrograde APERP, resulting in switch to nodal activation during entrainment.

Post-Pacing Sequence

- Methodology
  - Pace the ventricle at a CL 10–40 ms (usually 20 ms) faster than the TCL.
  - Once the atria are entrained at the pacing rate, the pacing is stopped.
  - The activation sequence at cessation of pacing is assessed.
- Interpretation
  - VAV or AHV response is seen with AVRT or AVNRT
  - VAAV or AAHV response is seen with AT or AVNRT with long HV
  - Pseudo-VAAV response:
    - VA time during pacing is longer than the pacing interval (long RP tachycardia)
      - Results in an apparent VAAV response at the cessation of pacing, during which the first A EGM is dependent on the second-to-last paced beat and the second A EGM is dependent on the last pacing beat. The timing of the 2 VA intervals should be consistent with that observed during ventricular entrainment.
      - In contrast, the VA timing in AT will not reflect the pacing VA interval.
    - VA time during AVNRT is negative (short RP tachycardia).
      - In typical AVNRT, the first A of the VAAV is conducted to the ventricle via the AVN and His bundle, producing a His EGM immediately prior to the simultaneous A and V EGMs, resulting in a VAHAV pattern.
      - In contrast, the first A of a VAAV response in AT is not conducted down the AVN, so there is no His EGM between the 2 A EGMs, resulting in a VAAHV pattern.

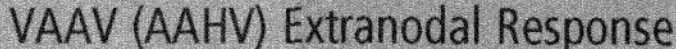

VAAV (AAHV) Extranodal Response

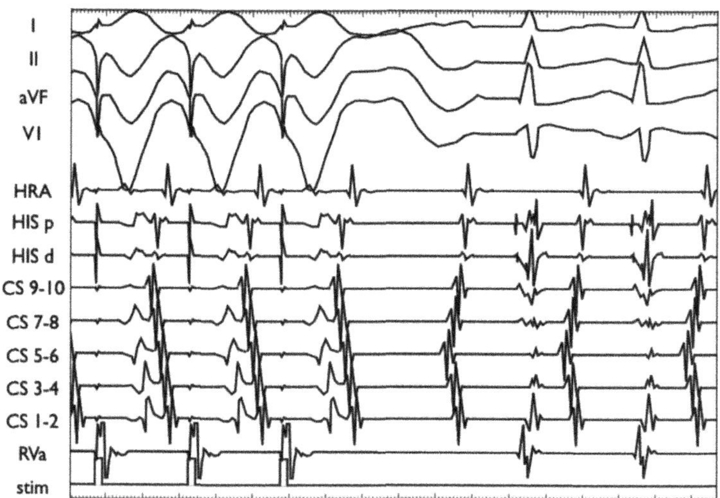

Ventricular entrainment during AT results 1:1: VA conduction with AT suppression. With cessation of ventricular pacing (V EGM) the last paced beat is conducted back to the atria (A EGM) followed by resumption of the first beat of tachycardia (A EGM), which then conducts back to the ventricle via the AVN (V EGM; VAAV response).

VAV (AHV) Nodal Response (AVNRT, AVRT)

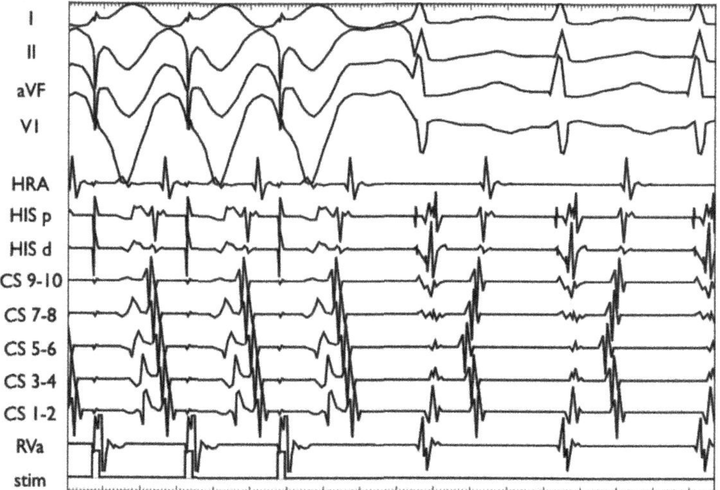

Ventricular entrainment during typical AVNRT results in 1:1 VA conduction. With cessation of ventricular pacing (V EGM), the last paced beat is conducted back to the atria (A EGM) by the fast pathway of the AVN, followed by anterograde conduction down to the ventricle via the slow pathway (V EGM; VAV response). A similar response is noted with AVRT, where the last beat is conducted back to the atria (A EGM) by the AP and then back down to the ventricle via the AVN (V EGM; VAV response).

Return Cycle Length Upon Discontinuation of Pacing

- Methodology
  - Pace the ventricle at a CL 10–40 ms (usually 20 ms) faster than the TCL.
  - Once the atria are entrained at the pacing rate, the pacing is stopped.
  - The time from the last ventricular pacing stimulus to the next V EGM in the RV catheter when tachycardia resumes is then assessed.
- Interpretation:
  - Post-pacing interval (PPI) – TCL
    - >115 ms: AVNRT, ORT (decremental or distant AP)
    - <115 ms: ORT
  - **Corrected PPI (cPPI)** = PPI – TCL – (AH_{RVP} – AH_{SVT})
    - >110 ms: AVNRT, ORT (decremental or distant AP)
    - <110 ms: ORT

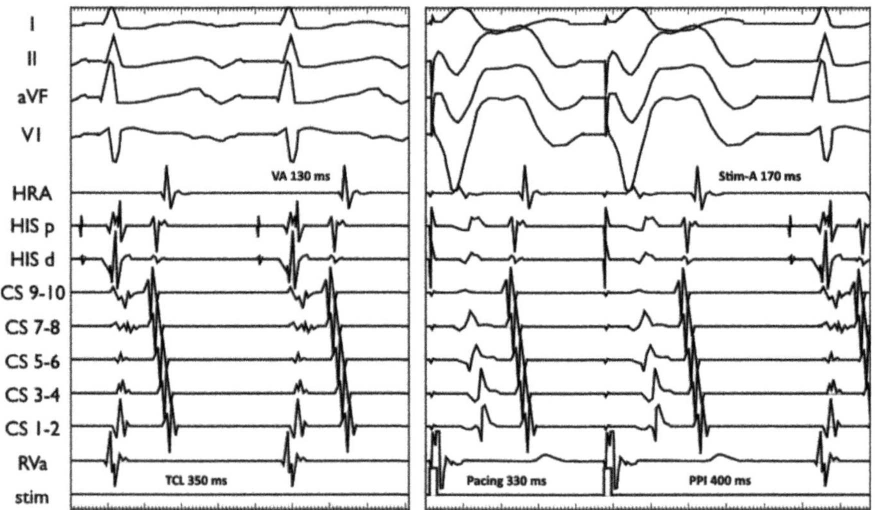

SVT entrainment via RV pacing at 330 ms (left panel: TCL 350 ms with a VA time of 130 ms). The SA–VA interval is 40 ms, and the PPI – TCL is 50 ms, consistent with an ORT using a right posteroseptal AP.

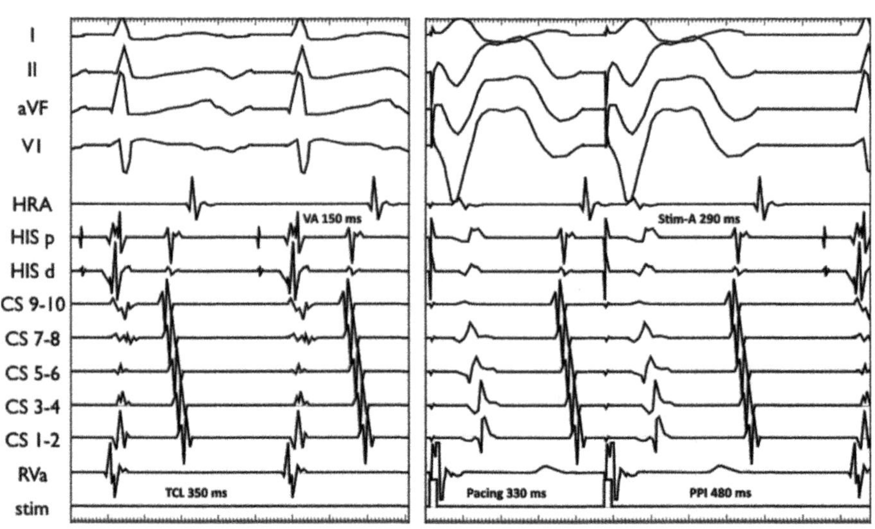

SVT entrainment via RV pacing at 330 ms (left panel: TCL 350 ms with a VA time of 150 ms). The SA–VA interval is 140 ms, and the PPI – TCL is 130 ms, consistent with atypical AVNRT.

VA Interval During Pacing

- Methodology
  - Pace the ventricle at a CL 10–40 ms (usually 20 ms) faster than the TCL.
  - Once the atria are entrained at the pacing rate, the pacing is stopped.
  - The VA interval is measured from the last pacing stimulus on the RV catheter to the last entrained HRA EGM (Stim-A_{RVP}) and is compared to the VA interval during tachycardia (VA_{SVT}).
- Interpretation
  - Stim-A_{RVP} – VA_{SVT}
    - <85 ms: ORT via septal AP (AVRT)
    - >85 ms: AVNRT, left AP, concealed decremental AP
  - Stim-A_{RVP} to VA_{SVT} ratio
    - 0.27–0.32: AVNRT
    - 0.9–1.08: posteroseptal AP
    - 0.94–1.29: anteroseptal AP

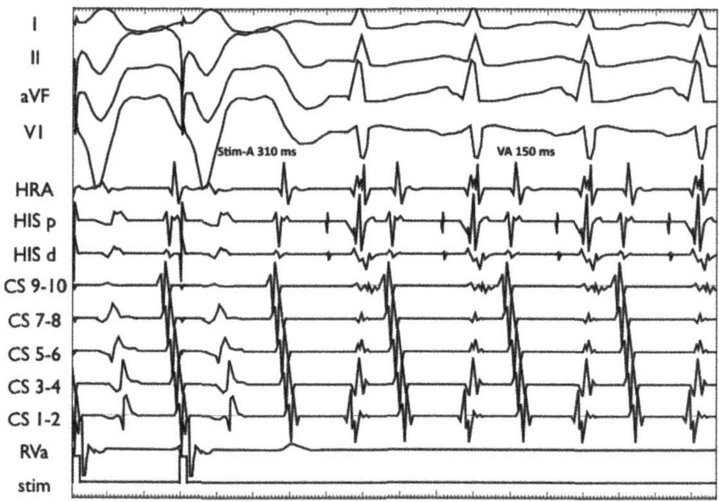

The **Stim-A_{RVP} – VA_{SVT}** interval is 160 ms, suggesting atypical AVNRT.

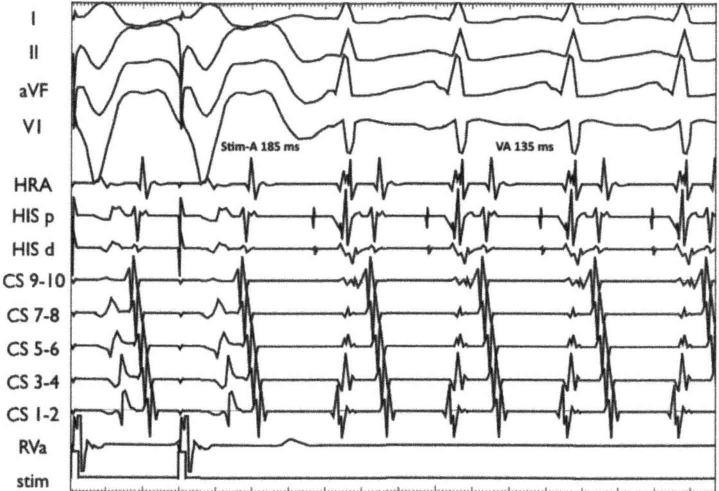

The **Stim-A_{RVP} – VA_{SVT}** interval is 50 ms, suggesting ORT from an anteroseptal AP.

VENTRICULAR PACING MANEUVERS DURING TACHYCARDIA

Differential RV Entrainment

- Entrainment at RVa and RV base is often used to differentiate atypical AVNRT from AVRT using a paraseptal decremental AP.
- Methodology
  - Pace the ventricle at a CL 10–40 ms (usually 20 ms) faster than the TCL at the RVa.
  - Once the atria are entrained at the pacing rate, the pacing is stopped.
  - Entrainment is then repeated at a CL 10–40 ms (usually 20 ms) faster than the TCL from the RV base.
- Interpretation
  - (cPPI – TCL) at the base – (cPPI – TCL) at the apex > 30 ms
    - Supports AVNRT or AT (shortest VA time is near apex)
  - **(Stim-A_{RVP} – VA_{SVT})** at the apex – **(Stim-A_{RVP} – VA_{SVT})** at the base < 0 ms
    - Supports AVNRT or AT

Parahisian Entrainment

- Entrainment with and without His capture is often used to differentiate atypical AVNRT from AVRT using a paraseptal decremental AP.
- Methodology
  - High-output pacing (i.e., 20 mA at 2.0 ms) at a CL 10–40 ms (usually 20 ms) faster than the TCL captures the septal RV myocardium and the His directly, resulting in retrograde AVN activation and anterograde ventricular activation with narrow QRS.
  - Entrainment is then repeated at a lower output such that the His is no longer invaded, and the ventricle captures with a wide left bundle branch block (LBBB) morphology QRS.
  - The Stim-A (with and without His capture) and the PPI – TCL are then assessed.
- Interpretation
  - Delta Stim-A (His loss – His capture)
    - >40 ms supports AVNRT
    - <40 ms supports AVRT
  - PPI – TCL (Stim to local V EGM) – Entrainment without His capture
    - >100 ms supports AVNRT, ORT (decremental or distant AP)
    - <100 ms supports ORT

Parahisian Entrainment in Tachycardia: AVNRT

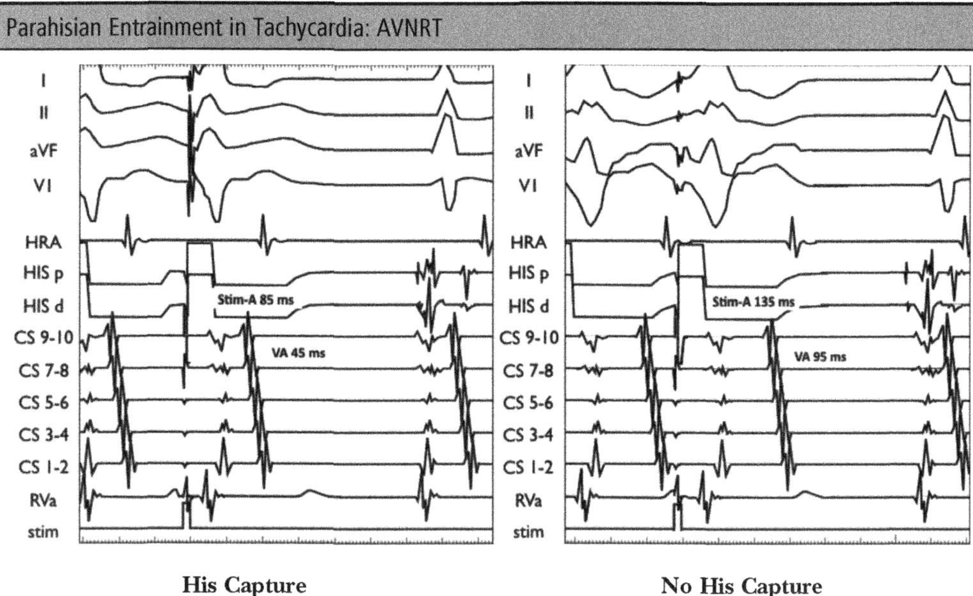

His Capture **No His Capture**

Narrow-complex tachycardia with earliest atrial activation in the proximal CS. Shown in the two panels are two separate entrainment maneuvers performed. In the **left panel**, there is His capture, and in the **right panel**, there is loss of His capture. The delta Stim-A with loss of His capture was 50 ms, consistent with AVNRT.

Parahisian Entrainment in Tachycardia: ORT via Posteroseptal AP

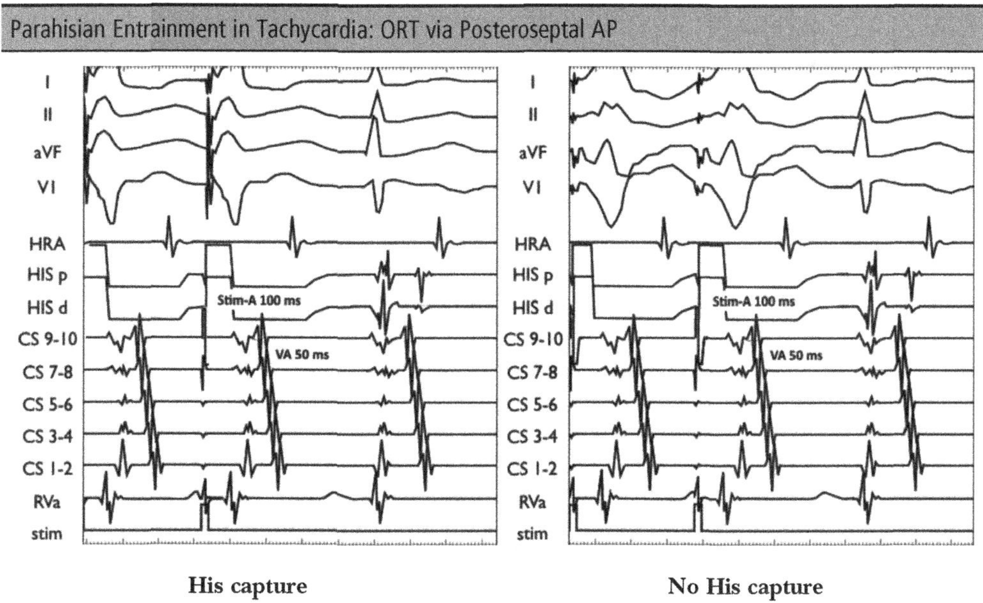

His capture **No His capture**

Similar pacing maneuvers are performed as above. In this case, the delta Stim-A (His loss – His capture) was 0 ms, consistent with AVRT (posteroseptal AP).

RV Burst Pacing

- Methodology
  - During tachycardia, the RVa is paced at 250–350 ms.
- Interpretation
  - If SVT continues and VA dissociated, it excludes AVRT.
  - If SVT terminates without A activation, it excludes AT.

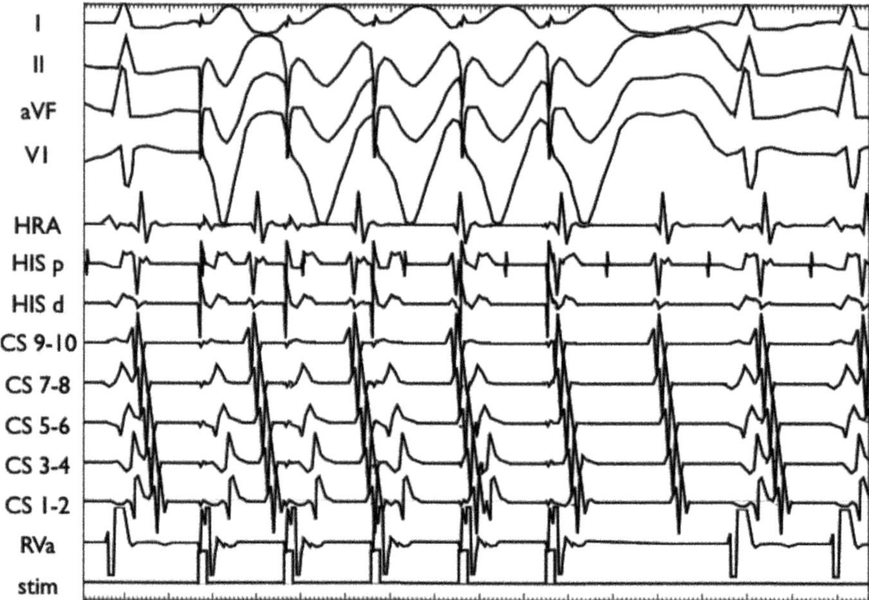

Burst pacing in the ventricle at 300 ms dissociates the ventricle without interrupting the tachycardia. Excludes AVRT as the tachycardia mechanism.

Diastolic Ventricular Extrastimuli

- His-synchronous VPB is used to identify the presence of a retrograde conducting AP (typically a septal AP), differentiating AVRT from atypical AVNRT.
  - Extrastimuli coincident with the His deflection cannot reach the atria via the AVN as the His bundle is refractory.
- Methodology
  - Measure the time from peak EGM on the RV catheter to His EGM on the His catheter.
  - During tachycardia, a single pacing stimulus is delivered at the above interval plus 20 ms and then delivered at progressively shorter coupling intervals (e.g., decrease by 10 ms).
- Measurements
  - The VPB that arrives closest to the timing of the anticipated His deflection is chosen.
  - The two atrial EGMs (preceding and following) are measured on the proximal CS and/or His.
- Interpretation
  - Tachycardia termination
    - Diagnostic of the presence of an AP as well as its participation in the tachycardia circuit

- Atrial advancement by a VPB
    - Proof of the existence of another route to the atria (i.e., retrograde AP); however, it does not confirm the AP as part of the tachycardia circuit
- **Atrial advancement by a VPB and the SVT resets** (i.e., early A advances the V with the subsequent AA interval remaining the same as the TCL)
    - This usually acts as confirmation of AP participation in the tachycardia.
    - Note: Tachycardia advancement (reset) may not be manifest despite AP participation in the tachycardia due to decremental AVN conduction.
    - Note: Tachycardia advancement may be present despite the lack of AP participation in the tachycardia (i.e., bystander AP) due to the advanced atrial beat entering the slow pathway and advancing AVNRT.
- Atrial delay by a VPB
    - Diagnoses the presence of a decremental AP that participates in tachycardia
- No response in atria
    - Non-diagnostic: Neither confirms nor excludes the presence of an AP

o Caveat
- CL variation or alternans makes His-synchronous VPB uninterpretable.

o Other observations
- **Pre-excitement index** (TCL – ESV CL needed to pre-excite atria)
    - <45 ms: Septal AP left free wall AP + LBBB
    - 45–75 ms: Right free wall
    - >75 ms: Left free wall
    - >100 ms: AVNRT

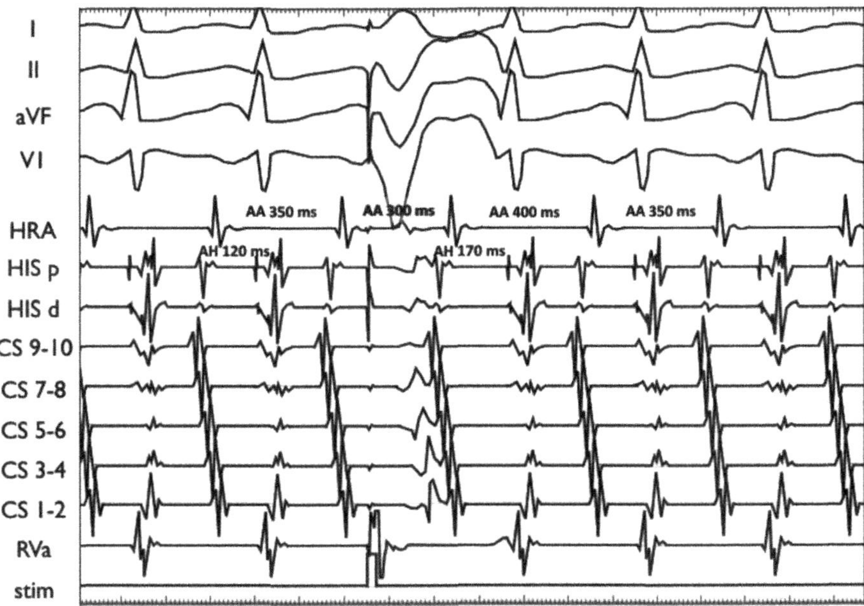

His-synchronous VPB advances the next A by 50 ms, confirming the existence of an AP (but not its involvement in tachycardia). Note: Concurrent AH prolongation (from 120 to 170 ms) means tachycardia is not advanced.

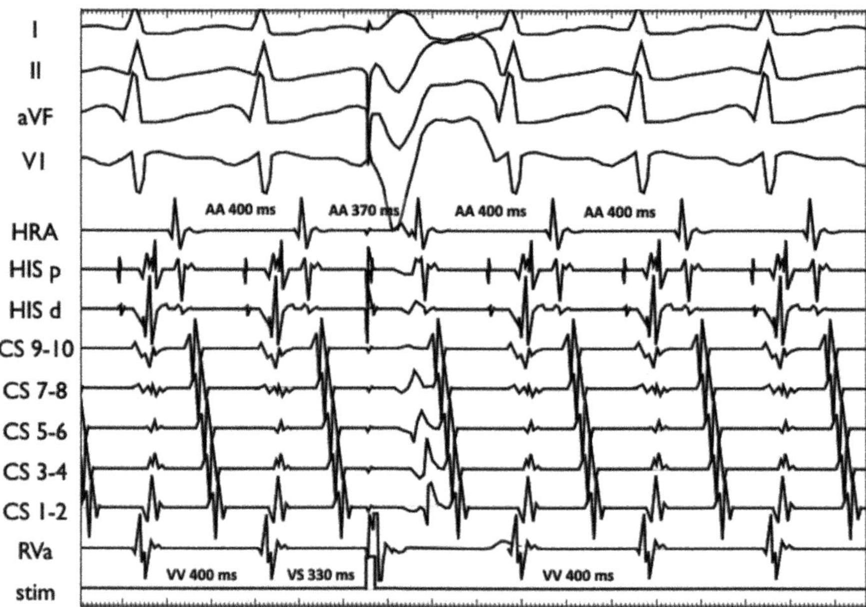

His synchronous VPB (delivered 70 ms early) advances the next A and tachycardia cycle by 30 ms (due to decrement in the AP), thus confirming the existence of an AP and its involvement in tachycardia.

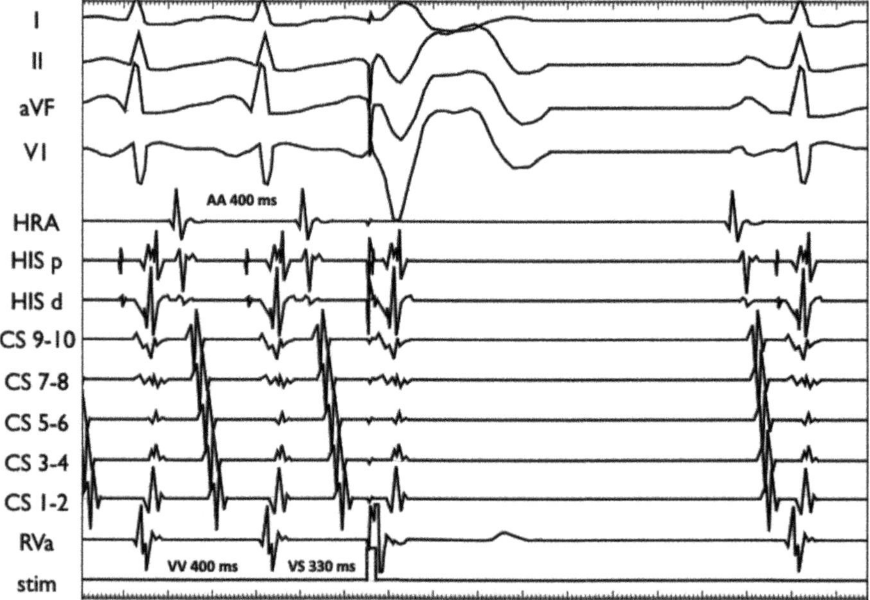

His synchronous VPB (delivered 70 ms early) terminates tachycardia without conducting to the atrium. This confirms the presence of an AP as well as its involvement in tachycardia (ventricle is a critical part of the circuit).

ATRIAL PACING MANEUVERS DURING TACHYCARDIA

Atrial Entrainment from Atrial Overdrive Pacing

- Methodology
  - Pace the atrium at a CL 10–40 ms (usually 20 ms) faster than the TCL.
  - Once the ventricles are entrained at the pacing rate, the pacing is stopped.
  - **Differential entrainment**: Consider repeating entrainment from multiple segments of the chamber of interest (for example, cavotricuspid isthmus [CTI], lateral RA, and septum for CTI-dependent flutter, or proximal and distal CS for LA).
- Interpretation
  - VA of first return beat
    - Fixed/linked VA timing (<10 ms of tachycardia VA) suggests AVNRT, ORT; excludes AT or junctional tachycardia (JT)
    - Variable VA timing suggests AT or JT
  - Post-pacing interval (PPI): TCL (Stim to local A EGM)
    - Concealed entrainment with PPI – TCL ≤20 ms: **In-circuit response**
    - Concealed entrainment with PPI – TCL >20 ms: **Bystander location**
    - Entrainment with fusion and PPI – TCL >20 ms: **Out-of-circuit response**
  - Post-pacing sequence
    - **AHA**: AVNRT, AVRT, AT
    - **AHHA**: Junctional ectopic tachycardia (JET)

AHA (AHVA) Response

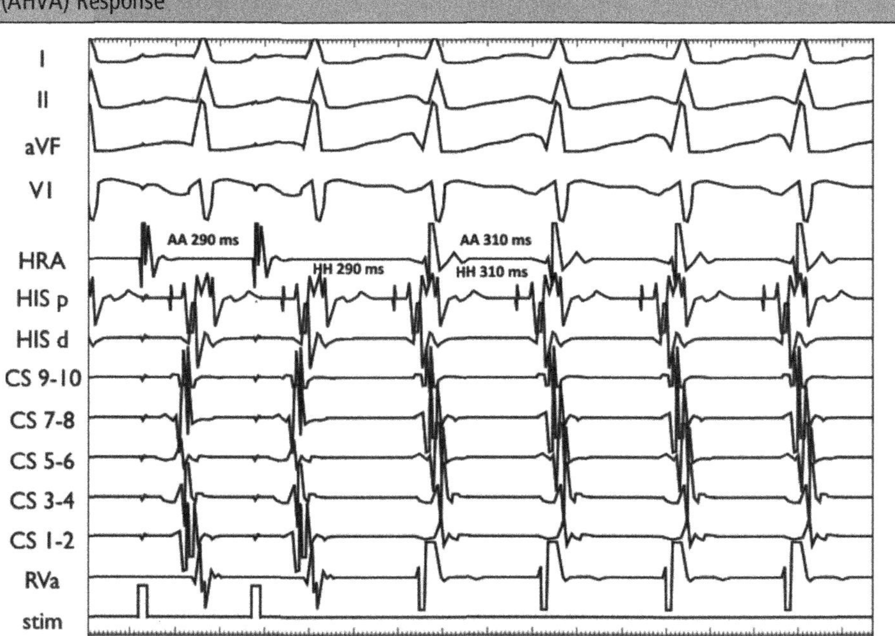

Atrial overdrive pacing is performed at 290 ms (TCL 310 ms). The HH intervals are noted, demonstrating the last advanced His signal. After cessation of pacing, an AHA response is observed.

AHHA Response

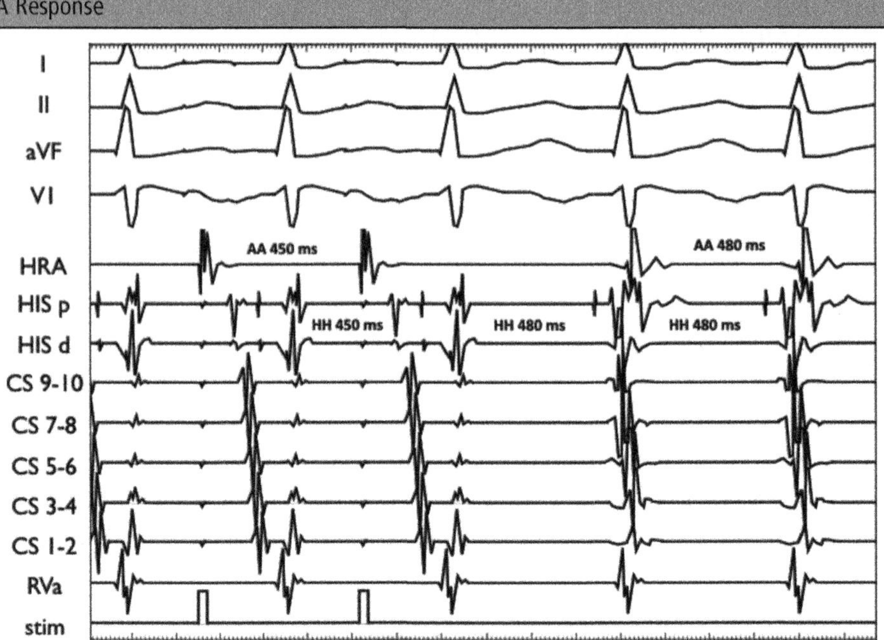

Entrainment of junctional tachycardia at 450 ms (TCL 480 ms). An AHHA response is observed after pacing.

Transient Atrial Overdrive Pacing

- Methodology
  - Pace the atrium at the longest CL that resulted in AV block.
  - Analyze the last AH interval before cessation of pacing.
- Interpretation
  - Tachycardia termination is AH dependent (short AH interval with termination compared to AH with tachycardia continuation), suggesting AVRT or AVNRT.

Diastolic Atrial Extrastimuli

- Useful to differentiate AVNRT from non-reentrant junctional tachycardia (i.e., narrow-complex tachycardia (NCT) with short VA)
- Methodology
  - Late-coupled premature atrial contraction (PAC) is delivered when the junction is refractory (timed to His refractoriness).
    - Advances (or delays) the subsequent His and resets the tachycardia: AVNRT
    - No effect on TCL: Junctional tachycardia
  - Early-coupled APC can help identify AVNRT or junctional tachycardia:
    - Advances the His with a short AH and terminates SVT: AVNRT (anterograde activation of the fast pathway renders it refractory to retrograde conduction)
    - Advances the His with a short AH and resets the tachycardia: Junctional tachycardia

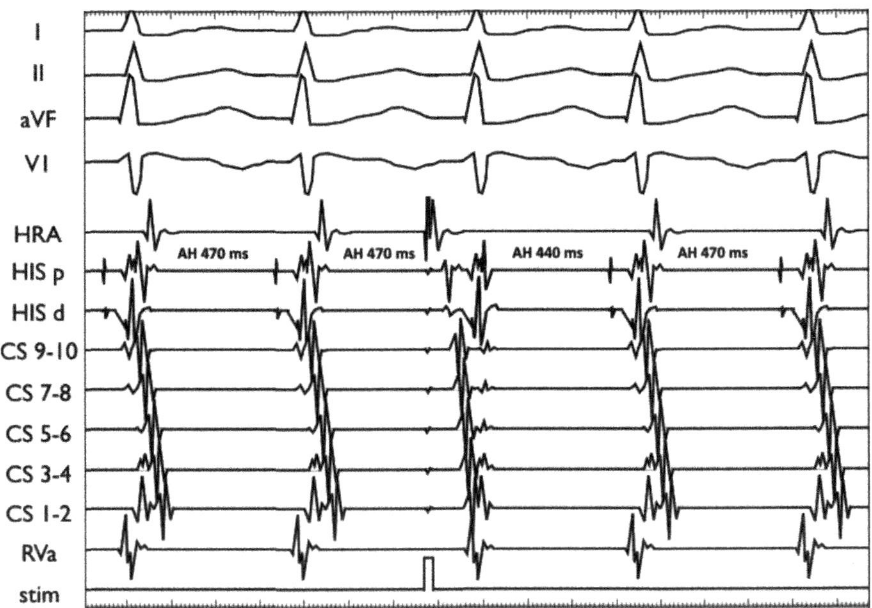

Premature atrial contraction (PAC) timed to junctional (His) refractoriness advances the next His by 30 ms, suggesting AVNRT as the mechanism.

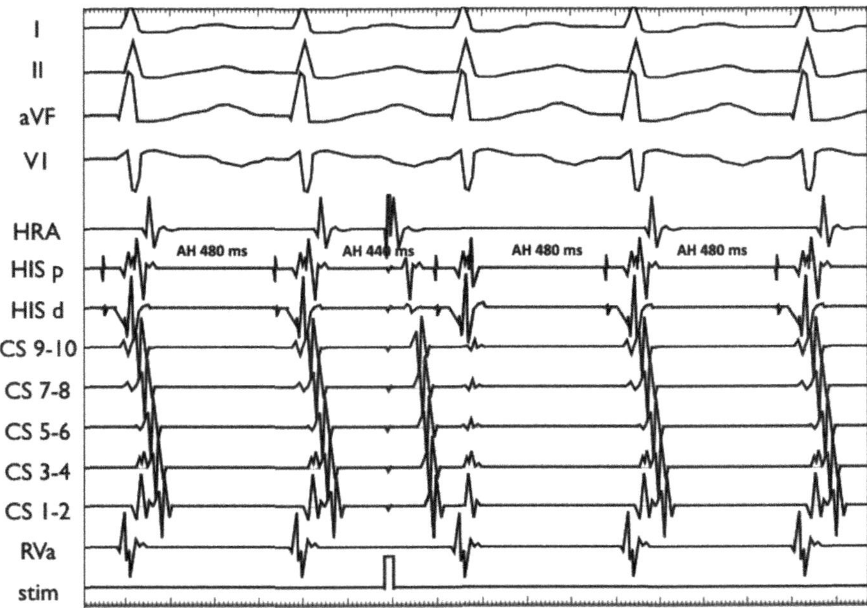

PAC timed to junctional (His) refractoriness advances the immediate His by 40 ms, suggesting JET as the mechanism.

PACING MANEUVERS DURING SINUS RHYTHM

Parahisian Pacing

- Parahisian pacing is useful to differentiate a septal AP from an anterior AVN retrograde exit site.
- Methodology
  - Position the catheter to record a retrograde His and atrial activation (S1A1 and H1A1).
  - Ventricular pacing at TCL is performed to the anterobasal RV septum 1–2 cm distal to the His bundle recording and adjacent to the proximal right bundle branch (HB-RB).
  - High-output pacing at TCL (i.e., 20 mA at 2.0 ms) captures the septal RV myocardium and the HB-RB directly, resulting in **anterograde** ventricular activation with narrow QRS and **retrograde** atrial activation via the AVN.
  - The process is repeated with low-output pacing at TCL (e.g., gradually reduce pacing output until the HB-RB is no longer invaded), resulting in ventricular captures with a wide LBBB morphology QRS.
- The timing and retrograde activation sequence between **HB-RB capture** and **non-capture** are examined.
- Interpretation
  - Classification of responses:

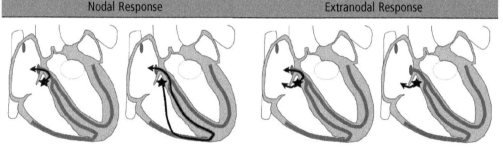

Nodal Response

Loss of HB-RB capture (right) forces the impulse to spread to the apex and up the right bundle to the AVN.

- S1A1 interval increases
  - Typically ≥50 ms
- H1A1 remains constant
  - Atria are still activated via His → AVN
- Retrograde atrial activation sequence
  - Should remain constant (retrograde AVN)

Extranodal Response

Loss of HB-RB capture (right) does not alter the atrial activation (still moves from RV septum → AP → RA).

- S1A1 interval
  - Unchanged or increases <40 ms
- H1A2 interval shortens
  - His activation is delayed (constant S1A1)
- Retrograde atrial activation sequence
  - Should change (switch from AVN to AP)

- Observations may include:
  - Identical retrograde atrial activation sequence
    - Nodal conduction (AVNRT, AT)
    - Exclusive AP conduction
  - Changes to the retrograde atrial activation sequence
    - Conduction switches from node to AP
    - Nodal conduction (switches from slow pathway to fast pathway)
  - Increased Stim-A (VA) interval
    - HA interval stable: Nodal conduction (AVNRT, AT), AP (decremental or distant)
    - HA interval decreases: AP
  - Decreased or unchanged Stim-A (VA) interval: AP
- Confounding factors:
  - Difficulty achieving consistent His bundle capture (catheter position varying with respiration)
  - Local A capture at the same time as His or V capture
  - RBBB

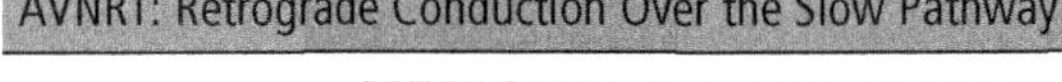

AVNRT: Retrograde Conduction Over the Slow Pathway

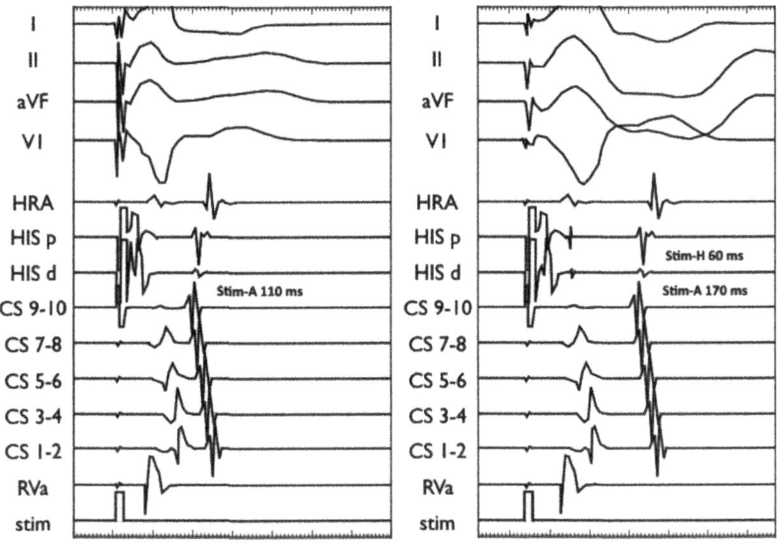

Left panel: Ventricular and HB-RB capture produce a relatively narrow QRS complex and early activation of the His bundle (buried within the V EGM on the His catheter).
Right panel: Loss of HB-RB capture results in widening of the QRS complex, an increase in the S-H interval (to 60 ms), and a 60 ms increase in the S-A interval (from 110 ms to 170 ms).

The stable **HA** interval (~100 ms) indicates that retrograde conduction was dependent on His bundle activation and not on ventricular activation (i.e., retrograde conduction occurs exclusively over the AVN).

Earliest atrial activation occurs on the proximal CS, suggesting that retrograde conduction occurs over the slow pathway.

AVRT: Anteroseptal Accessory AV Pathway

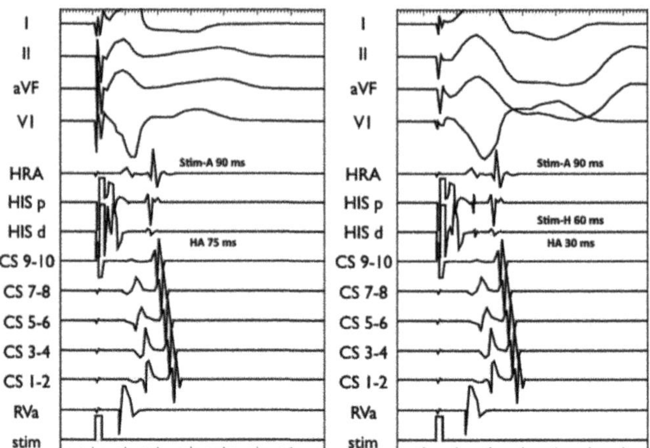

Left panel: Ventricular and HB-RB capture produce a relatively narrow QRS complex and early activation of the His bundle (buried within the V EGM on the His catheter).
Right panel: Loss of HB-RB capture results in widening of the QRS complex and an increase in the S-H interval (to 60 ms), but no change in the S-A interval (constant at 90 ms).

The stable **SA** interval (90 ms) but shorter delta **HA** interval (–45 ms) indicate that retrograde conduction was dependent on the timing of ventricular activation and not on the timing of the His bundle.

Earliest atrial activation occurs on the His, suggesting that retrograde conduction occurs over an anteroseptal accessory AV pathway.

AVRT: Midseptal Accessory AV Pathway

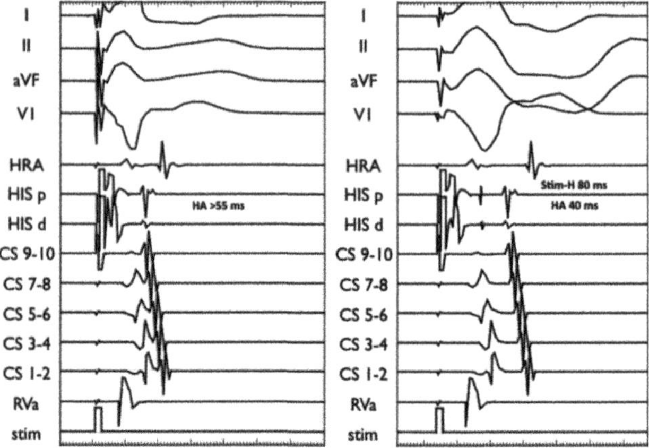

Left panel: Ventricular and HB-RB capture produce a relatively narrow QRS complex and early activation of the His bundle (buried within the V EGM on the His catheter).
Right panel: Loss of HB-RB capture results in widening of the QRS complex, a decrease in H-A interval (from 55 ms to 40 ms), and a slight change in atrial activation (shift from the AVN to a mid-septal AP).

Note: The loss of HB-RB capture is accompanied by a decrease in the H-A interval (from 55 ms to 40 ms) and a slight change in the atrial activation, indicating loss of retrograde activation by the AVN (fusion atrial activation by both the AVN and the AP during HB-RB capture but exclusive AP conduction during HB-RB non-capture).

Differential (Apical-Basal) RV Pacing

- Differential RV pacing is useful to differentiate an anteroseptal pathway from an anterior AVN exit site.
- Methodology
  - Pace the ventricle at the TCL from the RVa.
  - Once the atria are entrained at the pacing rate, the pacing is stopped.
  - Pacing is then repeated at the TCL from the RV base or RVOT.
- Interpretation
  - Classification of responses:

Nodal Response	Extranodal Response

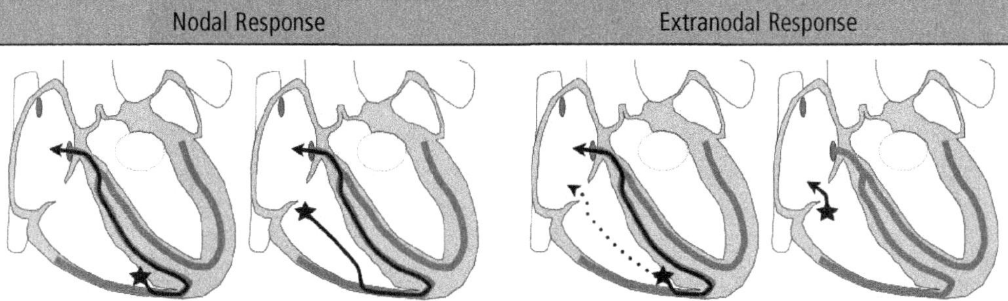

With exclusive retrograde AVN conduction, pacing from the base results in a longer VA/Stim-A time because the impulse must spread to the apex in order to enter the His-Purkinje system to return to the atria.	With a right-sided AP, pacing from the base results in a more direct atrial activation via the AP, resulting in a lessened (or similar) VA/Stim-A time when compared to apical pacing.

  - Observations may include:
    - Retrograde atrial activation sequence
      - Identical: Nodal response (AVNRT, AT), AP (decremental or distant)
      - Changes: AP, nodal (change from slow pathway to fast pathway)
    - Septal HA interval
      - Unchanged: Nodal response (AVNRT, AT), AP (decremental or distant)
      - <20–30 ms or negative: AP
    - VA intervals (Apex – Base)
      - <5–10 ms: Nodal response (AVNRT, AT), AP (decremental or distant)
      - >10 ms: AP
  - Caveats
    - Ensure low-output pacing to avoid right bundle branch/His capture.
    - Problems with RBBB and fasciculoventricular pathways may occur.

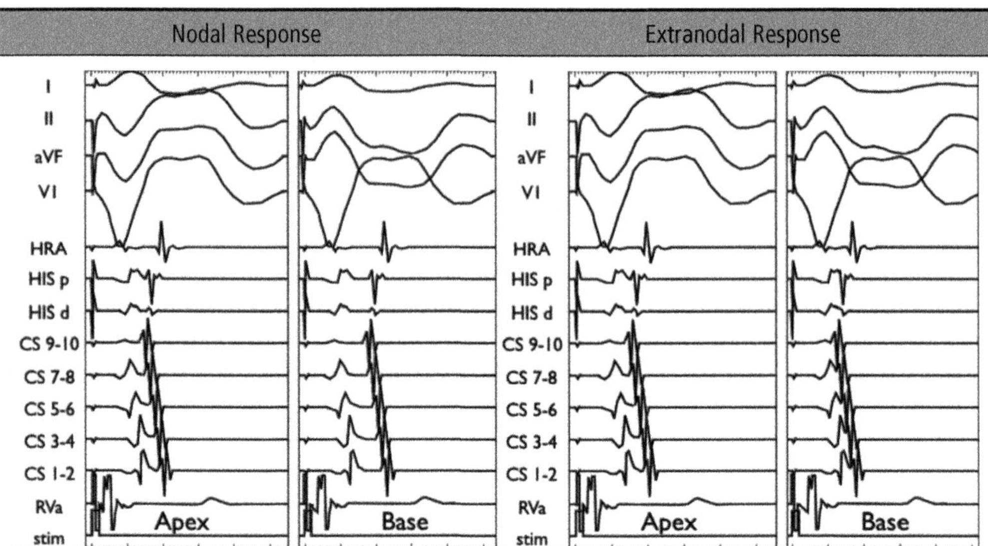

A longer VA time with change from apical to basal pacing suggests an absence of AP conduction.

No change in VA time with change from apical to basal pacing suggests posteroseptal AP.

Atrial Pacing at Tachycardia Cycle Length

- Atrial pacing at TCL is useful to differentiate an anteroseptal pathway from an anterior AVN exit site.
- Methodology
  - Pace the atrium at the TCL.
  - Compare the AH interval with atrial pacing to the AH interval during tachycardia.
- Interpretation
  - >40 ms difference: AVNRT
  - <20 ms difference: AP (septal)
  - <10 ms difference: AT

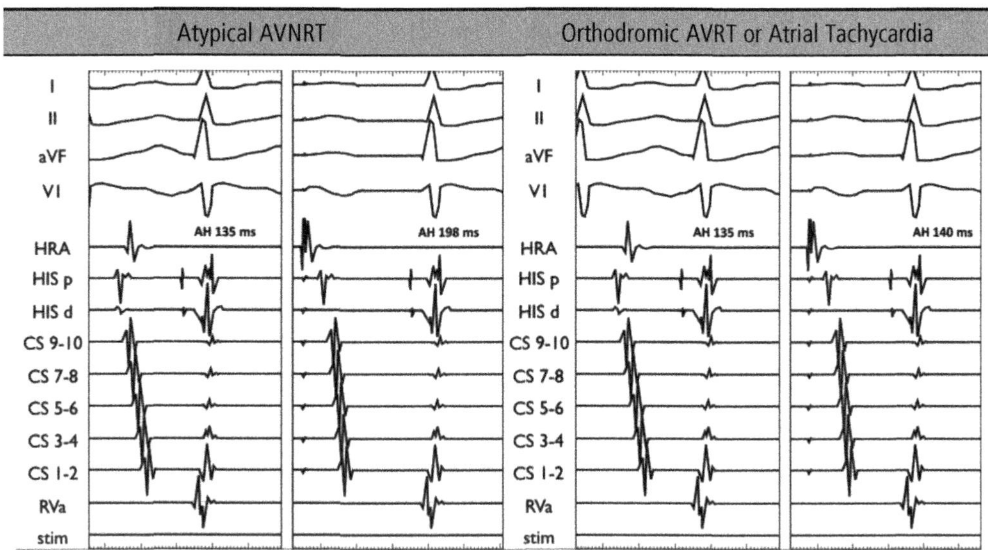

The AH interval is 135 ms during tachycardia (left) and 198 ms during atrial pacing at the TCL (right), leading to a delta AH of 63 ms.

The AH interval is 135 ms during tachycardia (left) and 140 ms during atrial pacing at the TCL (right), leading to a delta AH of 5 ms.

Ventricular Pacing at Tachycardia Cycle Length

- Useful to differentiate AVNRT from a JET
- Methodology
  - Pace the ventricle at the TCL.
  - Compare the HA interval with ventricular pacing to the HA interval during tachycardia.
- Interpretation
  - Negative delta HA: AVNRT
  - Positive delta HA: JET

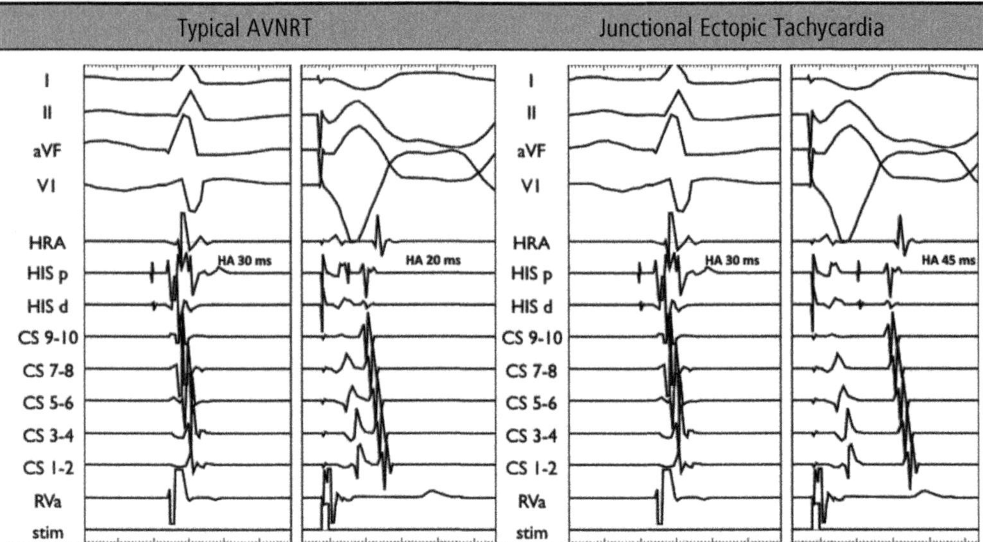

The HA interval is 30 ms during tachycardia (left) and 20 ms during ventricular pacing at the TCL (right), leading to a delta HA of –10 ms, suggesting AVNRT as the mechanism of tachycardia.

The HA interval is 30 ms during tachycardia (left) and 45 ms during ventricular pacing at the TCL (right), leading to a delta HA of 15 ms, suggesting JET as the mechanism of tachycardia.

Induction of Retrograde RBBB

- Methodology
  - Drive trains of 600 ms and 400 ms with 8 paced beats are followed by a coupled extrastimulus.
  - A retrograde RBBB is defined by a ≥50 ms increase in the retrograde V-H interval induced with a ≤20 ms decrease in the S1S2 coupling interval.
- Classification of responses:

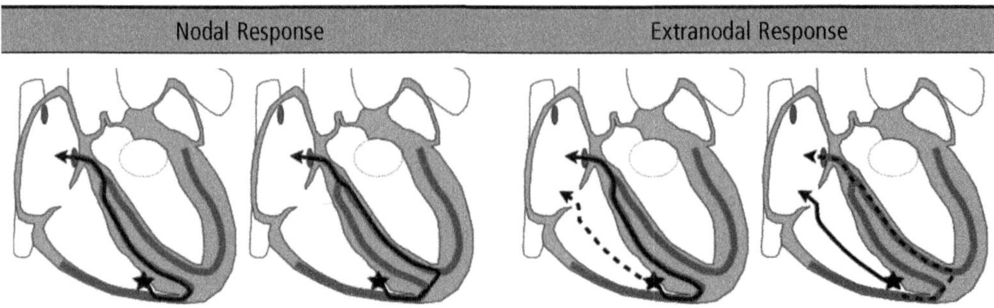

With exclusive retrograde AVN conduction, the induction of retrograde RBBB results in a prolongation of the VH interval >50 ms (the impulse must spread across the septum in order to enter the His-Purkinje system) with a concomitant increase in the VA interval by >50 ms.

With a right-sided AP, the induction of retrograde RBBB results in a prolongation of the VH interval by >50 ms (the impulse must spread across the septum in order to enter the His-Purkinje system). However, the VA time is unchanged as the atria are activated by a pathway.

- Interpretation
  - Increase in VH > Increase in VA: ORT
  - Increase in VH < Increase in VA: AVNRT

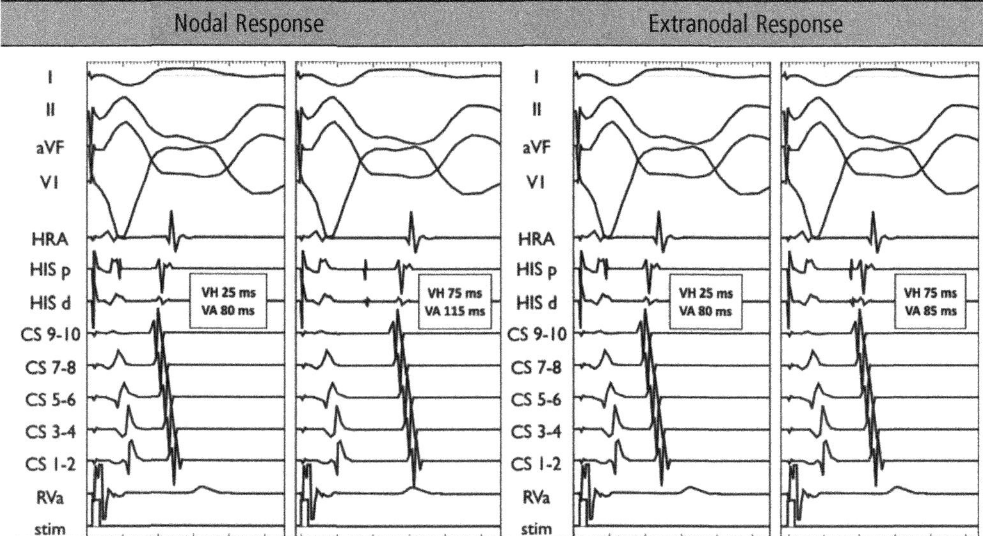

RV apical pacing at 600 ms with an S1S2 coupling interval of 360 ms results in a retrograde His 25 ms after the QRS with a VA interval of 80 ms. When the coupling interval is decreased to 340 ms, retrograde RBBB is induced (increased VH to 75 ms; delta VH of 50 ms) with concomitant prolongation of VA timing (115 ms; delta VA of 35 ms).

RV apical pacing at 600 ms with an S1S2 coupling interval of 360 ms results in a retrograde His 25 ms after the QRS with a VA interval of 80 ms. When the coupling interval is decreased to 340 ms, retrograde RBBB is induced (increased VH to 75 ms; delta VH of 50 ms) without altering VA timing (85 ms; delta VA of 5 ms).

EVALUATION OF SINUS NODE FUNCTION

Anatomy of the SA Node

- The SA node is a sub-epicardial collection of nodal cells within a matrix of connective tissue.
  - A conglomerate of specialized pacemaker cells (P cells) generate the normal cardiac rhythm.
  - Perinodal cells (T cells) allow the transmission of electrical impulses from the SA node to the RA.
- It is a comma-shaped structure 3 mm wide and 10 to 15 mm long.
  - The head is located on the crista terminalis lateral to the RA appendage near the junction of the RA and the SVC.
  - The tail extends downward along the crista terminalis toward the inferior vena cava.
- Sinus rate is modulated by:
  - Parasympathetic nervous system fibers (CN X: Vagus nerve)
  - Sympathetic nervous system fibers (T1–T4: Spinal nerves)

Sinus Node Automaticity

- Rapid extrinsic pacing suppresses SA node automaticity (phase 4 slope) by continually depolarizing the SA node faster than it can be intrinsically depolarized (overdrive suppression).
  - After cessation of pacing, there is a pause before the SA node begins spontaneously firing.
  - The interval from the last paced beat to the first sinus recovery beat is the sinus node recovery time (SNRT).
- Methodology
  - Pace the HRA at various CLs, then abruptly terminate pacing.
  - Start just below the baseline sinus CL (measured just before pacing onset) and pace for 30–60 s.
    - After cessation of pacing, there is normally a slight prolongation in the return CL (SNRT) followed by a return to the baseline sinus CL over 5–6 beats.
    - Note: Need to test over a wide range of intervals (600, 500, 400, 350, and 300 ms ± 800, 700 ms) due to potential for entrance block into the sinus node (results in less SA node penetration and potentially SNRT).
- Interpretation
  - SNRT: Normal values are <1500 ms.
    - Defined as the interval from the last paced beat to the first sinus recovery beat
  - Corrected sinus node recovery time (CSNRT): Normal values are <525–550 ms.
    - Calculated as: SNRT – baseline sinus CL (BCL)
  - SNRT/BCL ratio: Normal values are <160%.
    - Calcuated as: (SNRT ÷ BCL) × 100%
  - Total recovery time (TRT): Normal values are <5 seconds.
    - Defined as the interval between the cessation of pacing and the return to baseline sinus CL.
- Caveats
  - Sensitivity and specificity are only about 70% for detecting abnormal sinus node dysfunction.
  - The true SNRT is overestimated due to the time needed for the paced impulse to invade the sinus node and for the sinus impulse to escape.

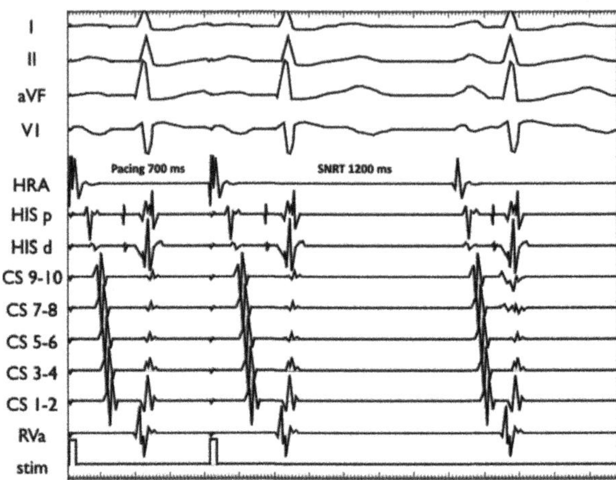

Pacing is performed from the HRA catheter at a CL of 700 ms. After cessation of pacing, the first sinus beat arrives after 1200 ms, and thus the SNRT is 1200 ms.

Sinoatrial Conduction Time (SACT)

- SACT measures the time it takes for a SA node impulse to travel through the perinodal tissue into the atria.
  - SACT detects delayed conduction between the sinus node and adjacent atrial tissue.
  - SACT focuses more on SA node exit block than decreased automaticity.
- Methodology
  - Technique depends on resetting the sinus node with a single extrastimuli delivered to the HRA.
  - Atrial extrastimuli are delivered at a range of coupling intervals to identify the zone of reset.
    - Start at 100 ms below sinus CL and then progressively decrease the coupling interval (A1A2) by 20 ms until **zone of reset** (range of A1A2 where A2A3 does not vary).
    - **SACT** = (return interval – BCL)/2 = (A2A3 – A1A1)/2
- Interpretation
  - Normal SACT is 50–125 ms.
  - Possible sinus node responses to atrial extrastimuli:

No Reset	Reset
A1A2 + A2A3 = 2 A1A1	A1A2 + A2A3 < 2 A1A1
The S2 impulse arrives late and collides with sinus beat outside the SA node (**no invasion**).	The S2 impulse arrives early enough to enter the SA node and reset it (**invasion**).

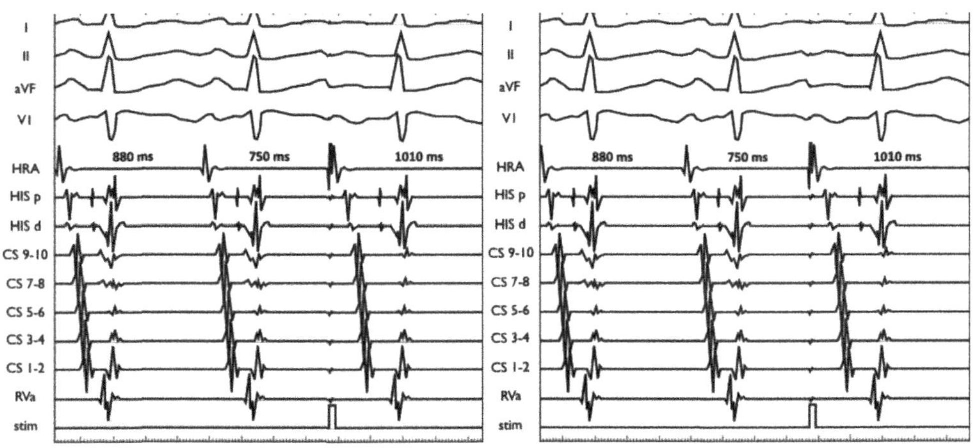

Interpolation	SA Echoes
A1A2 + A2A3 = A1A1	A1A2 + A2A3 < A1A1
The S2 impulse arrives too early to enter SA node. Next sinus beat arrives on time (blocked).	Very early the S2 impulse causes another ESA earlier than the next sinus beat (local reentry).

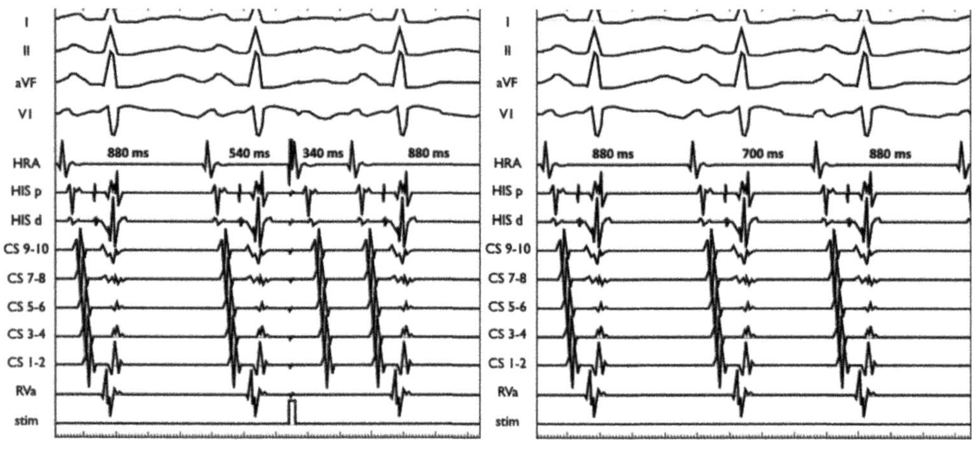

Intrinsic Heart Rate (IHR)

- SA node is richly innervated by sympathetic and parasympathetic fibers.
  - It can be difficult to determine if sinus bradycardia is due to intrinsic SA node disease or abnormal autonomic tone.
- Methodology
  - Pharmacologically block both ends of the autonomic nervous system and measure the IHR.
    - Sympathetic: Propranolol 0.2 mg/kg
    - Parasympathetic: Atropine 0.04 mg/kg
- Interpretation
  - Normal = 118.1 – (0.57 × age)
- Caveats
  - It is rarely necessary to perform this protocol.
  - The same results can be obtained through exercise testing (results in parasympathetic withdrawal).
    - Such findings indicate that chronotropic incompetence is due to intrinsic SA node disease.

EVALUATION OF ATRIOVENTRICULAR (AV) NODE FUNCTION

Anatomy of the AVN

- The AV conduction axis is a continuous system of histologically discrete cells that have their origin in the atrial myocardium and their insertion in the ventricular Purkinje cells.
  - The atrial components of this axis constitute the AVN.

- The AVN is positioned at the base of the atrial septum and set against the fibrofatty tissue of the AV junction in the upper part of the triangle of Koch.
  - The compact "knot" of randomly oriented AVN cell bundles breaks into two extensions that run toward the attachments of the tricuspid and mitral valves.
  - These bundles are surrounded on all sides by intermediate transitional cells.
- Functional anatomy involves:
  - Supranodal (AN or atrionodal) cells: Cells in the transitional region
    - Action potentials are intermediate between the fast/brief atrial AP and the slower nodal AP.
    - Delay in the supranodal cells account for 25%–60% of AV conduction delay.
    - Atrial-AN delay is independent of prematurity.
  - Midnodal (N or nodal) cells: "Most typical" AVN cells
    - Action potentials are slower rising and of longer duration (conduction velocity <2 cm/s).
    - Delay in the midnodal cells account for ~30% of AV conduction delay.
    - Delay is highly sensitive to the prematurity (decremental AP amplitude and upstroke).
  - Infranodal (NH or nodal-His) cells: Distal to the site of Wenckebach block
    - Action potentials are closer in appearance to the fast rising and long AP of the His bundle.
    - Delay in the infranodal cells account for only 5%–10% of AV conduction delay.
- Dromotropic control
  - Parasympathetic nervous system fibers (CN X: Vagus nerve)
    - Decrease the slope of phase 0 of the nodal APs, resulting in slower depolarization and reduced conduction velocity.
  - Sympathetic nervous system fibers (T1–4, spinal nerves)

Anatomy of the His-Purkinje System

- His bundle and bundle branches:
  - The proximal His bundle is located in the membranous atrial septum near the tricuspid valve.
  - The His bundle then penetrates the septum between the central fibrous body and the septal tricuspid valve leaflet to divide into the right and left bundle branches.
    - The **right bundle** is an insulated sheath of fibers that runs into the septum to the base of the RV papillary muscles and then fans out into the myocardium at the apex.
    - The **left bundle** begins in the membranous septum below the right and non-coronary aortic cusps and rapidly divides into the left anterolateral and right posteromedial fascicles.
  - Conduction velocity is 2 m/s.
- **Purkinje network**: Fans out through the ventricular endocardium, enabling rapid propagation of cardiac impulses (conduction speed 4 m/s, versus 0.5 m/s for the ventricular myocardium)

Baseline Intervals

- AH interval
  - The AH interval is the time needed for the impulse to travel across the AVN.
  - It is measured between the earliest rapid atrial deflection and the beginning of the His EGM on the His bundle catheter.
  - Normal: 55–125 ms
    - Note: The interval may vary by up to 20 ms based on autonomic tone.
- HV interval
  - The HV interval is the time taken for the cardiac impulse to travel from the His bundle through the His-Purkinje system to the ventricular myocardium.
  - It is measured between the onset of the HBE on the His bundle catheter and the earliest ventricular activation (on any catheter or surface lead).
  - Normal: 35–55 ms
    - Note: A minor delay in the His-Purkinje system results in a notching of the HBE, with significant delay causing a split HBE with separate early and late components.

HV Interval	Classification	Comment
<35 ms	Shortened	Ventricular pre-excitation Consider inadvertent RBBB recording
35–55 ms	Normal	
55–70 ms	Mild prolongation	Minimal clinical significance
70–100 ms	Moderate prolongation	Test for infrahisian block with: • Atrial pacing to <400 ms (± isoproterenol if limited by AV block) • Procainamide challenge: Positive test if HV >100 ms
>100 ms	Severe prolongation	High risk for complete heart block (25%/year)

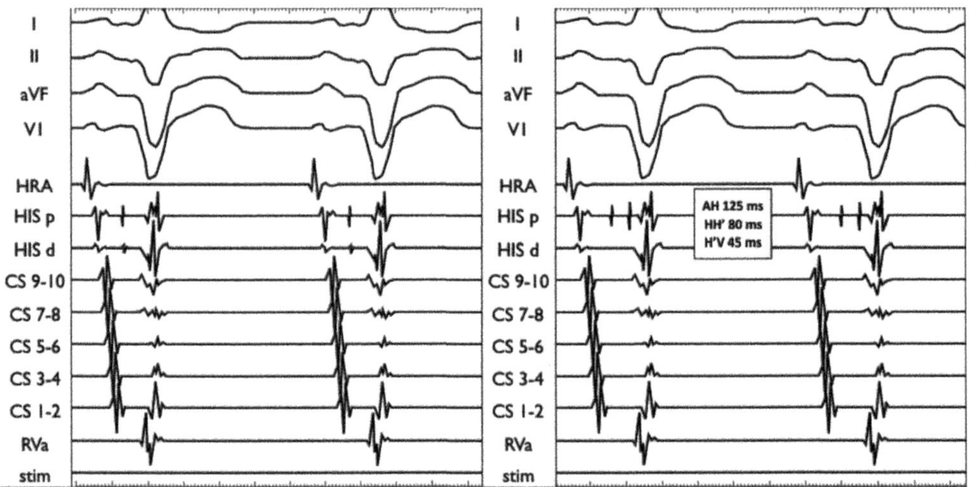

Infrahisian conduction delay as manifested by a prolonged HV interval (90 ms) and LBBB on the surface ECG.

Infrahisian conduction delay as manifested by a split His potential (HH′ interval of 80 ms). Note: The H′ to V interval is only 45 ms.

Conduction Curves and Incremental Pacing

- AVNERP
  - Longest atrial coupling interval (A1A2) that blocks in the AVN
- Anterograde AV block CL (AVBCL)
  - The longest pacing CL at which conduction through the AVN is blocked
  - Generally preceded by gradual AH prolongation during incremental pacing
- Wenckebach CL (WCL)
  - When the block occurs at the AVN level (atrial EGM without His or ventricular EGM), the AVBCL is known as the Wenckebach CL (WCL).

Classification and Definition of the Site of Conduction Disturbance

- Type 1: Progressive delay in the AVN with no change in infranodal conduction
  - Prolongation in the AH interval with no change in the HV interval
  - Loss of conduction at the level of the AVN (A EGM without subsequent His or V)
- Type 2: Early delay in the AVN, but at shorter coupling intervals, there is infranodal delay
  - Initial AH prolongation (similar to type 1)
  - With shorter coupling intervals, delay in the His-Purkinje system (aberrancy)
  - Loss of conduction in the atrium (loss of capture), AVN (AH block), or His-Purkinje (atrial and His EGM without V EGM)
- Type 3: Early delay in the AVN, but at shorter coupling intervals, there is sudden infranodal conduction delay (sudden increase in HV interval)
  - Loss of conduction first seen in His-Purkinje system (atrial and His EGM without V EGM)

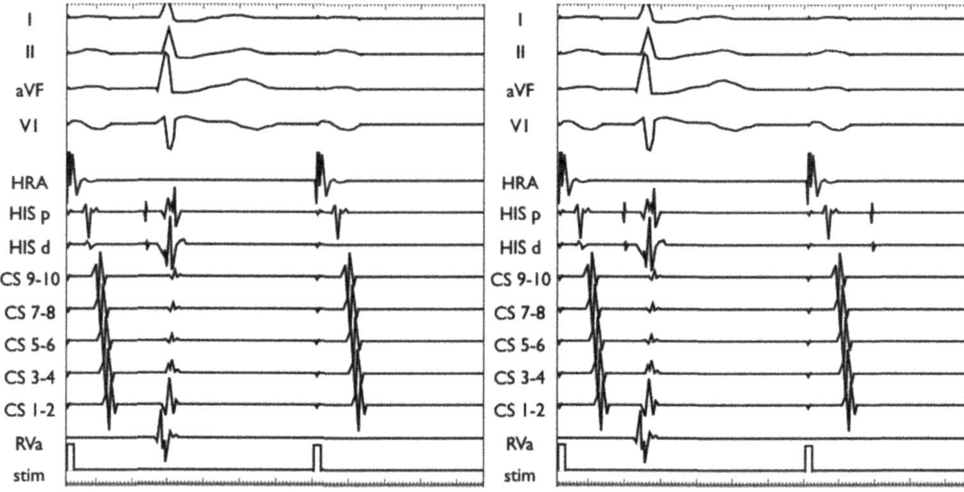

Type 1 Response: Pacing in the HRA leads to prolongation in the AH interval followed by loss of conduction at the level of the AVN (A EGM without subsequent His or V). Note the stability in the HV interval despite the changes in the AH interval (first and last paced beats).

Type 3 Response: Pacing in the HRA leads loss of conduction in the His-Purkinje system (A and His EGM without subsequent V). Note the stability in the AH interval.

Key References for Further Reading

- ACC/AHA/ESC Guidelines for the Management of Patients With Supraventricular Arrhythmias*—Executive Summary: A Report of the American College of Cardiology/American Heart Association Task Force on Practice Guidelines and the European Society of Cardiology Committee for Practice Guidelines (Writing Committee to Develop Guidelines for the Management of Patients With Supraventricular Arrhythmias). *Circulation.* 2003;108:1871–1909.
- American College of Cardiology/American Heart Association 2006 Update of the Clinical Competence Statement on Invasive Electrophysiology Studies, Catheter Ablation, and Cardioversion: A Report of the American College of Cardiology/American Heart Association/American College of Physicians Task Force on Clinical Competence and Training: Developed in Collaboration With the Heart Rhythm Society. *Circulation.* 2006;114:1654–1668.
- ACC/AHA/HRS 2006 Key Data Elements and Definitions for Electrophysiological Studies and Procedures: A Report of the American College of Cardiology/American Heart Association Task Force on Clinical Data Standards (ACC/AHA/HRS Writing Committee to Develop Data Standards on Electrophysiology). *Circulation.* 2006;114:2534–2570.
- Veenhuyzen GD, Quinn FR, Wilton SB, Clegg R, Mitchell LB. Diagnostic pacing maneuvers for supraventricular tachycardia: Part 1. *PACE.* 2011;34:767–782.
- Knight BP, Ebinger M, Oral H, Kim MH, Sticherling C, Pelosi F, et al. Diagnostic value of tachycardia features and pacing maneuvers during paroxysmal supraventricular tachycardia. *J Am Coll Cardiol.* 2000;36:574–582.
- Thomas KE, Josephson ME. The role of electrophysiology study in risk stratification of sudden cardiac death. *Prog Cardiovasc Dis.* 2008;51(2):97–105.

CHAPTER

3

Electrophysiology Study: Specific Approaches

APPROACH TO NARROW-COMPLEX TACHYCARDIA (NCT)

Indication for Diagnostic Electrophysiology Study (EPS)

- Patients with frequent or poorly tolerated NCT unresponsive to drug therapy
- Patients who prefer ablation to pharmacological therapy

Differential Diagnoses for Undiagnosed NCT

- Reciprocating tachycardia
  - Atrioventricular nodal reentrant tachycardia (AVNRT): Typical (50%–60%), Atpyical (5%–10%)
  - Atrioventricular reciprocating tachycardia (AVRT) (± Wolff-Parkinson-White syndrome): 30%
- Atrial tachycardia (AT)
  - Focal AT (including sinus node reentry): 10%
  - Macroreentrant AT (i.e., atrial flutter): 5%–10%
  - Automatic or junctional AT: <5%
- Ventricular tachycardia (VT; very rare)
  - Fascicular VT
  - Septal VT

Set-up for Diagnostic EPS

- Catheters
  - High right atrium (HRA): JSN quadripolar
  - Coronary sinus (CS): Deflectable or non-deflectable decapolar (± SL2 sheath)
  - His bundle: JSN or CRD2 quadripolar catheter
  - Right ventricular apex (RVa): JSN quadripolar catheter

The Clinical Cardiac Electrophysiology Handbook © 2016 Jason Andrade.
Cardiotext Publishing, ISBN: 978-1-942909-00-2.

- Access
  - Single groin (3 sheaths – one 7-Fr and two 5-Fr): His, RVa, and CS or HRA
  - Bilateral groin (7-Fr and 5-Fr in right groin; 7-Fr and 5-Fr in left groin): HRA, CS, His, RVa
  - Groin (7-Fr and two 5-Fr sheaths) and neck (5-Fr or 6-Fr): HRA, His, RVa via groin, CS via neck

Diagnostic Approach Consists of 5 Steps

- **Step 1**: Examine the surface electrocardiogram (ECG) during sinus rhythm and during tachycardia.
- **Step 2**: Identify arrhythmia substrate, with attention to:
  - Baseline intervals, anterograde conduction, and retrograde conduction
- **Step 3**: Induce and analyze tachycardia, focusing on:
  - Mode of initiation and termination
  - Atrioventricular (AV) relationship during tachycardia
  - Ventriculoatrial (VA) time and atrial activation sequence
  - Effect of bundle branch aberration
- **Step 4**: Undertake pacing maneuvers during tachycardia, with attention to:
  - Response to ventricular entrainment
  - Diastolic extrastimuli (His-synchronous ventricular premature beat [VPB] or premature atrial contraction [PAC])
  - Response to atrial overdrive pacing or extrastimuli (rarely)
  - Response to adenosine or antiarrhythmic drugs (AADs)
- **Step 5**: Perform pacing maneuvers in sinus rhythm.
  - Parahisian pacing
  - Differential pacing (RVa and base)
  - Pacing at tachycardia cycle length (TCL; atrial or ventricular)

Step 1: Examine the Surface 12-Lead ECGs

- 12-lead ECG during sinus rhythm may show any of the following:
  - Manifest pre-excitation indicates the presence of an anterograde-conducting accessory pathway (AP).
    - Favors the diagnosis of AVRT but is not diagnostic as the AP can be a bystander in up to 10%
  - The absence of pre-excitation does not exclude AVRT.
    - **Latent pre-excitation** occurs when anterograde activation is not manifest due to a relatively greater degree of atrioventricular nodal (AVN) conduction.
      - The relative balance of AVN and AP conduction is dependent on AVN conduction velocity, the AP conduction velocity, and the proximity of the AP to the atrial impulse.
      - In this case the delta wave may be revealed by intravenous (IV) adenosine testing or vagal maneuvers.
    - **Intermittent pre-excitation** suggests a relatively long anterograde effective refractory period (ERP).
    - **Concealed APs** are those with retrograde-only conduction.
      - The ECG shows no delta wave due to lack of anterograde activation, but these pathways can sustain orthodromic AVRT.

- 12-lead ECG or rhythm strips during tachycardia offers important information
  - The key is to identify the P waves (atrial activity) and their relationship to the QRS complex.
  - An AV ratio >1:1 is highly suggestive of atrial tachyarrhythmia (focal or macroreentrant).
    - Note: AVNRT rarely demonstrates an AV ratio >1:1 due to infranodal block
  - RP interval can help distinguish specific arrhythmia mechanisms.
    - Short interval (RP < PR) suggests the following:
      - AVNRT: P wave may be hidden in the QRS or slightly late
      - AVRT: P waves are usually just after the QRS complex
      - AT with concomitant AV block (PR interval = TCL)
    - Long interval (RP > PR) suggests the following:
      - AT
      - Atypical AVNRT
      - AVRT with slow-conducting accessory pathway
  - The mode of tachycardia initiation may also suggest a diagnosis.
    - Initiation following a sudden jump in PR interval suggests typical AVNRT.
    - Initiation following a VPB suggests AVRT; it is unusual with AVNRT or AT.
    - "Warm-up" suggests focal AT due to automaticity.
    - Sudden change in rate with no change in P-wave morphology suggests sinus node reentrant tachycardia (SNRT).
  - Tachycardia termination likewise may suggest a diagnosis.
    - Terminates with a P suggests AVNRT or AVRT (block in the AVN).
    - Terminates with a QRS suggests AT, atypical AVNRT, or atypical AVRT (block in the AP).
    - Terminates with a VPB suggests AVRT (block in the AP); it is very unusual with AVNRT or AT.
  - Other findings helpful in establishing a diagnosis include:
    - QRS alternans (beat-to-beat changes in QRS amplitude >1 mm) is more common with AVRT.
    - Repolarization abnormalities (ST depression or T-wave inversion) are more common with AVRT.
    - Bundle branch block during tachycardia:
      - Increased cycle length (CL; ≥25 ms) is diagnostic of AVRT using an ipsilateral AP.
      - No change in CL is seen with any supraventricular tachycardia (SVT), including ipsilateral AVRT (with compensatory AH interval shortening).
    - Continuous atrial activity (i.e., no isoelectric baseline) suggests macroreentry as the mechanism.
  - Response of tachycardia to vagal maneuvers/adenosine also helps establish a diagnosis.
    - Sudden termination with P (atrial activity) suggests AVNRT or AVRT.
    - Sudden termination with QRS (ventricular activity) suggests SNRT or AT.
    - Gradual slowing of atrial rate with reacceleration suggests focal AT.
    - Persisting AT with high-grade AV block suggests focal or macroreentrant AT.

Step 2: Identify Arrhythmia Substrate

- Obtain baseline intervals (see Table 3.1).

Table 3.1 Association of Baseline HV Interval with Differential Diagnosis

	AVNRT	AVRT	AT
HV Interval <35 ms (Pre-excitation)	Usually absent	Strongly predictive	Usually absent

- Assess the presence or absence of retrograde conduction (see Table 3.2).
  - Is retrograde conduction present? (If not, AVRT is unlikely.)
  - Is VA conduction normal (midline and decremental)?
  - Where is the earliest retrograde atrial activation?
  - What is the AP ERP? Can the AP support reentry?

Table 3.2 Association of Retrograde Conduction Findings with Differential Diagnosis

	AVNRT	AVRT	AT
Retrograde conduction	**Present or absent**	**Present** (if absent, AVRT unlikely)	**Present or absent**
Retrograde conduction	**Decremental**	**Non-decremental**	**Decremental**
Retrograde activation sequence	**Concentric** > Eccentric	**Eccentric** > Concentric	**Concentric** > Eccentric

- Assess the anterograde conduction (see Table 3.3).
  - Is there manifest pre-excitation? If so:
    - Determine AP anterograde conduction properties (i.e., accessory pathway ERP [APERP]/minimum pre-excited RR interval).
    - Determine AP location (earliest ventricular activation).
    - Identify whether the AP supports tachycardia.
  - Is there latent pre-excitation? If so:
    - Look for early ventricular activation activation on distal CS during anterograde conduction (sinus or atrial pacing).
    - Identify non-decremental AV conduction on the anterograde conduction curve.
    - Keep in mind the potential to unmask pre-excitation at shorter anterograde extrasystole coupling intervals, incremental pacing rates, pacing near the AP insertion site, or adenosine challenge.
  - Is there dual AVN physiology? Some clues include:
    - AH jump on the anterograde conduction curve
    - Atrial echoes or tachycardia

Table 3.3 Association of Anterograde Conduction Findings with Differential Diagnosis

	AVNRT	AVRT	AT
Anterograde activation sequence	Normal	Early ventricular activation	Variable (depends on foci)
Anterograde conduction	Decremental	Non-decremental	Decremental
Anterograde pacing	Dual AVN physiology	Manifest pre-excitation	

Step 3: Induce and Analyze Tachycardia

- Tachycardia initiation may identify diagnostic characteristics (see Table 3.4).

Table 3.4 Association of Induction Characteristics with Differential Diagnosis

	AVNRT	AVRT	AT
Induction (**extrastimuli or burst**)	**Atrial** (difficult from ventricle)	**Atrial or ventricular**	**Atrial** (never from ventricle)
Induction dependent on a critical AH interval	Strongly predictive	May be present (does not exclude)	May be present (does not exclude)
Typical induction pattern	Atrial impulse results in jump from fast pathway to slow pathway, resulting in AH delay and tachycardia initiation.	**1.** Atrial impulse results in block in AP with decremental AVN conduction (narrow QRS) and retrograde atrial activation via AP. **2.** Ventricular impulse results in retrograde AV block with atrial activation via AP.	Warm-up phenomenon

- Observations made during tachycardia episodes may identify key findings pointing to a specific diagnosis (see Table 3.5). The variables include:
  - AV relationship
  - VA timing
  - Atrial activation sequence
  - Additional factors

Table 3.5 Key Diagnostic Findings That May Be Observed During the Tachycardia Episode

	AVNRT	AVRT	AT
AV Relationship			
AV ratio	1:1	1:1	1:1 or ≥2:1
AV block during tachycardia (spontaneous, vagal maneuvers, adenosine, BB/ND-CCB)	**Sometimes** Usually terminates tachycardia Rarely 2:1 infrahisian AV block with continued tachycardia	**Terminates tachycardia** If tachycardia persists despite AV block, AVRT is excluded	**Strongly predictive** Uninterrupted tachycardia during AV block is typical of AT as the AVN **not** critical to the circuit
V > A	**Upper common pathway block** HA block (2:1 or Wenckebach)	**Nodofascicular pathway** Anterograde: His-Purkinje Retrograde: nodofascicular	**Junctional ectopic tachycardia** His precedes each V **1:2 tachycardia** Atrial impulse conducts down both AVN limbs (fast pathway and slow pathway), resulting in sequential ventricular activation

(Continued)

Table 3.5 (*Continued*)

	AVNRT	AVRT	AT
VA Timing			
Septal VA interval (earliest V on His or PCS to A on same channel)	≤70 ms (typical) >70 ms (atypical)	>70 ms (often >100) (≤70 ms **excludes**)	Variable (≤70 ms **does not exclude**)
HRA VA Interval (earliest V on His or PCS to A on HRA)	≤100 ms (typical) >100 ms (atypical)	>100 ms	Variable
Atrial Activation Sequence			
	Concentric > Eccentric	**Eccentric** > Concentric	**Eccentric** > Concentric
Other			
AH:HA Interval Ratio during tachycardia	>1 (slow-fast, slow-slow) <1 (fast-slow)		
CL variation during tachycardia	**Change in HH precedes** change in **AA** interval	**Change in HH precedes** change in **AA** interval	**Change in AA precedes** change in **HH** interval (AVN **is not** a critical part of the circuit)
Effect of bundle branch block on VA conduction time	**No effect** • increase ≥20 ms excludes	VA interval & TCL increase ≥20 ms indicates ipsilateral AP No effect if contralateral AP	No effect

- Tachycardia termination characteristics are also helpful in establishing a diagnosis (see Table 3.6).

Table 3.6 Association of Termination Characteristics with Differential Diagnoses

AVNRT	AVRT	AT
Ends with A (common) • Blocks in slow pathway Ends with V (uncommon) • Blocks in fast pathway	Ends with A (common) • Blocks in AVN Ends with V (uncommon) • Blocks in AP	Ends with V (common) • Normal AV conduction Ends with A • Effectively excludes AT

Step 4: Perform Pacing Maneuvers During Tachycardia

The various pacing maneuvers and outcomes in association with differential diagnoses are presented in Table 3.7.

Table 3.7 Response to Pacing Maneuvers During Tachycardia

	AVNRT	AVRT	AT
Ventricular Pacing in SVT			
RVa entrainment	**Entrainment** Yes	**Entrainment** Yes	**Entrainment** No
	Atrial activation timing • advanced only after complete ventricular capture	**Atrial activation timing** • advanced with partial ventricular capture (fusion)	
	Atrial activation sequence • pacing = tachycardia • if pacing ≠ tachycardia (AVNRT + bystander AP)	**Atrial activation sequence** • pacing = tachycardia • if pacing ≠ tachycardia (2nd AP)	**Atrial activation sequence** • pacing ≠ tachycardia
	Post-pacing sequence • VAV (atrial-ventricular) • AHAV (atrial-ventricular)	**Post-pacing sequence** • VAV (atrial-ventricular) • AHAV (atrial-ventricular)	**Post-pacing sequence** • VAAV • AAHV
	PPI – TCL (Stim to V EGM) ≥115 ms **cPPI = PPI – TCL – (AH_{RVP} – AH_{SVT})** ≥110 ms **Stim-A_{RVP} – VA_{SVT}** ≥85 ms **Stim-A_{RVP} / VA_{SVT}** 0.27–0.32	**PPI – TCL** (Stim to V EGM) <115 ms* **cPPI = PPI – TCL – (AH_{RVP} – AH_{SVT})** <110 ms* **Stim-A_{RVP} – VA_{SVT}** <85 ms* **Stim-A_{RVP} / VA_{SVT}** 0.9–1.08: posteroseptal AP 0.94–1.29: anteroseptal AP	
Parahisian entrainment	**PPI – TCL** (Stim to V EGM) ≥100 ms **Stim-A_{RVP} – VA_{SVT}** ≥75 ms	**PPI – TCL** (Stim to V EGM) <100 ms **Stim-A_{RVP} – VA_{SVT}** <75 ms	
Differential entrainment • from RVa and base	**cPPI – TCL (Base – Apex)** >30 ms **Stim-A (Apex – Base)** <0 ms (VA shorter at apex)	**cPPI – TCL (Base – Apex)** <30 ms **Stim-A (Apex – Base)** >0 ms (VA at base)	

* greater if left AP or concealed decremental AP

(*Continued*)

Table 3.7 (*Continued*)

	AVNRT	AVRT	AT
Burst RV pacing at 200–250 ms for 3–6 beats	**AV dissociation:** maybe May terminate	**AV dissociation:** excludes Should terminate	**AV dissociation:** present Termination **without** atrial activation **excludes AT**
Ventricular Extrastimulus			
His-synchronous VPB	No effect	**Atrial depolarization is:** • **Advanced**: Confirms AP exists If the subsequent V is advanced, then it confirms that the AP participates in SVT • **Delayed**: Confirms AP presence and role in tachycardia • **No effect**: Distant AP **Tachycardia termination** Diagnostic of orthodromic reentrant tachycardia (ORT)	No effect Termination **without** atrial activation **excludes AT**
Pre-excitement index	• >100–120 ms: AVNRT	• <45 ms: Septal AP • 45–75 ms: Right free wall • >75 ms: Left free wall	
Induction of right bundle branch block	VH increase (>50 ms) is < VA increase	VH increase (>50 ms) is > VA increase	VH increase (>50 ms) is < VA increase
Atrial Pacing in SVT			
Atrial entrainment at multiple atrial sites	Return VA: **Fixed/linked** (<10 ms of tachycardia VA CL)	Return VA: **Fixed/linked** (<10 ms of tachycardia VA CL)	Return VA: **Variable**
AV block CL	Termination is **Dependent** on AH interval	Termination is **Dependent** on AH interval	Termination is **Independent** of AH interval
Differential entrainment • from HRA and CS	Return VA CL: **Fixed/linked** (<10 ms of tachycardia VA)	Return VA CL: **Fixed/linked** (<10 ms of tachycardia VA)	Return VA CL: **Variable**

(*Continued*)

Table 3.7 (*Continued*)

	AVNRT	AVRT	AT
Atrial Extrastimulus			
Late coupled PACs (timed to when the septum is refractory; i.e., the A EGM on His catheter)	• No change (if A-His refractory) • Advances the His with long AH (enters circuit; i.e., too early) • Terminates tachycardia	• No change (if AP is refractory) • Advances the V (confirms AP); next His and A should be early • Terminates tachycardia	• No effect
Early coupled PACs	Advances the His with short AH → terminates SVT		Advances the His with short AH → SVT continues

Step 5: Perform Pacing Maneuvers During Sinus Rhythm

Table 3.8 Response to Pacing Maneuvers During Sinus Rhythm

	AVNRT	AVRT	AT
Parahisian Pacing			
His capture → V capture	**Retrograde atrial activation** • unchanged = nodal conduction • changes switch from slow pathway to fast pathway	**Retrograde atrial activation** • unchanged exclusive AP conduction • changes switch from AVN to AP	**Retrograde atrial activation** • unchanged nodal conduction
	Nodal response **SA interval** (VA) • increases (>50 ms)	**Extranodal response** **SA interval** (VA) • decreases • unchanged • increases (<40 ms)	**Nodal response** **SA interval** (VA) • increases (>50 ms)
	HA interval • unchanged	**HA interval** • decreases (septal AP) • unchanged (decremental AP)	**HA interval** • unchanged
Differential Pacing			
Pacing from RVa and base	**Atrial activation sequence** • unchanged • changes if jumps from slow pathway to fast pathway	**Atrial activation sequence** • changes	**Atrial activation sequence** • unchanged
	Septal HA interval • unchanged	**Septal HA interval** • <20–30 ms or negative	**Septal HA interval** • unchanged
	SA apex: Base (VA) • <5–10 ms	**VA apex: Base** (VA) • >10 ms	**VA apex: Base** (VA) • <5–10 ms

(*Continued*)

Table 3.8 (*Continued*)

	AVNRT	AVRT	AT
Atrial Pacing at TCL			
AH_{Pacing}: AH_{SVT}	>40 ms	<20 ms (septal AP)	<10 ms
Ventricular Pacing at TCL			
HA_{Pacing}: HA_{SVT}	Positive	Negative	–

Special Considerations

- Antidromic AVRT:
  - **QRS morphology during tachycardia:** Fully pre-excited
  - **Atrial activation**: Concentric
  - **Ventricular activation**: Advanced by PACs without involvement of the AVN (simultaneous to atrial activation near the AVN, or advances the ventricle more than the His)
  - **Retrograde His-Purkinje activation**: Right bundle (RB) and distal His activation precedes proximal His
- Pathway-to-pathway AVRT:
  - **Atria and ventricles:** Both obligatory parts of the circuit
  - **Atrial activation**: Eccentric
- AVNRT with bystander AP is diagnosed based on:
  - SVT with NCT that transitions to wide-complex tachycardia (WCT) without altering the CL or HH interval
  - Atrial extrastimuli that fail to advance the following:
    - Pre-excited QRS
    - Retrograde His
    - Subsequent atrial activation

APPROACH TO WIDE-COMPLEX TACHYCARDIA (WCT)

Indication for Diagnostic EPS

Diagnostic EPS is appropriate in patients with WCT in whom the diagnosis is unclear after clinical analysis, and for whom the correct diagnosis is essential for patient care.

- Differential diagnosis of unknown WCT includes the following:
  - VT
  - SVT with aberrancy
  - SVT with pre-excitation
    - Antidromic or pathway-to-pathway AVRT
    - AT or AVNRT with bystander AP

Set-Up for Diagnostic EPS

- 2–4 catheters (2× 5-Fr introducer and 2× 7-Fr introducer)
  - Right groin: HRA (JSN in 7-Fr), RVa (JSN in 5-Fr), and His (*if needed;* JSN or CRD2 in a 5-Fr)
  - Left groin: CS (*if needed;* deflectable decapolar in a 7-Fr)

The Diagnostic Approach Consists of 4 Steps

- **Step 1**: Obtain surface ECGs and clinical data
- **Step 2**: Identify arrhythmia substrate:
  - Baseline intervals, anterograde conduction, and retrograde conduction
- **Step 3**: Induce and analyze the tachycardia:
  - Comparison to clinical tachycardia
  - Mode of initiation and termination
  - AV relationship during tachycardia
  - VA time and atrial activation sequence
  - Effect of bundle branch aberration
  - His recording and HV interval
- **Step 4**: Assess response to pacing maneuvers during tachycardia:
  - Response to ventricular entrainment
  - Diastolic scanning with ventricular extrastimuli including His-synchronous VPB
  - Response to atrial overdrive pacing or extrastimuli
  - Pattern of tachycardia termination

Step 1: Obtain Surface ECGs and Clinical Data

- Clinical assessment should include the features described in Table 3.9.

Table 3.9 Clinical Features Suggestive of Tachycardia Mechanism

	VT	SVT with Aberrancy	Pre-excitation
Structural heart disease	Common	No relation	No relation
Carotid massage/vagal	No response	May terminate	May terminate
Cannon 'a' waves	May be present	Not seen	

- 12-lead ECG during sinus rhythm may show the following:
  - Manifest pre-excitation indicates an anterograde-conducting AP.
    - Suggests a diagnosis of SVT with pre-excitation (antidromic AVRT or pre-excitation AT/atrial fibrillation [AF])
  - Q waves in a coronary territory, suggests myocardial infarction (MI) as a substrate for VT.
  - A finding of baseline bundle branch block during sinus rhythm may be reproduced during tachycardia and may herald bundle branch reentry as the cause of VT.
- 12-lead ECG or rhythm strips during tachycardia may show the following:
  - Differentiation of VT from SVT with aberrancy or pre-excitation

Table 3.10 Key Diagnostic Findings That May Be Observed During the Wide-Complex Tachycardia Episode

	VT	SVT with Aberrancy	Pre-excitation
Onset			
Preceding beat	Ventricular	Atrial	Atrial
Preceding CL	Short	Long	–
Fixed coupling	Present	Generally absent	–
Warm-up phenomenon	Present	May be present	–
Progressive QRS width	–	Present	–
AV/VA Association			
AV dissociation	Rules in	Rules out	Rules out
Fusion/capture beats	Rules in	Rules out	Rules out
VA relationship	1:1 or ≥2:1	1:1	1:1
RP interval	Variable	Variable	Variable
QRS			
Initial QRS deflection	Differs from baseline QRS	Identical to baseline QRS	Same as delta wave
Axis (suggestive)	**1.** Change >40° from baseline **2.** Extreme axis deviation **3.** LBBB + RAD **4.** RBBB + LAD	Normal or mild deviation	Normal or mild deviation
QRS morphology	**Concordance** (positive or negative) Initial R wave ≥40 ms or R onset to S nadir >100 ms in ≥1 precordial lead **Atypical RBBB pattern** • Duration >140 ms • Positive concordance • Monophasic R in V1 • Biphasic QR or RS in V1 • Triphasic but R > r′ in V1 • S > R or QS in V6 **Atypical LBBB pattern** • Duration >160 ms • Negative concordance • R wave width >40 ms in V1 • Notched downstroke of S wave in V1-2 • >70 ms from onset to S nadir in V1-2 • Any Q in V6 (QR or QS pattern) QRS duration in tachycardia that is narrower than sinus rhythm is diagnostic of VT	Alternating LBBB/RBBB **RBBB pattern** Duration almost never >140 ms Typical RBBB Triphasic rSR′ in V1 or V6 R > S in V6 **LBBB pattern** Typical LBBB No R in V1 or small narrow R in V2 Monophasic R in V6 Septal Q in I and V6	**Positive concordance** if left posterior AP QRS duration and morphology depends on AP location

(*Continued*)

Table 3.10 (*Continued*)

	VT	SVT with Aberrancy	Pre-excitation
Rate and Regularity			
RR intervals	Slightly irregular (<0.04 ms)	Regular (usually)	Regular (usually)
Termination			
Compensatory pause	Complete	Incomplete	
Returning CL	Longer	No difference	

- **ECG criteria for differentiating SVT from VT based on a 12-lead ECG are as follows:**
  - **Wellen's criteria**: VT is favored in the presence of:
    - AV dissociation
    - Left axis deviation
    - Capture or fusion beats
    - QRS >140 ms
    - Precordial QRS concordance
    - RSR′ in V1, monophasic or biphasic QRS in V1, or monophasic QS in V6
  - **Brugada criteria** uses a stepwise approach wherein any answer of yes indicates VT:
    1. If RS complex is absent in all precordial leads (i.e., concordance): VT
    2. If the longest precordial RS interval is >200 ms in one or more precordial leads: VT
    3. If AV dissociation (or more QRS complexes than P waves) is present: VT
    4. If morphology criteria for VT are present in V1–V2 and V6: VT
       - RBBB-like QRS:
         - Monophasic R, QR, or RS in V1: VT
         - Triphasic QRS in V1 but first peak > second peak (RSr′): VT
         - R/S ratio <1.0, QS, or QR in V6: VT
       - LBBB-like QRS:
         - R >30 ms, >60 ms to S nadir, or notched S in V1 or V2
         - QR or QS in V6
    5. If none of the above is present: SVT
  - **Kindwall's criteria** for VT in LBBB include:
    - R wave in V1 or V2 >30 ms duration
    - Any Q wave in V6
    - Duration >60 ms from QRS onset to S wave nadir in V1 or V2
    - Notching on the downstroke of the S wave in V1 or V2

Step 2: Identify Arrhythmia Substrate

- Assess baseline intervals for pre-excitation.
- Assess anterograde conduction.
  - Is there manifest pre-excitation?
    - Determine the anterograde conduction properties of the AP.
    - Determine the AP location (earliest V).
    - Does the AP support tachycardia?

- Is there latent pre-excitation?
  - Early V activation on distal CS during anterograde conduction
  - Non-decremental AV conduction on the anterograde conduction curve
  - Unmasking of pre-excitation at shorter anterograde extrasystole coupling intervals, incremental pacing rates, pacing near the AP insertion site, or adenosine challenge
- Is there dual AVN physiology?
  - AH jump on the anterograde conduction curve
  - Atrial echoes or tachycardia

○ Assess retrograde conduction.
- Absence of VA conduction makes AVNRT and AVRT unlikely
- Presence of VA conduction:
  - Is VA conduction normal (midline and decremental)?
  - Where is the earliest retrograde A?
  - What is the APERP? Can the AP support reentry?

○ Other factors to look for include:
- Gap phenomena
- Parahisian pacing

Step 3: Induce and Analyze the Tachycardia

○ Tachycardia initiation can provide clues to the diagnosis, as seen in Table 3.11.

Table 3.11 Diagnostic Responses to Induction of Tachycardia

	VT	AVNRT	AVRT	AT
Induction (**extrastimuli or burst**)	**Ventricular** (difficult with A pacing unless fascicular VT)	**Atrial** (difficult with V pacing)	**Atrial or ventricular**	**Atrial** (never with V pacing)

- Inducibility of VT depends on the mechanism of the tachycardia:
  - Reentry (monomorphic VT): Ventricular pacing (burst or extrastimuli)
  - Automaticity (right ventricular outflow tract [RVOT], idiopathic left ventricular VT): Isoproterenol, epinephrine, atropine, exercise
  - Triggered activity: Multiple extrastimuli, burst pacing, and long-short sequences accompanied by isoproterenol, epinephrine, atropine, calcium, or aminophylline

○ Observations during tachycardia:
- Spontaneous or atrial pacing-induced AV dissociation may show that the atria are not part of the circuit.
- Examine the relationship between the His bundle and the ventricles; RB and distal His activation precede proximal His (retrograde activation by VT).

Table 3.12 Key Diagnostic Findings That May Be Observed During the Tachycardia Episode

	VT	AVNRT	AVRT	AT
AV Relationship				
AV relationship	1:1 or ≤2:1	1:1	1:1	1:1 or ≥2:1
V > A	Usually indicates VT	**Very rare** unless: Upper common pathway block (**HA block**)	**Essentially rules out AVRT** (except nodofascicular AP)	**Junctional ectopic tachycardia** His precedes each V **1:2 tachycardia**
VA Timing				
Septal VA interval (earliest V on His or PCS to A on same channel)	May be dissociated, stable (retrograde VA conduction), or variable (Wenckebach)	≤70 ms (typical) >70 ms (atypical)	>70 ms (usual >100 ms) (≤70 ms **excludes**)	Variable (≤70 ms ≠ **exclude**)
Atrial Activation Sequence				
	Dissociated or **Concentric** > Eccentric	**Concentric** > Eccentric	**Eccentric** > Concentric	**Eccentric** > Concentric
Other				
CL variation AA interval (HRA or CS) is compared to VV interval (RVa)	Change in **VV** interval precedes change in **AA**	**Change in HH/ VV** interval **precedes** change in **AA**	**Change in HH/ VV** interval **precedes** change in **AA**	**Change in AA** interval **precedes** change in **VV**
HV interval	• Negative • Shorter HV in tachycardia	**Positive**	**Positive** (negative with antidromic AVRT)	**Positive**
RB and His activation pattern	**RB precedes His**	**His precedes RB**	**ORT** (His precedes RB) **Antidromic AVRT** (RB precedes His)	**His precedes RB**
Bundle branch reentry	• H precedes every V • HV is stable • VV interval variations preceded by HH variations • Induction occurs with critical VH delay			

(Continued)

Table 3.12 (*Continued*)

	VT	AVNRT	AVRT	AT
Ventricular pacing at TCL (VH_{Pacing}: $VH_{Tachycardia}$)	<10 ms	>40 ms	<20 ms (septal AP)	<10 ms
His-Atrial time ($HA_{Tachycardia}$: HA_{Pacing})	Similar	Negative	Similar	Variable

- Tachycardia termination also offers diagnostic clues (see Table 3.13).

Table 3.13 Mode of Tachycardia Termination in Association with Specific Diagnoses

	VT	AVNRT	AVRT	AT
Termination	• Ends with A if VA conduction • Ends with V if no VA conduction	• Ends with A (common) due to block in the SP • Ends with V (rare) due to block in the FP	• Ends with A (common) due to block in the AVN • Ends with V (rare) due to block in the AP	• Ends with V (common) • Ends with A: Will exclude AT

Step 4: Assess Response to Pacing Maneuvers During Tachycardia

Table 3.14 Response to Pacing Maneuvers During Tachycardia

	VT	AVNRT	AVRT	AT
Ventricular Extrastimuli or Entrainment				
Post-pacing sequence	**Termination** VAV	VAV or VAHAV (atrial-ventricular)	VAV or VAHAV (atrial-ventricular)	VAAV or VAHAV
Atrial Pacing				
Atrial overdrive pacing CL 10–40 ms < TCL	AV dissociation or advancement of the V Does not terminate tachycardia	Entrainment ± termination Return VA CL: **Fixed** (<10 ms of tachycardia VA)	Entrainment ± termination Return VA CL: **Fixed** (<10 ms of tachycardia VA)	Entrainment ± termination Return VA CL: **Variable**
	QRS: Changes or narrows (capture or fusion)	**QRS:** No change unless bystander AP	**QRS:** No change unless multiple APs	**QRS:** No change unless bystander AP
		No constant QRS fusion	**Constant QRS fusion** if multiple APs	**No constant QRS fusion**
	AVVA response	AVA response	AVA response	AVA response

(Continued)

Table 3.14 (*Continued*)

	VT	AVNRT	AVRT	AT
Atrial extrastimuli	Advances V with a capture or fusion QRS complex	No pre-excitation	Pre-excites the ventricle	Pre-excites the ventricle
His-synchronous PAC		Return VA CL: **Fixed** (<10 ms of tachycardia VA)	Return VA CL: **Fixed** (<10 ms of tachycardia VA)	Return VA CL: **Variable**

Special Considerations

- **Antidromic AVRT** diagnosis is based on:
    - Fully pre-excited QRS morphology during tachycardia
    - **Atrial activation**: Concentric
    - **Ventricular activation**: Advanced by PACs without involvement of the AVN (simultaneous to atrial activation near the AVN or advances the ventricle more than the His)
    - **Retrograde His-Purkinje activation**: RB and distal His activation precedes proximal His
- **Pathway-to-pathway AVRT**:
    - Atria and ventricles are both obligatory parts of the circuit
    - **Atrial activation**: Eccentric
- **AVNRT with bystander AP**:
    - SVT with NCT that transitions to WCT without altering the CL or HH interval
    - Failure of atrial extrastimuli to advance the following:
        - Pre-excited QRS
        - Retrograde His
        - Subsequent atrial activation

PROGRAMMED VENTRICULAR STIMULATION

Indication for Electrophysiological Testing

- Remote MI and symptoms suggestive of VT (palpitations, pre-syncope, and syncope)
- To guide and assess the efficacy of VT ablation
- Evaluation of wide-QRS-complex tachycardia of unclear mechanism
- May be considered for risk assessment in non-ischemic cardiomyopathies (e.g., hypertrophic cardiomyopathy (HCM), arrhythmogenic cardiomyopathy (ARVC), and Brugada); however, the utility is limited (i.e., a high proportion of false positives/false negatives)

Set-Up for EPS

Set-up for EPS includes right groin: 2 catheters (JSN) moved between the HRA, His, and RVa.

Programmed Ventricular Stimulation

- **Extrastimulus testing** from the RVa
  - Testing consists of an 8-beat drive train (S1) followed by a single extrastimulus (S2).
    - The coupling intervals between the drive train and extrastimuli are progressively shortened by 10–20 ms until there is loss of capture (ventricular refractoriness).
    - The test is repeated at least two drive CLs (400, 600 ms ± 300–350 ms).
  - Double extrastimuli are brought in to ventricular refractoriness at the drive CLs.
    - S2 is left at 20–50 ms above ERP as S3 is decremented.
  - Triple extrastimuli are brought in to ventricular refractoriness at the drive CLs.
    - S2 and S3 are left at 20–50 ms above ERP as S4 is decremented.
- **Incremental pacing** consists of 8–12 incrementally paced beats brought in at 350 ms and decremented to ventricular refractoriness.
- **Burst pacing** consists of 5–10 paced beats near ventricular refractoriness.
- **If VT not induced**: Repeat protocol at RVOT.
- **If VT still not induced**: Repeat during an isoproterenol infusion (goal HR on isoproterenol of 110–140 bpm).
  - Note: An increasing number of extrastimuli and isoproterenol improve the sensitivity at the expense of specificity (i.e., 20%–30% of normal patients have polymorphic VT with triple extrastimuli). See Table 3.15.

Table 3.15 Sensitivity Versus Specificity

Factors Increasing Specificity of a Positive Study	Factors Increasing Sensitivity of a Positive Study
Duration >30 seconds (or >10 beats)	Non-sustained arrhythmia
Reproducible morphology (monomorphic)	Polymorphic VT or ventricular fibrillation (VF)
Inducible on single or double extrastimuli	Inducible with triple extrastimuli or incremental pacing
High pre-test probability	Low pre-test probability
CL ≥240 ms	

- Responses to programmed stimulation include the following:
  - **Non-inducible** (negative study)
  - **Repetitive ventricular response** (no clinical significance)
    - Single or short series of 3–5 ventricular beats following the extrastimulus
    - Similar morphology to the paced QRS due to local myocardial or bundle branch reentry
  - **Sustained monomorphic VT**
    - Specific finding regardless of the method of induction
  - **Non-sustained polymorphic VT or VF**
    - With triple or quadruple extrastimuli: Non-specific finding
    - With single or double extrastimuli: "Gray zone"
- **Arrhythmia termination**
  - **Hemodynamic collapse**: Urgent synchronized cardioversion
  - **Hemodynamic tolerance**: Burst pacing for 8–12 beats, 10–20 ms below tachycardia cycle
    - Note: The more aggressive the pacing intervention, the more likely it will accelerate the tachycardia or cause it to degenerate to VF.

PHARMACOLOGIC CHALLENGE FOR INHERITED ARRHYTHMIA SYNDROMES

Adrenaline (Epinephrine) Challenge

- Indication is for the evaluation of possible long QT syndrome (LQTS).
- Protocol:
  - 5 mL of 1:10,000 (0.5 mg) epinephrine is added to 45 mL of normal saline (total 50 mL) = 10 mcg/mL.
  - Baseline 12-lead ECG is performed and the infusion is started at 0.05 mcg/kg/min (0.3 mL/h/kg).
  - After 5 minutes, an ECG is performed, and the infusion is increased to 0.10 mcg/kg/min (0.6 mL/h/kg).
  - After 5 minutes, an ECG is performed, and the infusion is increased to 0.20 mcg/kg/min (1.2 mL/h/kg).
  - After 5 minutes, an ECG is performed and the infusion is discontinued. ECGs are then performed every 10 minutes for 30 minutes post infusion.
- Monitoring is undertaken as follows:
  - Continuous rhythm monitoring during infusion and for 1 hour post examination
  - Vital signs q5 minutes during infusion
- Endpoints for adrenaline termination are:
  - Systolic blood pressure falls below 80 mm Hg or exceeds 200 mm Hg
  - Non-sustained or polymorphic VT
  - ≥10 premature ventricular contractions per minute
  - Onset of T-wave alternans
  - Patient intolerance due to headache, nausea, abdominal pain, angina, or heart failure
- Antidote:
  - Metoprolol 2.5 to 5 mg IV over 1 minute if persistent symptoms after epinephrine discontinuation
- Interpretation of challenge requires that QT interval, heart rate, and corrected QT interval (QTc) should be measured at the end of each 5-minute period.
  - QTc prolongation of ≥50 ms is considered abnormal (i.e., consistent with LQTS).

Procainamide Challenge

- Indication is for the evaluation of Brugada syndrome.
- Protocol: Procainamide 15 mg/kg (to a maximum of 1 g) is infused at 50 mg/min.
  - Baseline 12-lead ECG and then every 10 minutes during infusion and then at conclusion, and every 30 minutes post infusion up to 1 hour.
- Monitoring includes:
  - Continuous rhythm monitoring during infusion and post examination
  - Vital signs q5 minutes during infusion
- Endpoints for procainamide termination are as follows:
  - Systolic blood pressure falls below 80 mm Hg
  - Non-sustained or polymorphic ventricular tachycardia
  - ≥10 premature ventricular contractions per minute
  - QRS widening ≥30% of baseline
  - Bradycardia or AV block (type 2 or 3)
- Antidote:
  - Isoproterenol 1–2 mcg/min

- Contraindications to the procainamide challenge are:
  - Bradycardia, advanced AV block, or bundle branch block
  - Hypertrophic cardiomyopathy
  - Heart failure left ventricular ejection fraction (LVEF) <35%
  - Pregnancy
  - Myasthenia gravis
  - Liver disease
- Interpretation
  - Induction of a type I Brugada pattern is considered a positive test.

Key References for Further Reading

- Veenhuyzen GD, Quinn FR, Wilton SB, Clegg R, Mitchell LB. Diagnostic pacing maneuvers for supraventricular tachycardia: Part 1. *PACE.* 2011;34:767–782.
- Knight BP, Ebinger M, Oral H, Kim MH, Sticherling C, Pelosi F, et al. Diagnostic value of tachycardia features and pacing maneuvers during paroxysmal supraventricular tachycardia. *J Am Coll Cardiol.* 2000;36;574–582.
- Thomas KE, Josephson ME. The role of electrophysiology study in risk stratification of sudden cardiac death. *Prog Cardiovasc Dis.* 2008;51(2):97–105.
- Obeyesekere MN, Klein GJ, Modi S, Leong-Sit P, Gula LJ, Yee R, et al. How to perform and interpret provocative testing for the diagnosis of Brugada syndrome, long-QT syndrome, and catecholaminergic polymorphic ventricular tachycardia. *Circ Arrhythm Electrophysiol.* 2011;4:958–964.
- Mitchell LB. The role of the transvenous catheter electrophysiologic study in the evaluation and management of ventricular tachyarrhythmias associated with ischemic heart disease. *Cardiac Electrophysiol Review.* 2002;6:458–462.

CHAPTER

4

Atrioventricular Nodal Reentrant Tachycardia

UNDERSTANDING AND MANAGING ATRIOVENTRICULAR NODAL REENTRANT TACHYCARDIAS (AVNRT)

General Information

AVNRT is a paroxysmal, narrow-complex tachyarrhythmia due to reentry involving 2 functionally and anatomically distinct pathways in the vicinity of the compact atrioventricular node (AVN).

Epidemiology and Clinical Features

- AVNRT accounts for 50%–60% of symptomatic paroxysmal supraventricular tachycardias (SVT)
- Females predominate (2:1 female:male).
- Symptom onset occurs between 30 and 50 years.
- Common symptoms include palpitations (neck pulsation), dizziness, syncope (10%).
- AVNRT is rarely associated with structural heart disease.

Anatomy

The AVN and its related structures lie along the interatrial septum in the **triangle of Koch**:

- The **apex** of the triangle is the atrioventricular (AV) component of the membranous septum containing the compact AVN and bundle of His.
- The **base** of the triangle is the coronary sinus (CS) ostium and the septal isthmus (tissue anteriorly from the CS os to tricuspid valve (TV) annulus).
- The **posterior margin** is the tendon of Todaro.
  - A fibrous continuation of the valve of the inferior caval vein (Eustachian valve)
- The **anterior margin** is the septal leaflet of the tricuspid valve.

The Clinical Cardiac Electrophysiology Handbook © 2016 Jason Andrade.
Cardiotext Publishing, ISBN: 978-1-942909-00-2.

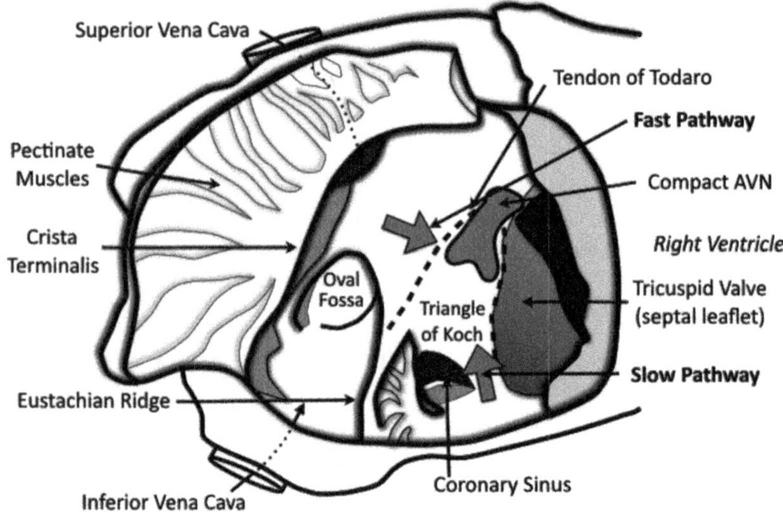

Pathophysiology (Mechanism)

Anatomic limbs of the reentrant circuit contain 2 alternative pathways.

- The fast pathway is located anteroseptal to the compact AVN at the apex of Koch's triangle (proximal to the usual His bundle recording position, and superior to the tendon of Todaro).
  - This pathway has the properties of rapid conduction with a long effective refractory period (ERP).
- The slow pathway is located posterior and inferior to the compact AVN (along the tricuspid annulus).
  - This pathway has the properties of slow conduction with a short ERP.
    - A late **slow-pathway potential** may be observed between the tricuspid valve and the CS ostium (i.e., within the septal isthmus).
  - **Rightward posterior extension** of the AVN (participates in most AVNRT)
    - Earliest retrograde activation is recorded between the tricuspid annulus and CS ostium.
  - **Leftward inferior extension** of the AVN
    - Earliest retrograde activation is recorded 2–4 cm inside the CS on the roof. Occasionally it is noted in the left atrium (LA) along the mitral annulus.

Classification

AVNRT can be divided into subtypes based on the anterograde and retrograde conduction.

- Slow-fast (or typical) AVNRT **is the most common subtype** (90%–95%).
  - **Retrograde conduction:** The **fast pathway** simultaneously activates both sides of the interatrial septum.
    - **Right atrial activation** is blocked along the Eustachian ridge.
    - **Left atrial activation** propagates inferiorly and laterally, CS roof → CS myocardium → CS ostium

- **Anterograde conduction:** Activation of the atrial myocardium between the tricuspid annulus and the CS ostium in the superior direction activates the atrial end of the **slow pathway**.
  - "Rightward inferior extension" (95%)
  - "Leftward inferior extension" (5%)
- Slow-slow AVNRT is often referred to as "atypical AVNRT."
  - Circuit has a counterclockwise "slow pathway" reentry as viewed in the right anterior oblique (RAO) projection.
  - **Retrograde conduction**: Slow pathway via the leftward inferior extension with activation progressing to the CS myocardium and LA
  - **Anterograde conduction:** Slow pathway via the rightward inferior extension with activation progressing to the common pathway (thus completing the circuit)
    - Passive LA activation → atrial septum → fast pathway (short AH interval)
    - Note: The fast pathway does not participate in the reentrant circuit.
- Fast-slow AVNRT is also referred to as "atypical AVNRT."
  - Circuit has a clockwise "slow pathway" reentry as viewed in the RAO projection.
  - Slow pathway via the leftward inferior extension with activation progressing to the CS myocardium and LA.
  - Slow pathway via the rightward inferior extension with activation progressing to the common pathway (thus completing the circuit)
    - Passive LA activation → atrial septum → fast pathway (short AH interval)
    - Note: The fast pathway does not participate in the reentrant circuit.

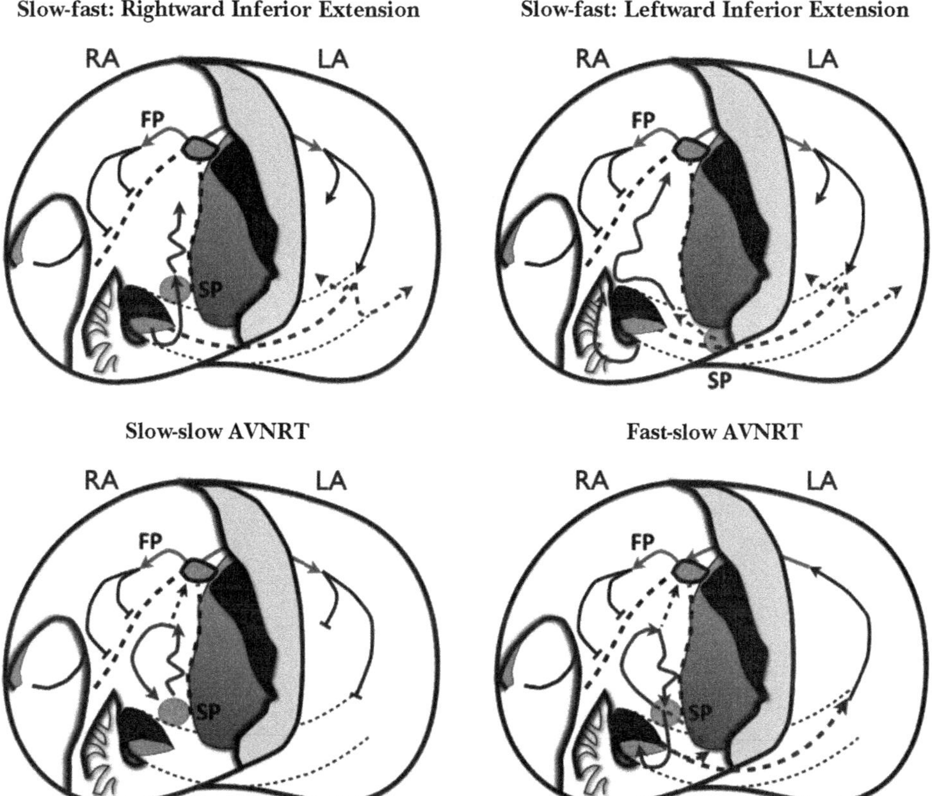

12-Lead Electrocardiogram (ECG)

Common characteristics include the following:

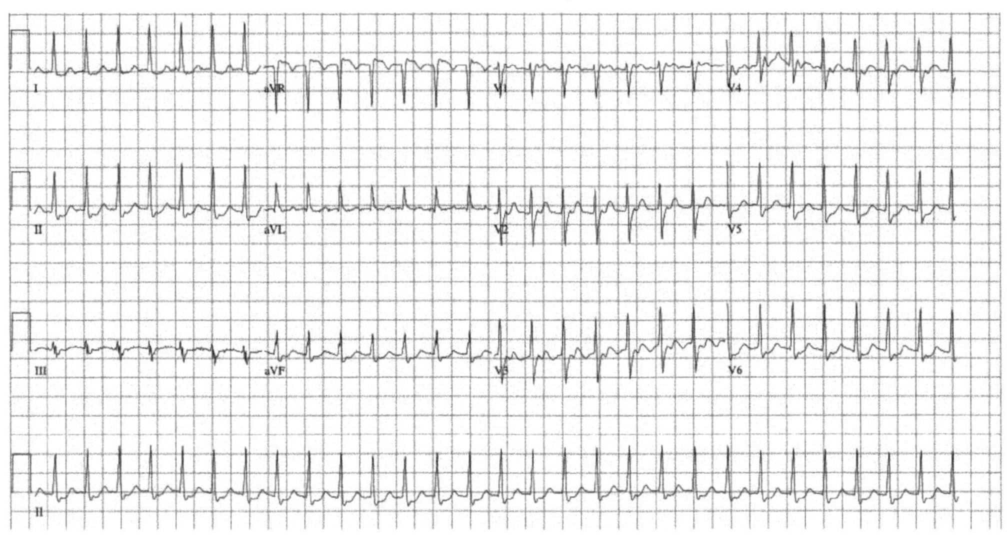

- Rate is typically 140–250 bpm, and rhythm is regular.
- In the P wave, retrograde atrial activation may not be appreciated (see Table 4.1).

Table 4.1 ECG Characteristics of AVNRT

	Typical (90%–95%)	Atypical (5%–10%)	
	"Slow-fast"	"Fast-slow"	"Slow-slow"
RP Interval*	Short	Long	Long
P waves	1. Absent (during QRS) 2. Late but within the QRS • pseudo r′ in V1 • pseudo S in II, III, aVF, V6	Negative P before the QRS • pseudo q in II, III, aVF, V6	Negative P after the QRS • pseudo S in II, III, aVF, V6

* The RP interval is dictated by the relative conduction velocity of the anterograde and retrograde limbs of the circuit and the HV interval.

- **QRS** is narrow unless conduction is aberrant or bundle branch block is present.
- **Onset/termination** is paroxysmal and initiated by an ectopic beat (atrial or ventricular).
- **Other**: Baseline ECG is often normal.

Other Investigations

- **24-hour Holter monitor**
  - Useful for diagnosis with episodes occurring more frequent than weekly

- Event recorder
  - Useful for diagnosis with symptomatic episodes occurring weekly to monthly
- Echocardiogram
  - Assessment of LV function and to exclude structural or congenital heart disease
- Electrophysiology study (EPS): See below.

Management

- The condition is not life threatening but can lead to symptoms.
  - Tachycardia-mediated cardiomyopathy may rarely occur (more often with atypical AVNRT).
- The goal of pharmacotherapy is to increase the refractory period and slow the conduction of AVN tissue.

Acute Management

- Includes the following options:
  - Vagal maneuvers: Valsalva, cough, ice water immersion, carotid sinus massage
  - Adenosine 6–18 mg intravenous push
  - Non-dihydropyridine calcium-channel blocker (ND-CCB) (preferred to β-blockers [BB], digoxin, amiodarone)
  - Direct current synchronized cardioversion (especially if unstable or signs of cardiogenic shock, angina, or heart failure)

Chronic Management

Table 4.2 Options for Chronic Management of AVNRT

	Poorly Tolerated AVNRT	Recurrent Symptomatic AVNRT	Infrequent Well-tolerated AVNRT
Vagal maneuvers	—	—	I
BB, ND-CCB	IIa	I	I
Digoxin	—	IIb	—
Flecainide, propafenone Sotalol	IIa	IIa (BB/CCB refractory)	I (pill-in-the-pocket)
Amiodarone	IIa	IIb	—
Catheter ablation	I	I	I

I: Should be performed; IIa: May be considered; IIb: Reasonable alternative; III: Not indicated.

- Nonpharmacologic therapy
  - Vagal maneuvers to terminate an episode as needed (described above)

- Pharmacologic therapy can be dichotomized into:
  - Chronic daily prophylaxis is used for patients with frequent symptoms.
    - BB, ND-CCB, and digoxin offer similar efficacy (30%–50% efficacy).
      - Wenckebach phenomenon in the slow pathway results in tachycardia termination.
    - Class Ic or Class III anti-arrhythmic drugs are second-line options.
      - Reserved for patients with refractory slow pathways that don't respond to typical AVN blocking agents.
  - "Pill-in-the-pocket" strategy is used for patients with infrequent but prolonged episodes (symptomatic but stable episodes that occur less than monthly).
    - Propranolol 80 mg and/or Diltiazem 120 mg > Flecainide 3 mg/kg
- Invasive therapy
  - Catheter ablation (slow-pathway modification) is preferred in most cases.

Electrophysiology Study (EPS)

Anterograde Conduction

- **Dual AVN physiology**
  - The presence of dual AVN physiology serves as evidence of multiple functionally and anatomically distinct conduction pathways.
  - **AH jump**: With a 10 ms decrease in the extrastimulus (A-A) coupling interval, there is a ≥50 ms increase in the AH interval.
    - This occurs when the fast pathway ERP is reached and conduction switches to the slow pathway.
    - At times, an AH jump may be observed during incremental atrial pacing.

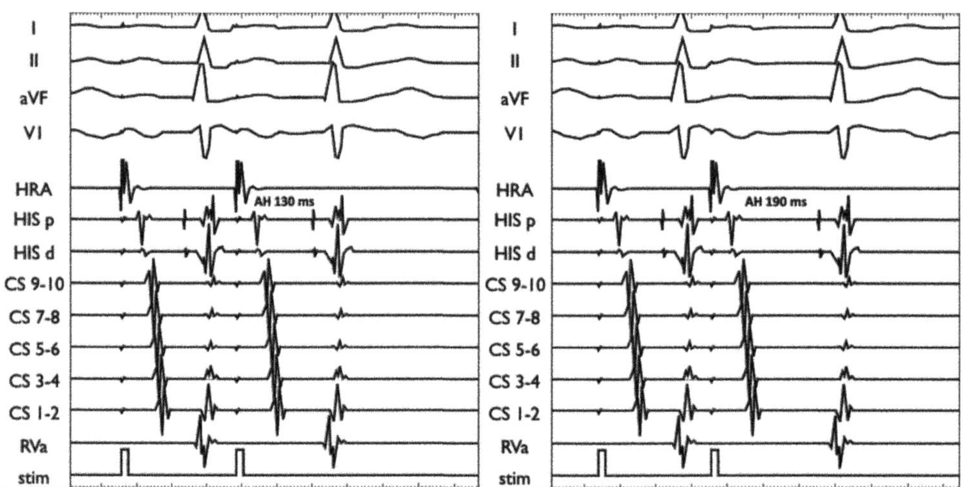

Programmed atrial stimulation. Drive train at 400 ms. In the left panel, an extrastimulus is delivered at a 260 ms coupling interval, resulting in an AH interval of 130 ms. In the right panel, the extrastimulus is delivered at a 250 ms coupling interval, resulting in an AH interval of 190 ms.

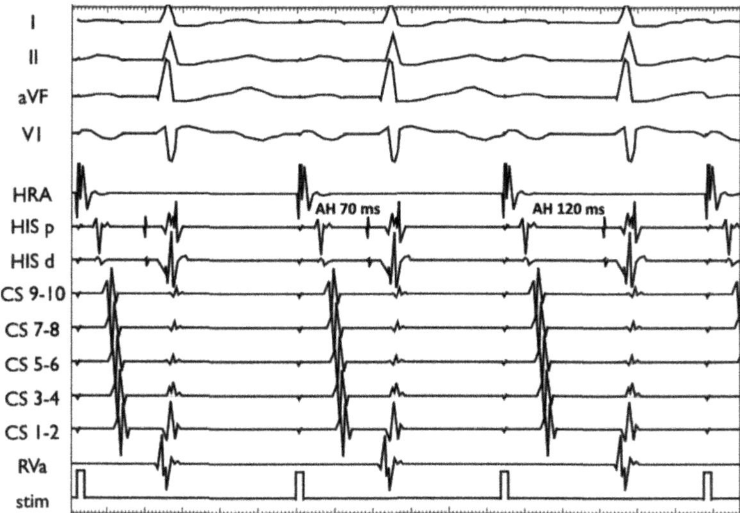

Incremental atrial pacing is performed from a high right atrial (HRA) catheter. With a 10 ms decrease in the pacing cycle length (CL), the AH interval increases from 70 ms to 120 ms.

- **Two-for-one response**: A single atrial impulse results in 2 His-ventricular depolarization
    - Due to simultaneous anterograde conduction through both the fast and slow pathways
    - May lead to **non-reentrant dual atrioventricular nodal tachyarrhythmia**, whereby a non-tachycardic atrial impulse results in tachycardia due to the presence of 2 ventricular impulses for every atrial impulse

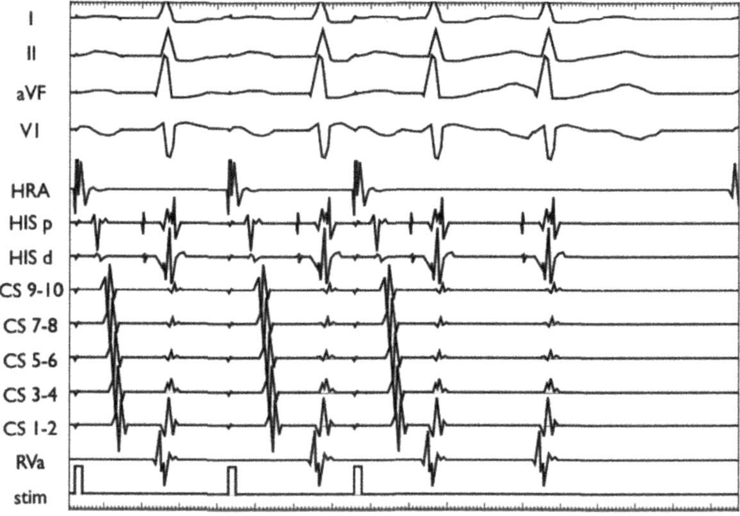

Programmed atrial stimulation. Drive train at 400 ms. An extrastimulus is delivered at a 250 ms coupling interval, resulting in simultaneous conduction to the ventricle via the fast pathway and the slow pathway.

- **Typical AVN echo**
  - Typical AVN echo is a premature atrial depolarization that conducts anterograde down the slow pathway.
    - In the presence of sufficient conduction delay, the fast pathway is able to recover its excitability and conduct the impulse retrograde back to the atria, with near-simultaneous atrial (A) and ventricular (V) depolarization.
    - It confirms the presence of dual AVN physiology and retrograde fast pathway conduction.
  - Tachycardia (or echo) zone defines the range of premature beats that induce reentrant tachycardia.
    - The zone is measured from the fast pathway ERP to the slow pathway ERP.
    - The wider the tachycardia (or echo) zone, the more likely it is that a premature impulse will fall within that zone and induce reentrant tachycardia.

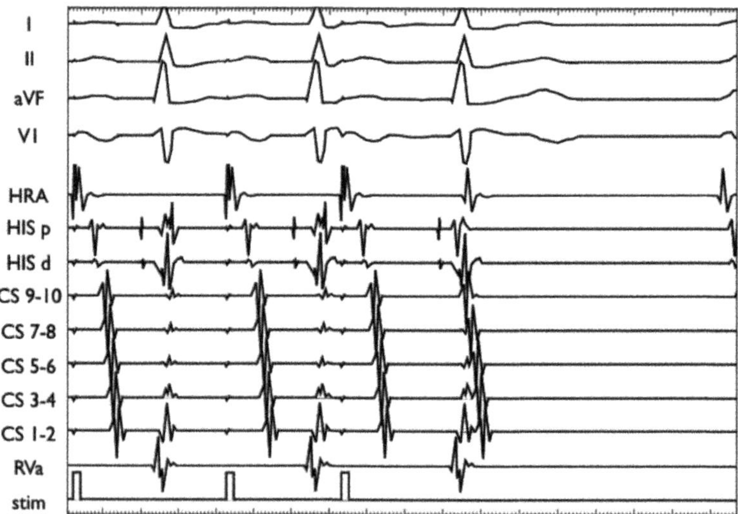

Programmed atrial stimulation. Drive train at 400 ms. An extrastimuli delivered at a 250 ms coupling interval results in an AH jump followed by a typical AVN echo beat.

Retrograde Conduction

- VA conduction should be present and midline (concentric).
  - Caveats:
    - Retrograde conduction may not be midline with bystander accessory pathway (AP).
    - Ventriculoatrial (VA) conduction will not be present in patients with retrograde block between the ventricle and lower common pathway.
- Dual retrograde AVN pathways are a less common cause of VA jump.
  - At long coupling intervals, ventricular extrastimuli are conducted up the His-Purkinje system and exit the node via the fast pathway in the atria.
    - Short VA time (<70 ms on His bundle electrogram (EGM) or <100 ms on HRA EGM)
    - Earliest activation at the His bundle catheter ("concentric activation")

- With progressive ventricular extrastimulus prematurity, decremental VA conduction is observed.
  - In the presence of dual retrograde AVN pathways, there is a VA interval jump as retrograde fast pathway ERP is reached and conduction shifts to the slow pathway.
  - As the atrial insertions of the fast and slow pathways differ, the earliest retrograde activation may shift from the His catheter (fast pathway) to the proximal CS (slow pathway).
  - This shift can be followed by an "atypical" echo.
- Note: **Infrahisian delay** is the more common cause of VA jump.
  - With progressive prematurity of ventricular extrastimuli, there may be a sudden increase in the VA interval due to block in the His-Purkinje system below the AVN.
  - After retrograde right bundle branch block ([RBBB]; retrograde right bundle branch ERP), the impulse must travel across the interventricular septum in order to enter the conduction system via the left bundle, and subsequently travel to the His and AVN.
  - This prolongation in the VH interval may reveal a retrograde His potential, which is normally hidden within the ventricular EGM.

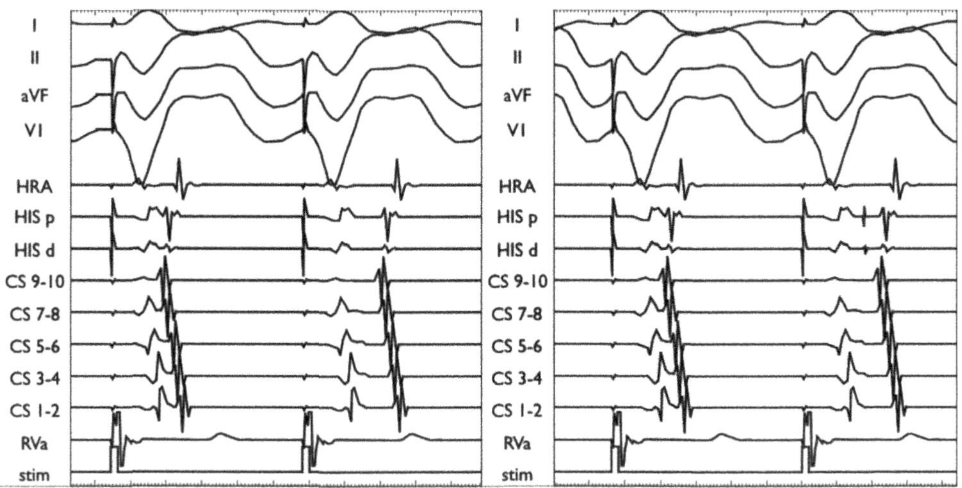

VA jump during decremental ventricular pacing. In the left panel, the retrograde conduction "jumps" from the fast pathway to the slow pathway as the ventricular pacing CL is decreased. In the right panel, the "jump" observed is due to infrahisian delay (as manifested by a prolongation in VH time with the emergence of a retrograde His potential).

Tachycardia Induction

- Performed by rapid atrial overdrive pacing or atrial extrastimuli
  - This results in block in the fast pathway with the impulse switching to the slow pathway.
    - The delay allows retrograde conduction to occur in the fast pathway and induction of tachycardia.
  - It may require atropine or isoproterenol infusion to facilitate induction.

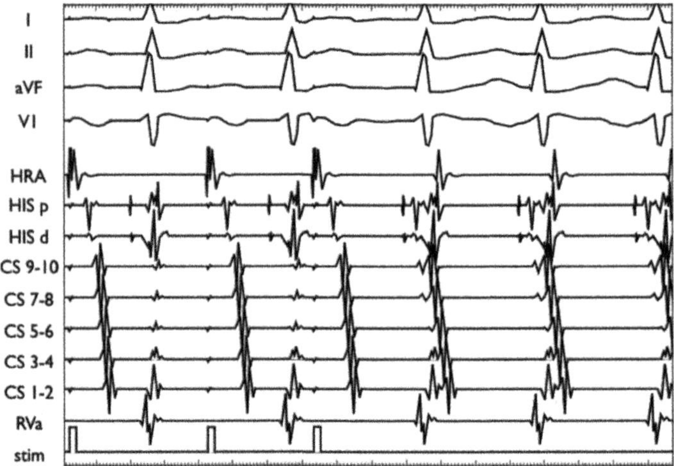

AVNRT initiation during programmed atrial stimulation. Drive train at 600 ms followed by a single atrial extrastimuli at 440 ms results in AH jump and tachycardia initiation (concentric atrial activation with VA timing <70 ms).

Observations During Tachycardia

- **Short VA time** (e.g., ≤70 ms on His bundle catheter or ≤100 ms on HRA catheter)
- **Concentric activation**
  - **Anterior exit:** Earliest activation is in the anterior septum (His catheter).
  - **Posterior exit:** Earliest activation is in the posterior septum (proximal CS).
- **Spontaneous conduction block**:
  - The atria, ventricles, and bundle branches are not necessary components of the tachycardia circuit; therefore, it is possible to see spontaneous AV block (more atrial than ventricular depolarizations), spontaneous VA block (more ventricular than atrial depolarizations), and bundle branch block without any alteration in the tachycardia cycle length (TCL).

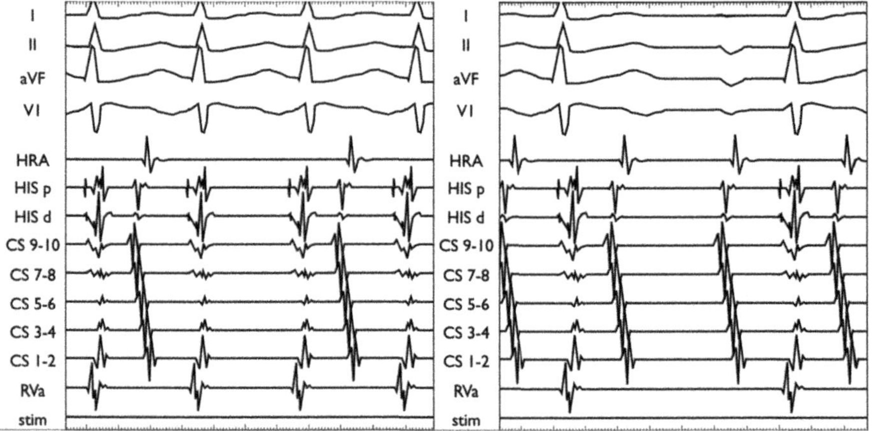

Atypical AVNRT: Anterograde conduction via the fast pathway and retrograde conduction via the slow pathway. Atrial activation is concentric with a long VA time. In the left panel, there is 2:1 upper common pathway block; each His is followed by a ventricular EGM, but only every second His is followed by an atrial EGM. In the right panel, there is 2:1 lower common pathway block; each His EGM is followed by an A EGM, but only every second His is followed by a V EGM.

Maneuvers During Tachycardia

- Late-coupled atrial extrastimuli
  - Used to differentiate atypical AVNRT from from atrioventricular reciprocating tachycardia (AVRT) (i.e., narrow-complex tachycardia [NCT] with long VA)
  - Two possible responses to late coupled atrial extrastimuli
    - No effect on TCL: Does not enter the circuit (encounters refractory tissue and is blocked)
    - Resets the tachycardia: Conducts down the slow pathway (advances the His with a long AH), and back up the fast pathway
- Early coupled atrial extrastimuli
  - Used to differentiate AVNRT from from non-reentrant junctional tachycardia (i.e., NCT with short VA)
  - Terminates the tachycardia: Conducts down the fast pathway (advances the His with short AH), making it refractory to retrograde depolarization

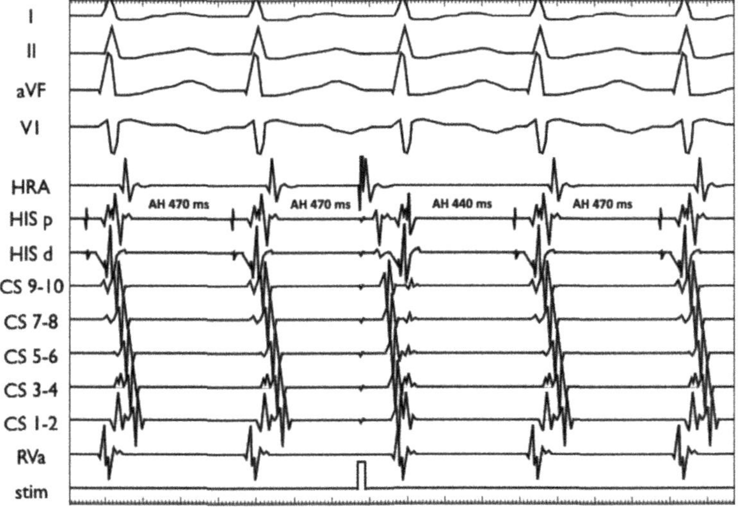

A premature atrial complex timed to junctional (His) refractoriness advances the next His by 30 ms, indicating AVNRT as the tachycardia mechanism.

- Premature ventricular impulses (His-synchronous ventricular premature beat [VPB])
  - Used to differentiate atypical AVNRT from AVRT
  - The timing of the atrial activation (A EGM) and TCL after a premature ventricular impulse timed to junctional (His) refractoriness is examined
    - For AVNRT, there should not be any response unless the VPB is very early (e.g., >100 ms).

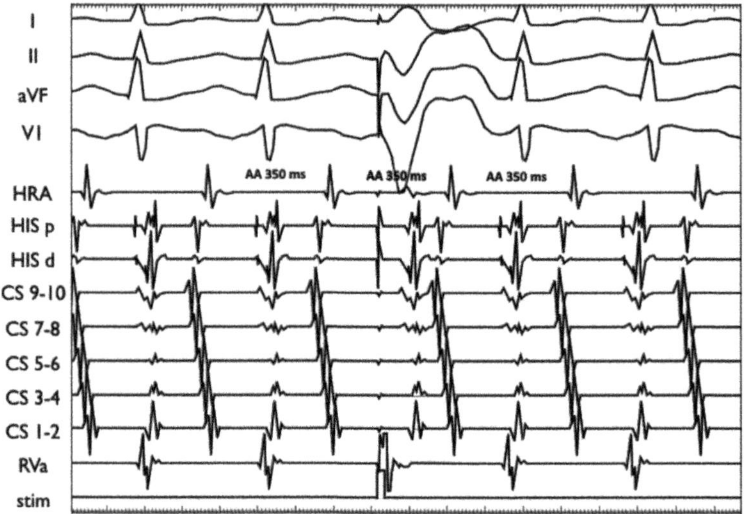

His-synchronous VPB does not affect the timing of the next A or tachycardia cycle.

- Entrainment via ventricular overdrive pacing
  - Used to distinguish AVNRT from atrial tachycardia (AT) and AVRT using a paraseptal AP.
  - VA activation should be similar during pacing and tachycardia.
  - With termination of pacing:
    - A **VAV** (or AHAV) response is observed.
    - The return CL has baseline VA timing intervals (fixed coupling).
    - **PPI – TCL** (Stim to V EGM) ≥115 ms
    - **cPPI** = (PPI – TCL) – (AH_{RVP} – AH_{SVT}) ≥110 ms
    - **Stim-A_{RVP} – VA_{SVT}** ≥ 85 ms

Entrainment via Ventricular Overdrive Pacing from the Right Ventricular Apex (RVa)

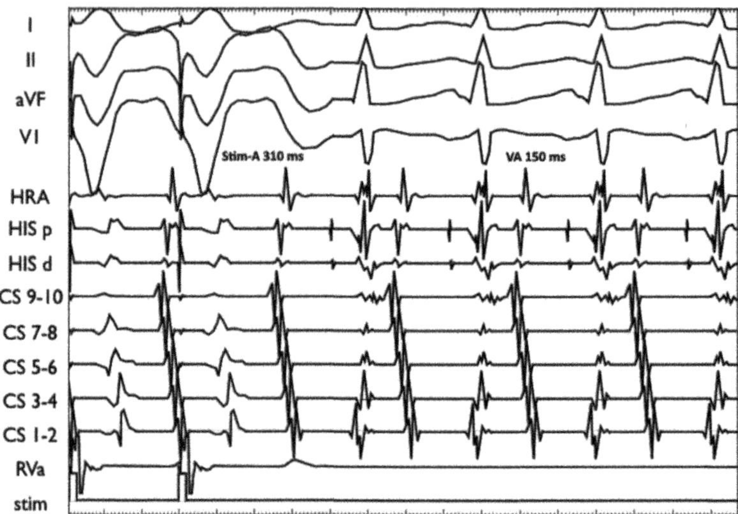

Supraventricular tachycardia (SVT) entrainment via ventricular overdrive pacing from the RVa results in 1:1 VA conduction. After cessation of pacing, the EGM response is atrial-ventricular (VAV or VAHV) consistent with atypical AVNRT. The VA interval on first post-paced ventricular beat is <10 ms different from the tachycardia VA (VA linking).

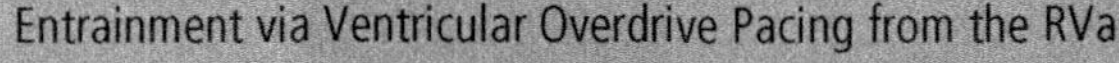

Entrainment via Ventricular Overdrive Pacing from the RVa

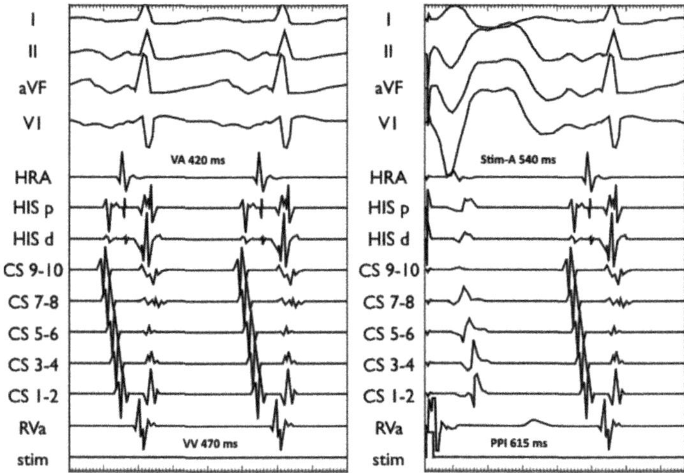

SVT entrainment via ventricular overdrive pacing from the RVa is performed at 440 ms (TCL 470 ms with a VA time of 420 ms). The ventriculo-atrial (VA_{SVT}) interval and TCL are measured immediately before entrainment (left panel). After cessation of pacing, the stimulus-atrial ($Stim\text{-}A_{RVP}$) interval is measured from the last pacing stimulus to the last entrained HRA EGM, and the post-pacing interval (PPI) is measured from the last pacing stimulus to the return cycle right ventricular (RV) EGM (right panel). The ($Stim\text{-}A_{RVP}$) – VA_{SVT} interval is 120 ms, and the PPI – TCL is 145 ms, consistent with atypical AVNRT.

- Entrainment via atrial overdrive pacing
  - Entrainment via atrial overdrive pacing is used to differentiate AVNRT from AT.
  - With termination of pacing:
    - The VA of first return beat should demonstrate fixed VA timing (<10 ms of tachycardia VA) in AVNRT and orthodromic AVRT (effectively excludes atrial or junctional tachycardia).
    - The post-pacing sequence should be **AHA** in AVNRT.

Entrainment via Atrial Overdrive Pacing from the HRA

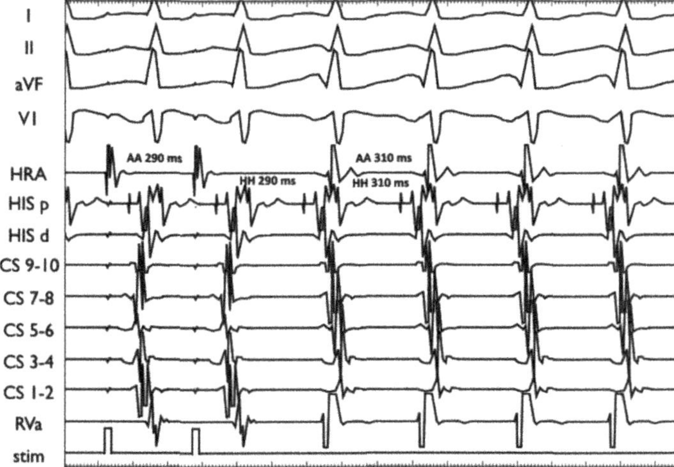

Atrial overdrive pacing is performed at 290 ms (TCL 310 ms). The HH intervals are noted, demonstrating the last advanced His signal. After cessation of pacing, an AHA response is observed.

- Differential RV entrainment
  - Entrainment at RVa and RV base is often used to differentiate atypical AVNRT from AVRT using a paraseptal decremental AP.
  - Interpretation:
    - [PPI – TCL (base)] – [PPI – TCL (apex)] >30 ms
    - [Stim-A – VA (apex)] – [Stim-A – VA (base)] <0 ms
- Parahisian entrainment
  - Entrainment with and without His capture is often used to differentiate atypical AVNRT from AVRT using a paraseptal decremental AP.
  - Interpretation:
    - Delta SA (His loss – His capture) > 50 ms
    - **PPI – TCL** (Stim to local V EGM) ≥ 100 ms

Parahisian Entrainment in Tachycardia: Atypical AVNRT

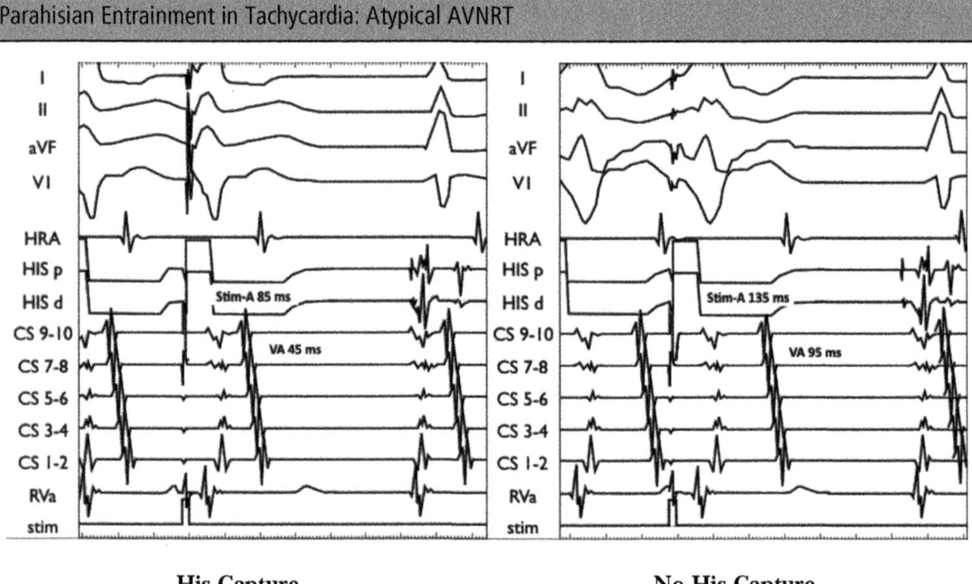

His Capture **No His Capture**

NCT with a long VA time and earliest atrial activation in the proximal CS (CL 420 ms). Shown in the 2 panels are 2 separate entrainment maneuvers performed at 400 ms. In the **left panel**, there is His capture; in the **right panel**, there is loss of His capture. The delta SA with loss of His capture was 110 ms (480–370 ms), consistent with AVNRT.

Maneuvers in Sinus Rhythm

- Parahisian pacing
  - Useful to differentiate an anteroseptal pathway from an anterior AVN exit site
  - Interpretation: **Nodal response**
    - The retrograde atrial activation sequence is unchanged.
    - The Stim–A interval increases (>50 ms), but the His bundle–atrial interval is stable.

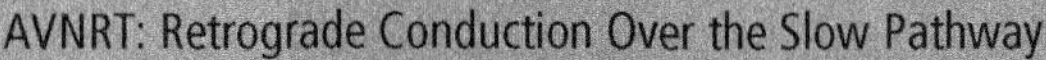

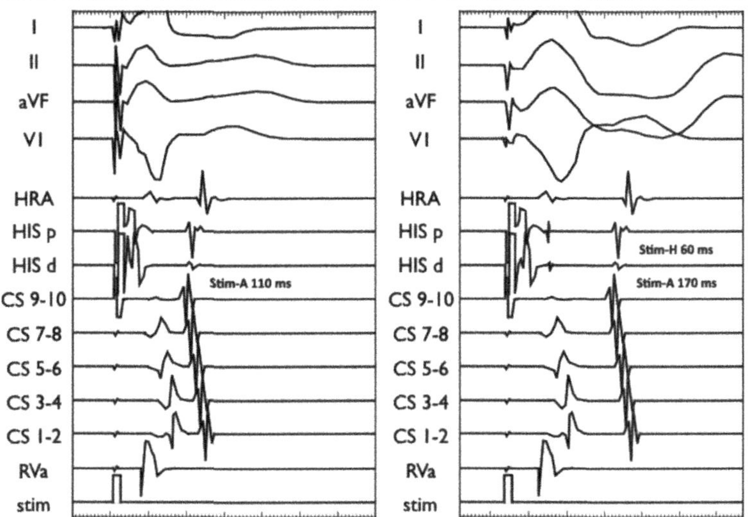

Left panel: Ventricular and HB-RB capture produce a relatively narrow QRS complex and early activation of the His bundle (buried within the V EGM on the His catheter).
Right panel: Loss of HB-RB capture results in widening of the QRS complex, an increase in the SH interval (to 60 ms), and a 60 ms increase in the SA interval (from 110 ms to 170 ms).

The stable **HA** interval (~100 ms) indicates that retrograde conduction was dependent on His bundle activation and not on ventricular activation (i.e., retrograde conduction occurs exclusively over the AVN).

Earliest atrial activation occurs in the proximal CS, suggesting that retrograde conduction occurs over the slow pathway.

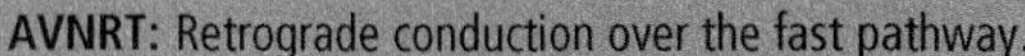

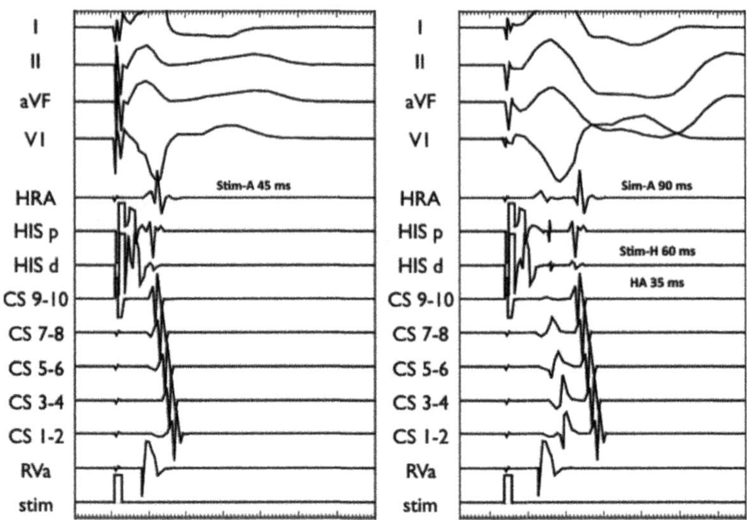

Left panel: Ventricular and HB-RB capture produce a relatively narrow QRS complex and early activation of the His bundle (buried within the V EGM on the His catheter).
Right panel: Loss of HB-RB capture results in widening of the QRS complex and a 45 ms increase in the S-H interval (from 15 ms to 60 ms) and the S-A interval (from 45 ms to 90 ms).

The stable **HA** interval (30 ms) indicates that retrograde conduction was dependent on His bundle activation and not on local ventricular activation (i.e., retrograde conduction exclusively over the AVN).

Earliest atrial activation occurs on the His catheter, suggesting retrograde conduction over the fast pathway.

- Differential (apical-basal) pacing
  - Useful to differentiate an anteroseptal pathway from an anterior AVN exit site
  - In the absence of AP conduction, the basal pacing impulse must travel to the apex, then invade the His-Purkinje system before returning to the atrium.
    - This results in a longer Stim-A time from the RV base than from the RVa (SA Apex:Base <10 ms).
    - Retrograde atrial activation sequence is unchanged.
    - Septal HA interval is unchanged.

Differential Pacing from the RVa and Base

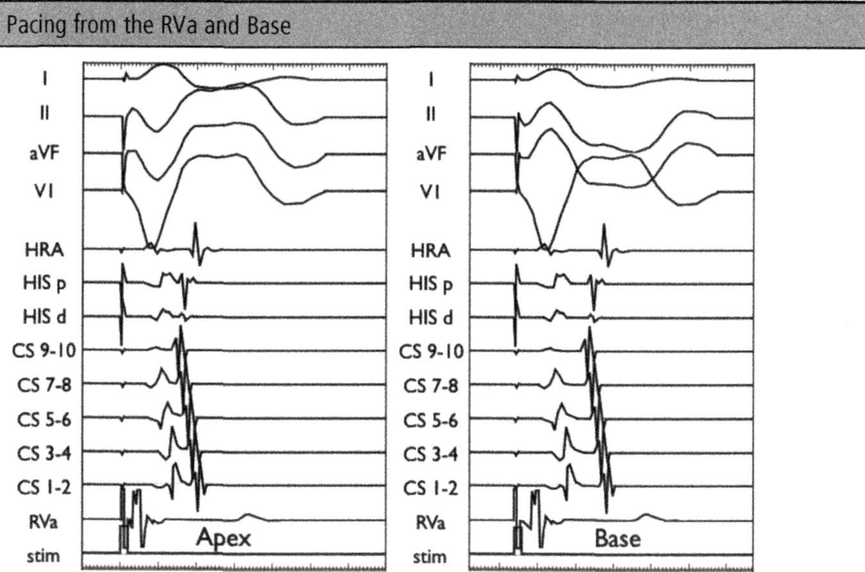

Longer VA time with basal pacing suggests an absence of AP conduction (nodal response).

- Atrial pacing at TCL
  - Interpretation: AH time in pacing is longer than in tachycardia (>40 ms).

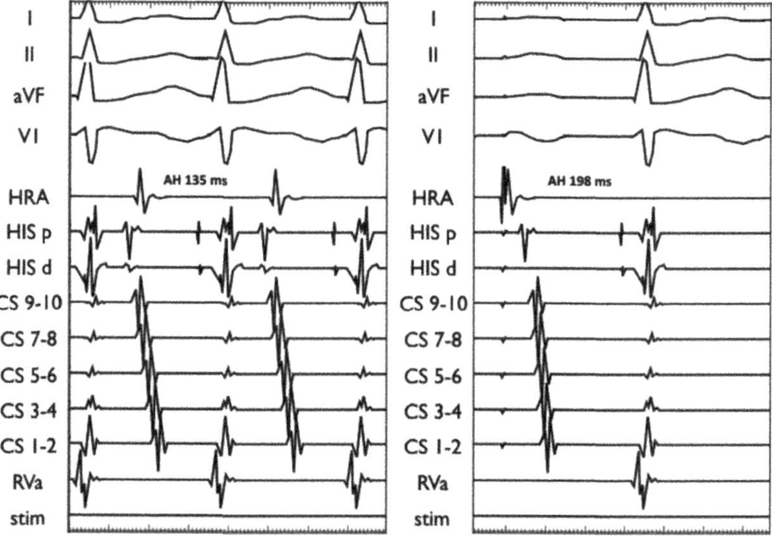

A comparison of AH intervals during atypical AVNRT (left panel) and HRA pacing at the TCL (right panel). The AH interval is 135 ms during tachycardia (left panel) and 198 ms during atrial pacing (right panel), leading to a delta AH of 63 ms.

- Ventricular pacing at TCL
  - Interpretation: VA (and HA) time in pacing is longer than in tachycardia.

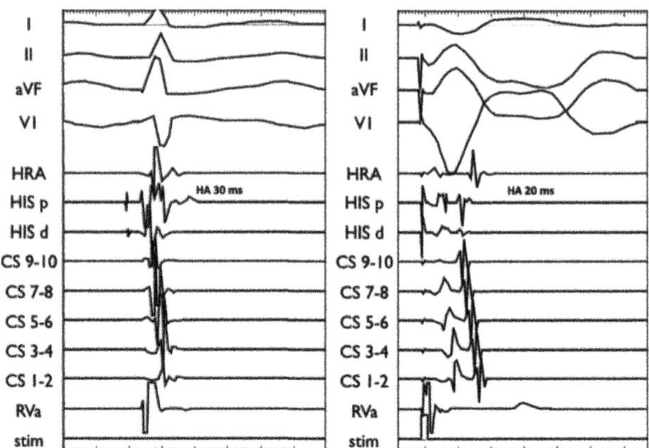

A comparison of HA intervals during AVNRT (left panel) and ventricular pacing at the TCL (right panel). The HA interval is 30 ms during tachycardia (left panel) and 20 ms during ventricular pacing (right panel), leading to a delta HA of –10 ms.

- Induction of retrograde RBBB
  - There is usually no change in VA timing or TCL.
  - The increase in VH approximates (or is shorter than) the increase in VA.

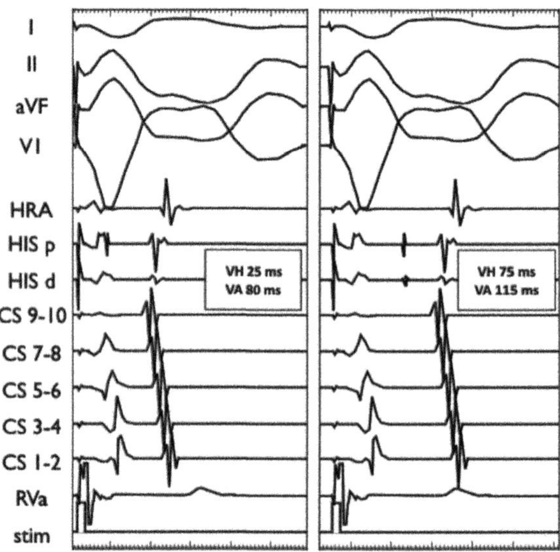

RV apical pacing at 600 ms with an S1S2 coupling interval of 320 ms results in a retrograde His 25 ms after the QRS with a VA interval of 80 ms. When the coupling interval is decreased to 300 ms, retrograde RBBB is induced (increased VH to 75 ms; delta VH of 50 ms) with prolongation of VA timing (115 ms; delta VA of 35 ms).

Table 4.3 Localizing the AVNRT Circuit

	VA (His)	VA (HRA)	AH:HA During Tachy	Earliest Retrograde Atrial Activation
Slow-fast AVNRT				
• Rightward inward extension (90%)				Inferoseptal TV-CS
• Leftward inward extension (<10%)	<70 ms	<100 ms	>1	CS roof
• Left atrial/left septal (<10%)				Left septal His EGM, dCS
Slow-slow	>70 ms	>100 ms	>1	CS roof (60%) Inferoseptal TV-CS (40%)
Fast-slow (5%–10%)	>70 ms	>100 ms	<1	Inferoseptal TV-CS (75%) CS floor (25%)

DIFFERENTIATING ATRIOVENTRICULAR NODAL REENTRANT TACHYCARDIAS FROM OTHER TACHYCARDIAS

The characteristics differentiating AVNRT from perinodal AT and AVRT (septal AP) are presented in Tables 4.4 and 4.5, respectively. Differentiating AVNRT from junctional tachycardia is discussed separately.

Table 4.4 Differentiating AVNRT from Perinodal AT

	AVNRT	AT (Perinodal)
Anterograde pacing	Dual AVN physiology	
Arrhythmia induction	**Atrial extrastimuli or burst** (difficult with V pacing)	**Atrial extrastimuli or burst** (never with V pacing)
AV relationship during tachycardia	1:1 (Rarely 2≥1 or 1≤2)	1:1 or 2≥1
AV block during tachycardia (vagal, adenosine, verapamil, or extrasystoles)	**Sometimes** • usually terminates tachycardia • rarely 2:1 infrahisian AV block with continued tachycardia	**Strongly predictive** Uninterrupted tachycardia during AV block is typical of AT • AVN **not** critical to circuit • rarely terminates tachycardia
Septal VA interval during tachycardia (earliest V on His or PCS to A on same channel)	≤70 ms (typical) >70 ms (atypical)	Variable (≤70 ms ≠ **exclude**)
HRA VA interval during tachycardia (earliest V on His or PCS to A on HRA)	≤100 ms (typical) >100 ms (atypical)	Variable
Atrial activation during tachycardia	**Concentric** > Eccentric	**Eccentric** > Concentric

(*Continued*)

Table 4.4 (*Continued*)

	AVNRT	AT (Perinodal)
CL variation during tachycardia	Change in HH interval precedes change in AA interval • Delay in anterograde AVN (critical part of circuit)	Change in AA interval precedes change in HH interval (AVN not critical part of circuit)
Tachy termination (spontaneous)	Ends with A (common) • Blocks in slow pathway Ends with V (uncommon) • Blocks in fast pathway	Ends with a V (common) • normal AV conduction Ends with an A • effectively excludes AT
RVa entrainment	**Able to entrain** • Yes	**Able to entrain** • No
	Atrial activation sequence • Pacing = tachycardia	**Atrial activation sequence** • Pacing ≠ tachycardia (usually)
	Post-pacing sequence • VAV (atrial-ventricular) • AHAV (atrial-ventricular)	**Post-pacing sequence** • VAAV • AAHV
Burst RV pacing at 200–250 ms for 3–6 beats	May have AV dissociation May terminate	AV dissociation is common Termination **without** atrial activation **excludes AT**
Atrial entrainment	Return VA CL: **Fixed/linked** (<10 ms of tachy VA)	Return VA CL: **Variable** (usually >10 ms of tachy VA)
Differential entrainment • from HRA and CS	Return VA CL: **Fixed/linked** (<10 ms of tachy VA)	Return VA CL: **Variable** (usually >10 ms of tachy VA)
Early-coupled PACs	Advances the His with short AH → terminates SVT (fast pathway refractory)	Advances the His with short AH → SVT continues
	Return VA CL: **Fixed/linked** (<10 ms of tachy VA)	Return VA CL: **Variable**
Atrial pacing at TCL in sinus • $AH_{Pacing} - AH_{SVT}$	>40 ms	<10 ms

AVNRT vs. AVRT (Septal AP)

- ECG findings help to differentiate AVNRT from AVRT.
  - Presence of pseudo r′ or pseudo S suggests AVNRT.
  - >20 ms increase in RP interval between V1 and III indicates posterior AVNRT.
  - AV block or AV dissociation can be either AVNRT or AT.
  - Lengthening in TCL or VA interval with bundle branch block indicates ipsilateral AVRT.

Table 4.5 EPS Characteristics Distinguishing AVNRT from AVRT

	AVNRT	AVRT
HV interval <35 ms (sinus)	Usually absent	**Strongly predictive**
Retrograde conduction	**Decremental**	**Non-decremental** (if conduction via the AP)
Retrograde activation sequence	**Concentric** > Eccentric	**Eccentric** > Concentric (depends on AP location)
Anterograde activation sequence	Normal	**Early ventricular activation** (if manifest pre-excitation)
Anterograde pacing	Decremental AV conduction Dual AVN physiology	Non-decremental AV conduction Manifest pre-excitation
Arrhythmia induction	**Atrial extrastimuli or burst** (difficult with V pacing)	**Atrial extrastimuli or burst** **Ventricular extrastimuli or burst**
AV block during SVT	**Sometimes**	**Terminates tachycardia**
Septal VA interval in SVT (earliest V on His or PCS to A on same channel)	≤70 ms (typical) >70 ms (atypical)	>70 ms (often >100) (≤70 ms **excludes**)
HRA VA interval in SVT (earliest V on His or PCS to A on HRA)	≤100 ms (typical) >100 ms (atypical)	>100 ms
Atrial activation in SVT	**Concentric** > Eccentric	**Eccentric** > Concentric
Effect of bundle branch block on VA time in SVT	No effect (↑ ≥25 ms excludes)	VA interval and TCL ↑ ≥25 ms • indicates ipsilateral AP No effect if contralateral AP
RVa entrainment in SVT	**Atrial activation timing** • Advanced only after complete ventricular capture	**Atrial activation timing** • Advanced with partial ventricular capture (fusion)
	PPI – TCL (Stim to V EGM): ≥115 ms **cPPI = PPI – TCL – (AH_{RVP} – AH_{SVT})**: ≥110 ms **Stim-A_{RVP} – VA_{SVT}**: ≥85 ms **Stim-A_{RVP} / VA_{SVT}**: 0.3	**PPI–TCL** (Stim to V EGM): <115 ms **cPPI = PPI – TCL – (AH_{RVP} – AH_{SVT})**: <110 ms **Stim-A_{RVP} – VA_{SVT}**: <85 ms **Stim-A_{RVP} / VA_{SVT}**: 1.0
Parahisian entrainment in SVT	**PPI – TCL** (Stim to V EGM): ≥100 ms **Stim-A_{RVP} – VA_{SVT}**: ≥75 ms	**PPI–TCL** (Stim to V EGM): <100 ms **Stim-A_{RVP} – VA_{SVT}**: <75 ms
Differential entrainment in SVT from RVa and base	**cPPI – TCL (Base – Apex)**: >30 ms **Stim-A (Apex – Base)**: <0 ms (VA shorter at apex)	**cPPI–TCL (Base – Apex)**: <30 ms **Stim-A (Apex – Base)**: >0 ms (VA shorter at base)

(Continued)

Table 4.5 (*Continued*)

	AVNRT	AVRT
Burst RV pacing at 200–250 ms for 3–6 beats	May have AV dissociation May terminate	AV dissociation **excludes** Should terminate
His-synchronous PVC in SVT	No effect	**Atrial depolarization** • **Advanced**: Confirms AP exists • **Delayed**: Confirms AP and role in SVT **Tachycardia termination** • Confirms AP and role in SVT
	Pre-excitement index (PEI) • >100–120 ms: AVNRT	**PEI** • <45 ms: Septal AP
Induction of retrograde RBBB with pacing (↑ VH interval >50 ms)	VH increase < VA increase	VH increase > VA increase
Parahisian pacing in sinus	**Retrograde atrial activation** • Unchanged: Nodal conduction • Changes: Switch from slow pathway to fast pathway	**Retrograde atrial activation** • Unchanged: AP conduction • Changes: Switch from node to AP
	Nodal response • **SA interval** increases (>50 ms) • **HA interval** unchanged	**Extranodal response** • **SA interval** increases (<40 ms) • **HA interval** decreases (septal AP)
Differential pacing from RVa and base in sinus	**Atrial activation sequence** • Unchanged (node)	**Atrial activation sequence** • Changes (AP to node) • Unchanged (AP)
	Septal HA interval • Unchanged	**Septal HA interval** • <20–30 ms or negative
	SA Apex – Base (VA) • <5–10 ms	**VA Apex – Base** (VA) • >10 ms
Atrial pacing in sinus at TCL • $AH_{Pacing} - AH_{SVT}$	>40 ms	<20 ms (septal AP)
Ventricular pacing in sinus at TCL $HA_{Pacing} - HA_{SVT}$	Positive	Negative

AVNRT vs. Junctional Ectopic Tachycardia (JET)

- JET presents with a junctional rhythm with gradual onset and termination (70–130 bpm).
  - Narrow QRS tachycardia with AV dissociation is also characteristic.
  - RR interval may be irregular.
  - Substrate includes anterograde conduction with normal HV and AH conduction curves.
- JET is usually induced via isoproterenol > rapid A or V pacing.
  - Observations during tachycardia may find earliest atrial activation in any of the anteroseptal, posteroseptal, or midseptal locations.
- Maneuvers in tachycardia include:
  - Late-coupled atrial extrasystole delivered when the junction is refractory (timed to His refractoriness)
    - If the maneuver advances (or delays) the subsequent His and resets the tachycardia, this supports AVNRT.
    - No effect on TCL supports diagnosis of JET.
- Early-coupled APC advances the His with a short AH.
  - If this activates the fast pathway anterograde and renders it refractory to retrograde conduction, it terminates SVT, and the diagnosis is AVNRT.
  - If this resets the tachycardia, the diagnosis is JET.
- Atrial overdrive pacing
  - AHA response at termination of entrainment: AVNRT
  - AHHA response at termination of entrainment: JET
- Maneuvers in sinus rhythm include assessment of the difference in HA interval during RV basal pacing vs. tachycardia:
  - Positive: AVNRT
  - Negative: JET

CATHETER ABLATION OF ATRIOVENTRICULAR NODAL REENTRANT TACHYCARDIA

Indications

- For treatment of AVNRT that is symptomatic, recurrent, or refractory to medical therapy

Anticipated Success

- >93%–96% acute success rate
- ~5%–10% 1-year recurrence of conduction
  - Fast-slow, 1.2%
  - Slow-fast, 0.4%
  - Slow-slow, 6%

Anticipated Complications

- Complete heart block occurs in 1%–2% if the slow pathway is targeted (up to 20% if fast pathway targeted).
- The remainder of anticipated complications is similar to that observed for all ablation procedures.

Patient Preparation

- Stop all antiarrhythmic drugs (AAD) for 3–5 half-lives before the procedure.
- Conscious sedation is preferred to general anesthesia due to the risk of arrhythmia non-inducibility.

Set-Up

- General set-up is similar to SVT.
- Ablation catheters of choice are the following:
  - Non-irrigated radiofrequency (RF): D-curve (medium/blue), or F-curve (large/orange) ± guiding sheath
  - Cryocatheter (6 mm): blue or orange

Slow Pathway Mapping and Approaches

- Electroanatomic approach:
  - The ablation catheter is positioned at the level of the CS ostium between the CS and the tricuspid valve.
    - Small A EGM with a large, sharp V EGM (A:V ratio of 1:2 to 1:10).
    - The A EGM on the ablation catheter should occur 20–30 ms later than that seen in the His.
- Slow pathway potential ablation approach:
  - Mapping in the posterior portion of the triangle of Koch with the proximal unipolar electrode can lead to the detection of a slow pathway potential.
  - At a good ablation site:
    - An initial small, far-field atrial potential is generated by the RA posterior to the Eustachian ridge.
    - This is followed by an isoelectric interval and then the sharp slow pathway potential.
    - Lastly, a large, sharp ventricular potential (generated by the ventricular myocardium under the atrial myocardium in the muscular AV septum) is seen.
  - Note: Late timing of the slow pathway potential during sinus rhythm (i.e., after activation in the proximal CS) may be explained by conduction block at the Eustachian ridge.
    - The sinus impulse enters the triangle of Koch either from the inferior right atrium (extension of activation from the crista terminalis) or from the LA via the CS.
- Tricuspid annulus to CS ostium line approach:
  - Create a linear lesion between the tricuspid annulus and the anterior edge of the CS ostium (at the level of the middle of the CS ostium).
    - Start on the ventricular aspect of the TV annulus identified by recording a slow pathway potential.
    - Deliver RF energy until the atrial potential on the unipolar EGM is markedly diminished.
    - Continue pulling the catheter back until the ablation electrode reaches the apical edge of the CS ostium.

Ablation (Slow Pathway Modification)

RF Ablation (Non-Irrigated)

- Use 25 to 45 W (electrode temperature <60°C) at sites distant to compact AVN.
  - Reduce power to 20–25 W when approaching the CS ostium.
- If superior location (near AVN), start at 10–15 W and titrate up.
- At successful sites, a "slow" junctional rhythm with 1:1 retrograde VA conduction (via fast pathway) emerges within seconds of RF application due to enhanced automaticity in heated tissues.
  - Immediately terminate RF if a loss of 1:1 conduction or a fast junctional rhythm is observed:
    - Suggests injury to the compact AVN or fast pathway.
    - Heralds impending complete heart block.
  - Continue RF energy until 15–20 seconds after cessation or slowing of the junctional rhythm.
- If no effect:
  - Re-evaluate the procedural endpoint (see below) prior to delivering further ablation.
  - Junctional rhythm may not be universally observed and slow pathway modification may have been successful.
  - If not, progressively perform ablation from the initial inferior-posterior position to a more anterior-superior position.
- Note: Avoid delivering RF energy near the floor of the CS ostium due to injury to the coronary artery.

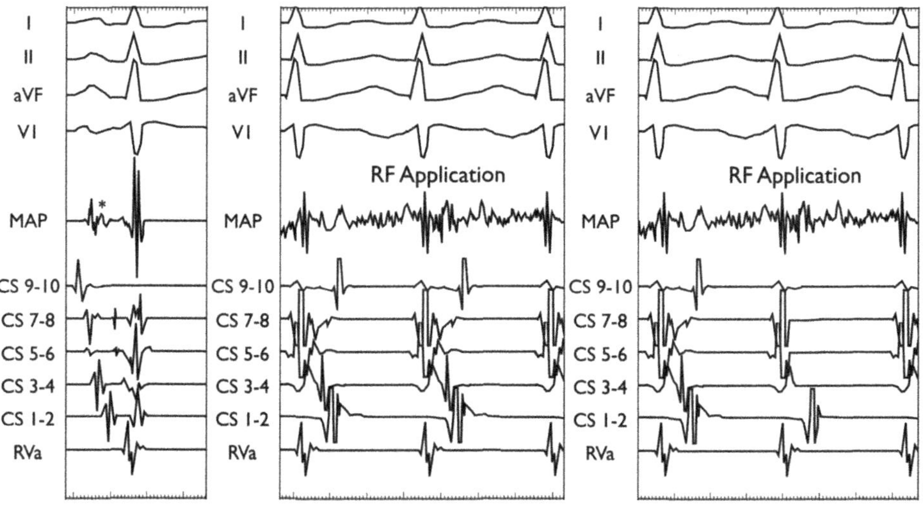

Left panel: The ablation catheter is positioned at the level of the CS ostium, between it and the tricuspid valve. There is a large V and small A EGM with a slow pathway potential (*) slightly earlier than the anticipated His.
Middle panel: RF application results in a junctional rhythm with a 1:1 AV ratio due to anterograde conduction via the His-Purkinje system (V) and retrograde conduction to the atria (A) via the fast pathway. This response suggests that this is a successful ablation site, and is usually observed within a few seconds.
Right panel: Similar to the middle panel, RF application results in a junctional rhythm with a 1:1 AV ratio due to anterograde conduction via the His-Purkinje system (V). On the second beat, there is retrograde block due to fast pathway injury. This is an indication for immediate termination of ablation.

Cryoablation

- The ideal site is similar to that used with RF except slightly more proximal and more cranial (larger A:V ratio).
  - Cryoablation may require ablation within the CS ostium.
- For the first 60–90 seconds during the cryoapplications, the AH interval should be monitored.
  - Terminate ablation if the AH interval increases by >25%–30% from baseline.
  - If the AH interval is stable, then begin testing anterograde conduction during ablation.
    - Terminate ablation if the arrhythmia is still inducible.
    - If not, continue the ablation for the full 4 minutes and then retest.

Determinants of Success

- The determinants of success depend on the ease of inducibility of tachycardia prior to ablation.
- Ideally, all of the criteria listed below should be achieved (if possible):
  - Elimination of inducible tachycardia (rest and with isoproterenol stimulation)
    - Tachycardia elimination is a satisfactory endpoint if it was easily inducible prior to ablation.
    - Single slow-fast atrial echo complexes are allowed (i.e., slow pathway modification).
  - Elimination of 1:1 anterograde conduction over the slow pathway during decremental atrial pacing
    - Increase in the AV block CL
    - Inability to create long AH intervals during atrial overdrive pacing
  - Elimination of the AH jump that was present prior to RF application (i.e., slow pathway ablation)
    - This is the target of ablation in patients where tachycardia was not inducible prior to ablation.

CATHETER ABLATION OF ATYPICAL ATRIOVENTRICULAR NODAL REENTRANT TACHYCARDIA SUBSTRATES

"Leftward Inferior Extension" Slow-Fast AVNRT (5%)

- The target is the atrial end of the leftward inferior extension along the anterior-superior edge of the proximal CS roof (2–4 cm inside).
- Avoid positioning the catheter perpendicular to the CS roof during ablation at the CS ostium.
  - The fast pathway may be injured by direct injury or catheter movement into a high-risk location.

"Left Atrial Insertion" Slow-Fast AVNRT (<1%)

- The initial target is the atrial end of the leftward inferior extension.
- If unsuccessful, target the atrial end of the slow pathway in the LA close to the inferolateral mitral annulus.
  - This target can be identified by the "**resetting response**": During AVNRT, a late atrial extrastimulus (**after** the onset of retrograde atrial activation) delivered to the inferolateral mitral annulus advances the next His by 10 ms, followed by tachycardia reset (HH interval equal to TCL).
  - The resetting response indicates that the pacing site is located close to the atrial end of the slow pathway.
  - Ablation at the site of resetting frequently produces accelerated junctional rhythm with retrograde fast pathway conduction (slow pathway automaticity) and eliminates the tachycardia.
  - Note: Ablation at this site is not successful if the extrastimulus fails to advance the next His.

Slow-Slow AVNRT

- The initial target is the retrograde slow pathway conduction (**earliest retrograde atrial activation** of the tachycardia), typically at the proximal CS roof.
  - Ablation should result in termination of the tachycardia (continue ablation for a full minute).
  - Monitor for 1:1 retrograde VA conduction (via fast pathway).
  - Consider pacing the atrium at a CL slightly slower than the tachycardia in order to avoid significantly displacing the catheter with termination of the tachycardia.
- If unsuccessful, target anterograde slow pathway conduction by performing ablation of the rightward inferior extension between the tricuspid annulus and CS ostium.
  - Note: During ablation at this site, accelerated junctional rhythm frequently is associated with VA block because retrograde fast pathway conduction is either absent or poor in most patients with slow-slow AVNRT.

Fast-Slow AVNRT

- The initial target is retrograde slow pathway conduction (**earliest retrograde atrial activation** during tachycardia), typically the region between the inferoseptal tricuspid annulus and the CS ostium.
  - Note: Avoid delivering RF energy near the floor of the CS due to injury to the coronary artery.
  - Ablation should result in termination of the tachycardia (continue ablation for a full minute).
  - Monitor for 1:1 retrograde VA conduction (via the fast pathway) as per above.
  - Consider pacing the atrium at a CL slightly slower than the tachycardia in order to avoid significantly displacing the catheter with termination of the tachycardia.
- If unsuccessful, ablate the anterograde slow pathway region and use the elimination of slow pathway conduction as a determinant of success if it was present at the beginning of the procedure.

Key References for Further Reading

- Katritsis DG, Camm AJ. Atrioventricular nodal reentrant tachycardia. *Circulation.* 2010;122:831–840.
- Delacrétaz E. Supraventricular tachycardia. *N Engl J Med.* 2006;354:1039–1051.
- Gonzalez-Torrecilla E, Almendral J, Arenal A, Atienza F, Atea LF, del Castillo S, et al. Combined evaluation of bedside clinical variables and the electrocardiogram for the differential diagnosis of paroxysmal atrioventricular reciprocating tachycardias in patients without pre-excitation. *J Am Coll Cardiol.* 2009;53:2353–2358.
- Veenhuyzen GD, Quinn R, Wilton SB, Clegg R, Mitchell LB. Diagnostic pacing maneuvers for supraventricular tachycardia: Part 1. *PACE.* 2011;34:767–782.
- Knight BP, Ebinger M, Oral H, Kim MH, Sticherling C, Pelosi F, et al. Diagnostic value of tachycardia features and pacing maneuvers during paroxysmal supraventricular tachycardia. *J Am Coll Cardiol.* 2000;36:574–582.
- Nakagawa H, Jackman WM. Catheter ablation of paroxysmal supraventricular tachycardia. *Circulation.* 2007;116:2465–2478.
- Schwagten B, Van Belle Y, Jordaens L. Cryoablation: How to improve results in atrioventricular nodal reentrant tachycardia ablation? *Europace.* 2010;12:1522–1525.
- De Sisti A, Tonet J. Cryoablation of atrioventricular nodal reentrant tachycardia: A clinical review. *PACE.* 2012;35:233–240.

CHAPTER

5

Accessory Pathways

UNDERSTANDING AND EVALUATING ACCESSORY PATHWAYS (APs)

General Information

The ventricles are normally insulated from the atria by a fibrofatty connective tissue skeleton that also contains the valvular structures.

- In certain cases, an extranodal bypass tract (or accessory pathway, AP) connects the atrial and ventricular myocardium across the atrioventricular (AV) groove, bypassing the atrioventricular node (AVN).
- Such an AP allows for electrical activation of the ventricular myocardium before the impulse arrives via the AVN/His-Purkinje conduction system, causing pre-excitation.

Anatomy and Pathophysiology

Most APs have rapid, non-decremental conduction similar to myocardium or His-Purkinje tissue.

- **Bidirectional conduction** is present in most bypass tracts.
  - Bidirectional conduction could result in orthodromic or antidromic atrioventricular reciprocating tachycardia (AVRT) and pre-excited atrial arrhythmias/atrial fibrillation (AF).
- **Anterograde conduction** could result in antidromic AVRT and pre-excited atrial arrhythmias/AF. It can be:
  - **Manifest**: Anterograde conduction down AP results in pre-excitation on electrocardiogram (ECG).
  - **Latent**: Anterograde activation is not manifest due to relatively greater degree of AVN conduction. The relative balance of AVN and AP conduction is dependent on:
    - AVN conduction velocity (vagal maneuvers, premature atrial complexes [PAC], and adenosine increase pre-excitation by decreasing AV conduction)
    - AP conduction velocity (increased pre-excitation with rapid conduction)
    - The proximity of the bypass tract to the atrial impulse; for example, a sinus node impulse reaches the AVN or a right-sided AP earlier than it would a left-sided AP.
  - **Intermittent:** Suggests a relatively long anterograde effective refractory period (ERP)

The Clinical Cardiac Electrophysiology Handbook © 2016 Jason Andrade.
Cardiotext Publishing, ISBN: 978-1-942909-00-2.

- **Retrograde**: Exclusive retrogradely conducting pathways are called concealed APs.
  - No delta wave is seen due to lack of anterograde activation.
  - Orthodromic AVRT is possible, but pre-excited atrial arrhythmias/AF cannot occur.

Types of APs

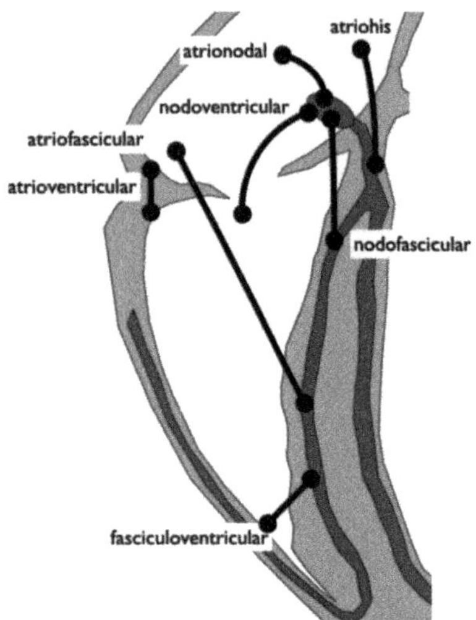

- **Atrioventricular** (bundle of Kent; Wolff-Parkinson-White syndrome [WPW])
  - Bypass tract along the AV groove connects atrial and ventricular myocardium (bypassing the AVN/His-Purkinje system).
  - **ECG**: Short PR interval with wide QRS/delta wave (if manifest)
  - **Electrophysiology study (EPS)**: Short HV interval (if manifest)
- **Atrionodal** (James fibers; Lown-Ganong-Levine syndrome)
  - Bypass tract connects the atrium to the distal compact AVN.
  - **ECG**: Short PR interval with normal QRS
  - **EPS**: Short AH interval
- **Intranodal** (James fibers; Lown-Ganong-Levine syndrome)
  - Specialized fibers in node
  - **ECG**: Short PR interval with normal QRS
  - **EPS**: Short AH interval
- **Atriohisian** (Brechenmacher fibers; Lown-Ganong-Levine syndrome)
  - Bypass tract connects the atrium to the His bundle
  - **ECG**: Short PR interval with normal QRS
  - **EPS**: Short AH interval
- Other
  - **Atriofascicular**: Atrium (anterolateral tricuspid valve [TV] annulus) to distal Purkinje fibers (right bundle near right ventricular apex [RVa])
  - **Nodofascicular**: AVN to distal Purkinje fibers (intranodal connection)
  - **Nodoventricular**: AVN to ventricular myocardium
  - **Fasciculoventricular**: His bundle to ventricular myocardium

12-Lead ECG

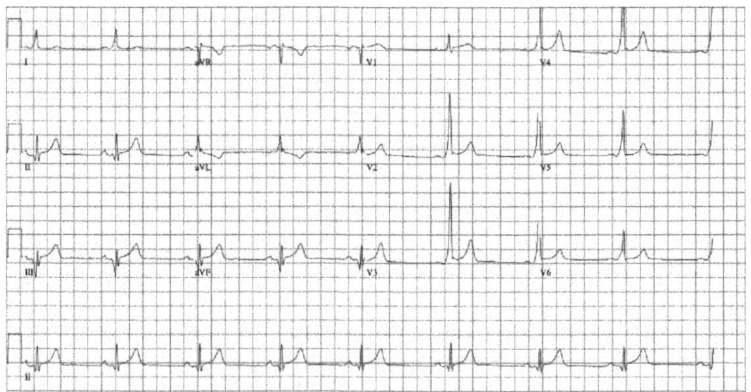

- ECG criteria for for pre-excitation are as follows:
  - PR interval <120 ms (adults) or 90 ms (children)
  - QRS duration >120 ms (adults) or 90 ms (children)
  - Delta wave seen in most leads (slurred initial upstroke of QRS complex)

Localizing the AP

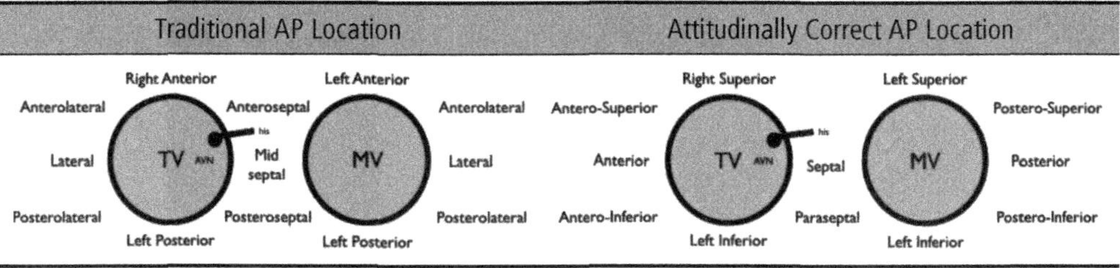

AP Localization via Delta Wave and QRS Morphology

- Rule of thumb: A negative delta wave points to the AP.
- First step:
  - Left free wall: Negative delta in lateral leads (I, aVL) and positive in V1 (R > S)
  - Right free wall: Positive delta in V1 with transition in V5 (R > S)
  - Septal: V1 is isoelectric or negative but transitions by V2
- Next step:
  - For free wall:
    - Positive delta in aVF suggests anterior location
    - Negative delta in aVF suggests posterior location
  - For septal:
    - Positive delta in aVF suggests anteroseptal or mid septal (R > S in III suggests anteroseptal)
    - Negative delta in aVF suggests posteroseptal (V1 delta negative = right; positive = left)

AP Localization via Retrograde P-Wave Morphology

- First step:
  - Left free wall: Negative P wave in lateral leads (I, aVL)
  - Right free wall: Negative P wave in V1 with positive P wave in lateral leads (I, aVL)
  - Septal: Demonstrate P wave characteristics that are not consistent with the above
- Next step:
  - Positive P wave in aVF suggests anterior location.
  - Negative P wave in aVF suggests posterior location.
- Note: Identification of the atrial insertion may suggest the presence of multiple APs if it differs from the location identified by AP localization via delta wave/QRS morphology.

Other Investigations

- 24-hour Holter and exercise stress test:
  - AP is deemed to be at lower risk if intermittent pre-excitation (abrupt loss of delta wave) is observed.
- Echocardiogram:
  - Used for assessment of left ventricular function and to exclude structural or congenital heart disease.
  - Exclude Ebstein's anomaly: Found in 10%–15%, and is associated with multiple right-sided pathways.
- Drug challenge using intravenous (IV) procainamide 10 mg/kg over 5 min or ajmaline 1 mg/kg over 3 min.
  - Look for an abrupt disappearance of anterograde AP conduction (rarely used).
- Electrophysiology testing:
  - Facilitates an evaluation of AP conduction properties (AP refractory period).
    - Adjunctive use of isoproterenol (0.02 mcg/kg/min) can be used to assess whether the AP is high risk (results in 20–30% reclassification). Isoproterenol will: (1) reduce the accessory pathway effective refractory period (APERP) by 60–90 ms, (2) increase the potential for 1:1 AV conduction at shorter cycle lengths, and (3) facilitate a higher risk shortest pre-excited RR interval (SPERRI) in AF.
  - Facilitates pathway localization ± ablation.

Management

- Lifestyle limitations:
  - Driving: No restrictions unless the patient has experienced syncope.
    - In that case, driving restricted until the disease is controlled.
  - Sports: No restriction; however, care should be used with dangerous environments such as climbing, motorsports, or downhill skiing.
- The risk of "prophylactic" catheter ablation may outweigh the benefits in asymptomatic individuals.
  - Only perform EPS for patients with high-risk occupations (commercial driver, pilot, competitive athlete, scuba diver).
    - Post-ablation: May resume competitive sports after 1–3 months
  - For everyone else, counsel to seek medical attention if they experience symptoms (palpitations, presyncope).

Prognosis and Risk Stratification

Sudden Cardiac Death (SCD)

- Epidemiology:
  - 0.05%–0.1% annual risk; 3.4% lifetime risk
- SCD is usually due to rapidly conducted AF resulting in ventricular fibrillation.
  - Risk is proportional to the anterograde refractory period of the AP.
  - High-risk features:
    - Highly functional AP (Anterograde APERP, SPERRI during AF or shortest 1:1 anterograde conduction is ≤250 ms)
    - History of symptomatic (or inducible) AVRT
    - Multiple APs
    - Mid-septal or right-sided pathway
    - WPW associated with Ebstein's anomaly
    - Male gender
  - Low-risk features (all suggest that the AP has a long refractory period):
    - Intermittent spontaneous loss of pre-excitation in sinus rhythm
    - Sudden loss of delta wave with increased HR (e.g., on stress testing or Holter monitoring)
    - Loss of pre-excitation with Class Ic drugs (i.e., procainamide, ajmaline)
    - SPERRI during AF >300 ms
    - No history of symptomatic arrhythmias (if >35 years old)

Key References for Further Reading

- Fox DJ, Klein GJ, Skanes AC, Gula LJ, Yee R, Krahn AD. How to identify the location of an accessory pathway by the 12-lead ECG. *Heart Rhythm.* 2008;5:1763–1766.
- Obeyesekere MN, Leong-Sit P, Massel D, Manlucu J, Modi S, Krahn AD, et al. Risk of arrhythmia and sudden death in patients with asymptomatic preexcitation: A meta-analysis. *Circulation.* 2012;125:2308–2315.
- Wellens HJ. When to perform catheter ablation in asymptomatic patients with a Wolff-Parkinson-White electrocardiogram. *Circulation.* 2005;112:2201–2216.

CHAPTER

6

Atrioventricular Reciprocating Tachycardia

ARRHYTHMIAS ASSOCIATED WITH ACCESSORY PATHWAYS (APs)

- AV reciprocating/reentrant tachycardia (85%)
  - See below.
- Supraventricular tachycardia with pre-excited QRS complexes
  - Atrial tachycardia, atrial flutter (AFL), or atrioventricular nodal reentrant tachycardia (AVNRT)
    - **Electrocardiogram (ECG)**: Regular, wide-complex tachycardia with QRS morphology similar to pre-excitation
  - Atrial fibrillation (5%–15%)
    - **ECG**: Irregular, wide-complex tachycardia with variable QRS morphology (QRS morphology varies beat-to-beat depending on the degree of fusion between AP and the AV node [AVN] conduction).

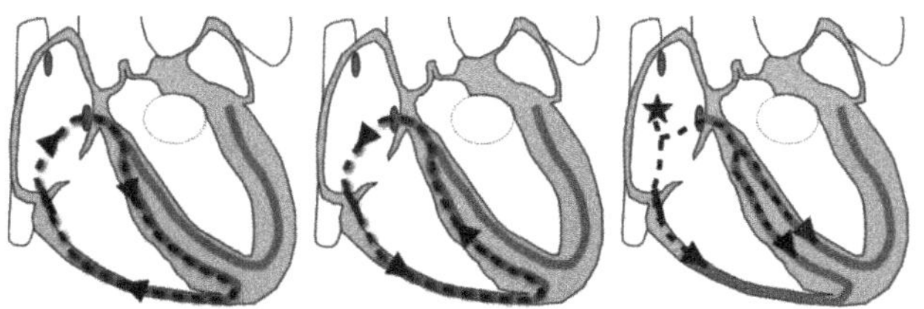

Orthodromic AVRT   Antidromic AVRT   Pre-excited atrial tachycardia

ATRIOVENTRICULAR RECIPROCATING TACHYCARDIA (AVRT)

General Information

- AVRT is a paroxysmal, regular, narrow-complex tachyarrhythmia due to a macroreentrant circuit involving the atria and ventricles, which are connected via an accessory pathway (AP).
  - During tachycardia, a **long RP** interval may be observed.
  - The baseline ECG may demonstrate evidence of pre-excitation.

Epidemiology and Clinical Features

- 30% of symptomatic paroxysmal supraventricular tachycardia (PSVT)
- Males predominate overall
  - Orthodromic AVRT: Relatively more common in men
  - Antidromic AVRT (rarer): Relatively more common in women
- Symptom onset typically in 20s (or younger)
- Palpitations, dizziness, syncope (10%)
- Rarely associated with structural heart disease

Table 6.1 Classification of AVRT

	Orthodromic (95%)	Antidromic (5%)	Pathway–Pathway
Anterograde conduction	AVN	AP	AP
Retrograde conduction	AP	AVN	AP

12-Lead ECG

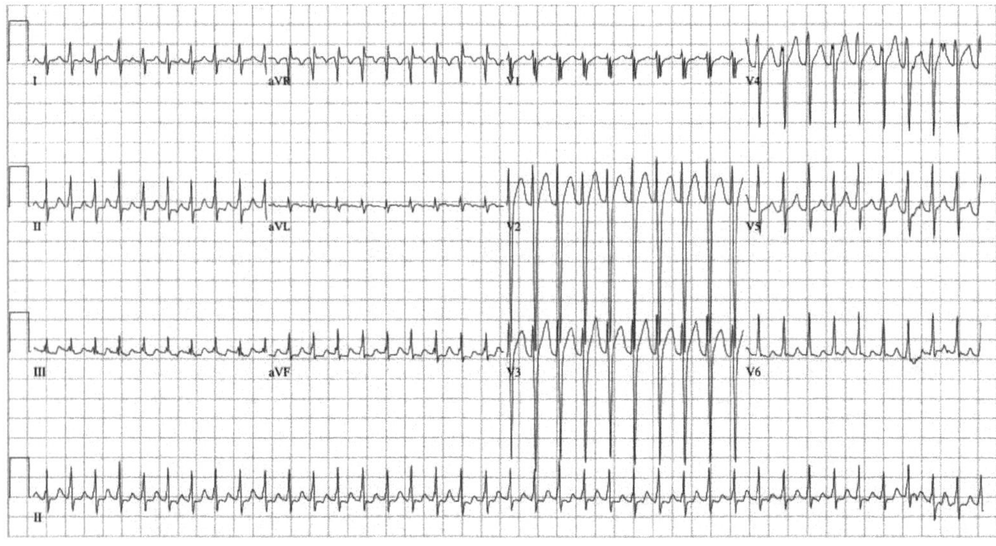

- Rate: Usually 140–250 bpm
- Rhythm: Is regular
- The P wave, PR interval, and QRS are variable.
  - They depend on the AP location, AVN conduction time, and direction of conduction.
  - Negative P wave in I and aVL (left-sided reentrant pathway with LA involvement)

Table 6.2 Differentiation of AVRT Mechanisms by QRS Width and RP Interval

	Orthodromic	Antidromic	Pathway-Pathway
QRS width	Narrow	Wide	Wide
RP interval	Long	Short	Long

- Onset/termination: Paroxysmal
  - Usually preceded by an ectopic beat (atrial or ventricular)
- Other
  - The baseline ECG may show pre-excitation (manifest APs).
  - A sudden decrease in the tachyarrhythmia rate coincident with the development of bundle branch block (BBB) suggests that the involved bundle branch and the AP are on the same side of the heart, and are both involved in the tachyarrhythmia circuit.

Other Investigations

- **24-hour Holter monitor**
  - Useful for diagnosis with episodes occurring more frequent than weekly
- **Event recorder**
  - Useful for diagnosis with symptomatic episodes occurring weekly to monthly
- **Echocardiogram**
  - Assessment of LV function and to exclude structural or congenital heart disease
- **Electrophysiology study (EPS)**: See below.

Management

Acute Management

- Narrow-complex tachycardia (orthodromic)
  - Vagal maneuvers, adenosine, non-dihydropyridine calcium-channel blocker (preferred)
  - B-blockers, digoxin, amiodarone (alternate)
  - DC cardioversion (especially if unstable)
- Wide complex
  - DC cardioversion (especially if unstable)
  - Ibutilide, flecainide or procainamide (preferred)
    - Slows conduction and/or causes block over the AP
  - AVN targeting agents
    - Effective for antidromic or orthodromic AVRT
    - Ineffective with pathway-pathway AVRT and pre-excited atrial tachyarrhythmias, as the AVN is not a component of circuit
    - Should be avoided in atrial fibrillation (AF) with pre-excited conduction
  - Adenosine should be avoided.
    - May precipitate AF with rapid ventricular response

Chronic Management

Table 6.3 Management of AVRT

	Poorly Tolerated AVRT	Well Tolerated AVRT	WPW with AF	Infrequent AVRT (No Pre-excitation)	Asymptomatic Pre-excitation
Surveillance	—	—	—	I	I
Vagal maneuvers	—	—	—	I	—
β-blocker	IIb	IIa	—	I (pill-in-the-pocket)	—
ND-CCB	III	III	—	I (pill-in-the-pocket)	—
Flecainide, propafenone	IIa	IIa	—	IIb	—
Sotalol, amiodarone	IIa	IIa	—	IIb	—
Ablation	I	I	I	IIa	IIa

I: Should be performed; IIa: May be considered; IIb: Reasonable alternative; III: Not indicated.
ND-CCB: Non-dihydropyridine calcium-channel blocker.

- Non-pharmacologic therapy
  - Vagal maneuvers
- Pharmacologic therapy
  - Chronic daily prophylaxis is used for patients with frequent symptoms.
    - Class Ic or III antiarrhythmic drugs (AADs) (preferred)
      - Alter the conduction through the AP and the AVN via class 1c (flecainide, propafenone) and class III (sotalol, amiodarone) AADs.
      - Alter the conduction through the AP alone (rarely used) via class Ia (quinidine, procainamide, disopyramide) AADs
      - Note: This may result in increased arrhythmia by increasing the antero-grade refractory period, thus increasing the tachycardia zone.
    - β-blocker, non-dihydropyridine (ND)-calcium-channel blocker (ND-CCB), digoxin
      - AVN agents; second-line due to their lack of direct effect on the AP
  - The "pill-in-the-pocket" strategy is used for patients with infrequent but prolonged episodes (symptomatic but stable episodes that occur less than monthly).
    - Propranolol 80 mg and/or diltiazem 120 mg > flecainide 3 mg/kg
- Invasive therapy
  - Catheter ablation is preferred in most cases.

ATRIOVENTRICULAR REENTRANT TACHYCARDIAS

Electrophysiology Study

Baseline Intervals

- Enhanced AVN conduction (Lown-Ganong-Levine: Atrionodal, atriohisian)
  - AH interval in sinus rhythm of ≤60 ms (normal: 80–120 ms in most subjects)
  - Shortened atrioventricular nodal refractory times
    - 1:1 conduction between atrium and His bundle are maintained during right atrial pacing at cycle lengths (CLs) below 300 ms.
  - Abnormal responses to decremental atrial pacing
    - AH prolongation ≤100 ms at the shortest 1:1 conduction when compared to the sinus rhythm value
- Manifest pre-excitation
  - Short HV interval (<35 ms)
  - Short local AV times: The earliest ventricular (V) EGM will be observed near the AP

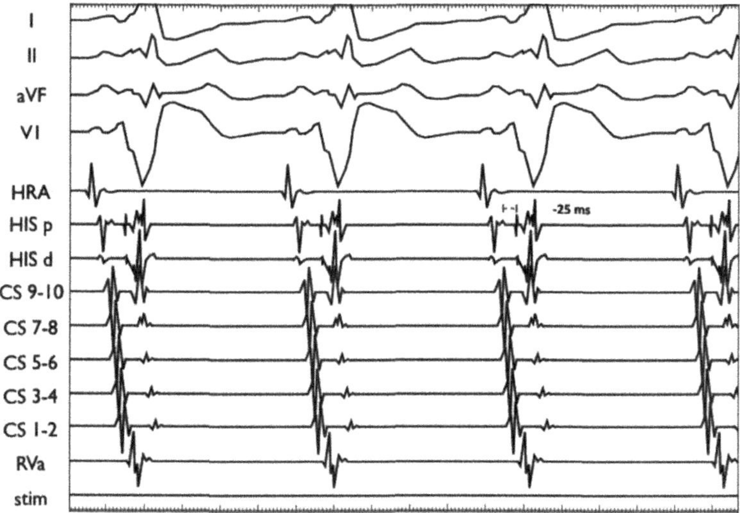

Manifest pre-excitation from a right lateral AP (HV –25 ms).

Anterograde Conduction

- Decremental atrial pacing (DAP)
  - For manifestat or latent APs, the degree of pre-excitation depends on the anterograde conduction properties of the AP and the relationship between the AP and the AVN conduction velocities.
    - Note: For concealed APs, the anterograde conduction will be via the AVN.
  - Decremental conduction through the AVN with DAP results in **AH interval prolongation** with a relative shift in ventricular activation to favor the AP, which is associated with:
    - Shortening in the **HV interval** (via AP)
    - Widening of the **QRS complex** (increased pre-excitation)

- Conduction through the AP is generally non-decremental (90%) and continues until the point of block in the AP (the AP ERP).
  - Note: If the AP ERP is longer than the AVN ERP, then pre-excitation disappears (long AH, normal HV and narrow QRS), and conduction continues to decrement through the AVN until the AVN ERP is reached.
  - Note: If the AP ERP is shorter than AVN ERP, the AV block occurs when AP ERP is reached.

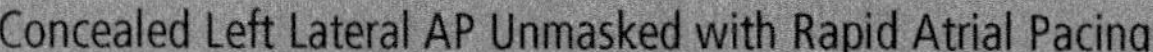

Concealed Left Lateral AP Unmasked with Rapid Atrial Pacing

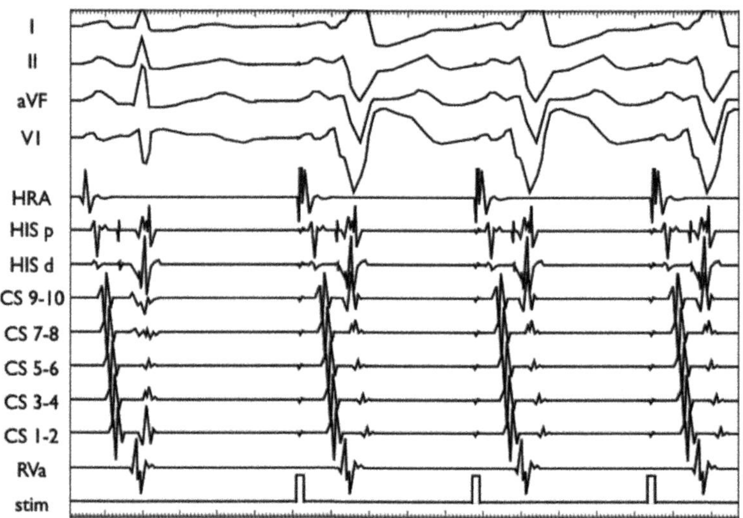

With increased atrial pacing rates, the impulse slows in the AVN (increasing AH interval), allowing increasing degrees of ventricular activation via the AP (HV shortening with manifest pre-excitation). Note the persistence of a short local AV time on the distal CS catheter, which is located near to the AP insertion.

- Anterograde conduction curve
  - Discontinuous as conduciton shifts from the AVN to AP (or vice versa)

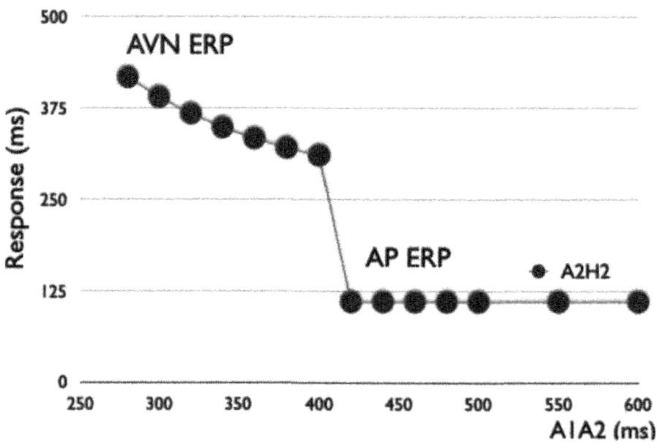

Retrograde Conduction

- Must be present to complete the AVRT circuit
  - If the pathway only conducts anterograde, the retrograde conduction will be via the AVN.
  - If the pathway conducts retrograde, then retrograde conduction may be:
    - Decremental via the AVN
    - Non-decremental via AP
- Atrial activation sequence
  - Generally **eccentric** with the earliest atrial activation at a site other than the AVN:
    - Left lateral AP (55%): Distal coronary sinus (CS) → proximal CS → His bundle EGM (HBE) → high right atrial (HRA)
    - Right free wall AP (10%): HRA → HBE → proximal CS → distal CS
    - Posteroseptal AP (35%): Proximal CS → HBE → distal CS → HRA
  - Can be concentric
    - **Anteroseptal AP** (5%): Atrial insertion site is near the normal AVN exit.
      - HBE → proximal CS → distal CS and HRA
      - Note: AP will not display decremental conduction properties.
    - **Distant AP** (e.g., left lateral AP with right ventricular apical pacing)
      - Normal atrial activation occurs via the AVN before the impulse is able to conduct via the AP.
      - Activation should shift from **concentric to eccentric** with decremental conduction in the AVN, ventricular pacing near the AP insertion site, or through the use of drugs that slow or block AVN conduction (e.g., adenosine, verapamil).
    - **Slowly conducting AP**:
      - The conduction velocity of the AP is slower than that of the AVN.
    - **Poorly conducting AP**:
      - The ERP of the AP occurs at a longer CL than the AVN ERP.
    - **Atriofascicular AP**:
      - Normal atrial activation via AVN (no retrograde AP conduction)

Tachycardia Induction

- Tachycardia can be induced with atrial or ventricular overdrive pacing or extrastimuli.
- Orthodromic AVRT
  - Anterograde induction
    - Increasingly rapid atrial pacing or extrastimuli results in AH prolongation (pre-excited QRS).
    - An AP block before an AVN block allows conduction exclusively down the AVN (narrow QRS).
    - If conduction is slow enough through the AVN (or with ipsilateral BBB) the AP can recover and conduct retrograde; this results in an "atrial echo" (completed loop).
    - If the AVN has recovered, then the echo may conduct anterograde; doing so facilitates the induction and perpetuation of tachycardia.

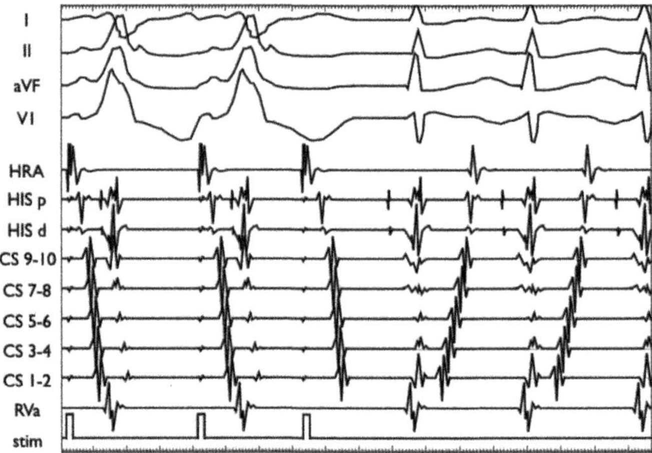

- Retrograde induction (orthodromic)
  - The same principles apply as above.
  - Increasingly rapid ventricular pacing or extrastimuli result in a retrograde AVN block with continued retrograde AP conduction.
  - If the AVN has recovered, then it may conduct the impulse anterograde.

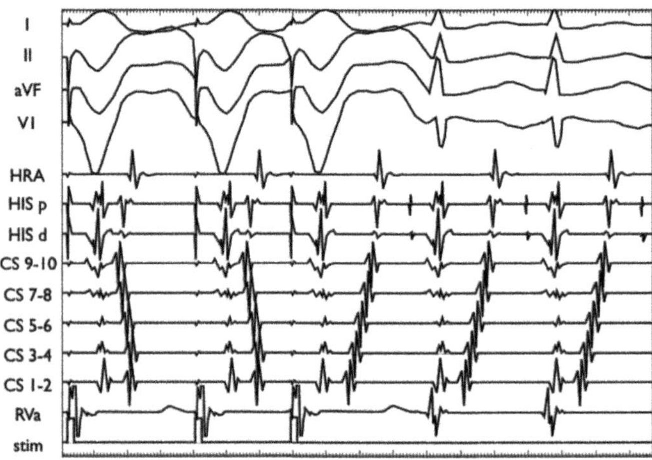

- Antidromic AVRT
  - The same principles apply as above (except reversed).
  - Anterograde induction
    - An AVN block allows conduction exclusively down the AP (wide pre-excited QRS).
    - If the conduction is slow enough, the AVN can recover and conduct retrograde.
    - If the AP has recovered, then the wave of depolarization may conduct anterograde down the AP.
  - Retrograde induction
    - A retrograde AP block allows conduction exclusively down the AVN.
    - If conduction is slow enough, the AP can recover and conduct anterograde.
    - If the AVN has recovered, then it may conduct the impulse retrograde to the atria.

- Concealed bypass tracts
  - The initiation of macroreentry may be more difficult.
  - Even through there is no manifest pre-excitation, the AP usually has some degree of **concealed conduction**. (anterograde penetration of an atrial impulse), rendering the AP refractory to retrograde conduction.
  - To initiate macroreentry, the impulse must occur early enough so that concealed conduction into the bypass tract is blocked.
    - It is facilitated by pacing near the bypass tract, which allows more time for the AP to recover.

Observations During Tachycardia

- VA relationship
  - Obligatory 1:1 relationship (unless nodo-fascicular or nodo-ventricular AP; may have V > A)
- Long VA time (e.g., >70 ms on His bundle catheter or >100 ms on HRA catheter)
  - Atria and ventricles are activated in series
- Atrial activation
  - Concentric or eccentric (see above under retrograde conduction)
- Spontaneous variations in TCL
  - Usually has a constant VA interval
  - CL wobble is usually due to the variation in AVN conduction.
- Spontaneous BBB alters the TCL and VA timing (prolonged by ≥25 ms)
  - Ipsilateral BBB forces conduction to pass via the contralateral bundle branch and then cross the interventricular septum before returning to the AP. This results in an increase in the TCL and VA time.

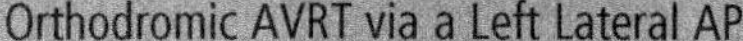
Orthodromic AVRT via a Left Lateral AP

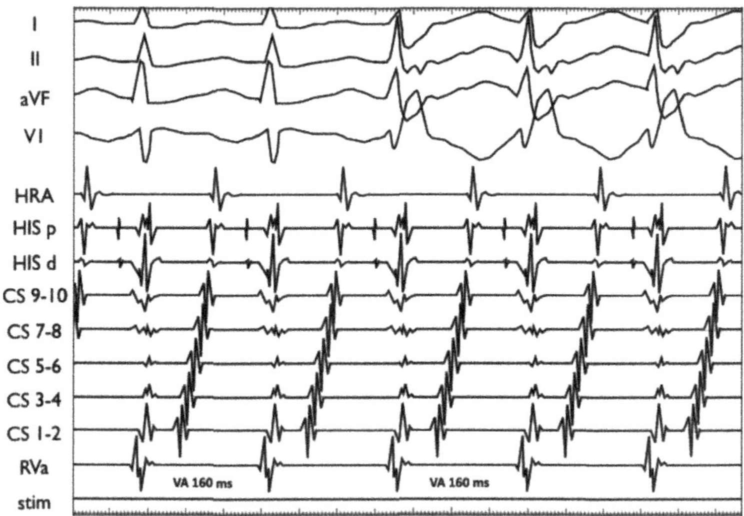

The development of right bundle branch block (RBBB) does not affect the VA timing nor CL, indicating that the right bundle was not part of the circuit.

Orthodromic AVRT via a Left Lateral AP

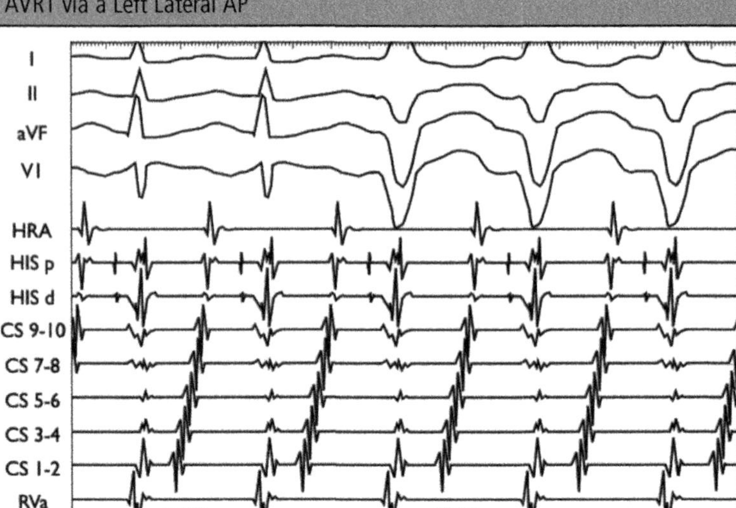

The development of left bundle branch block (LBBB) results in a prolongation of the Tachcyardia CL and VA timing (30 ms) and CL indicating that the left bundle is part of the tachycardia circuit.

Maneuvers During Tachycardia

- Premature ventricular impulses (His-synchronous ventricular premature beat)
  - Used to differentiate atypical AVNRT from AVRT via a septal AP.
  - The timing of the atrial activation (A EGM) or TCL after a premature ventricular impulse timed to junctional (His) refractoriness is examined.
    - For AVRT, the His synchronous VPB can advance the next atrial activation, delay the next atrial activation, terminate the tachycardia, or exert no effect.

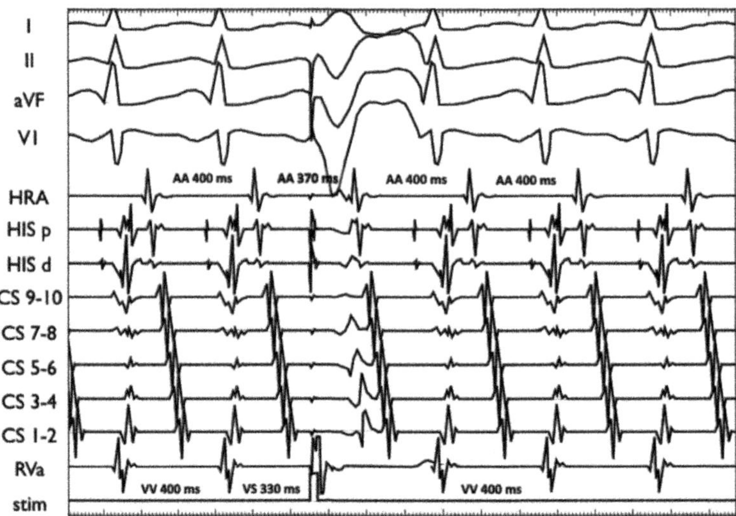

His-synchronous premature ventricular contraction (PVC; delivered 70 ms early) advances the next A and tachycardia cycle by 30 ms (due to decrement in the AP), thus confirming the existence of an AP (but not its involvement in tachycardia).

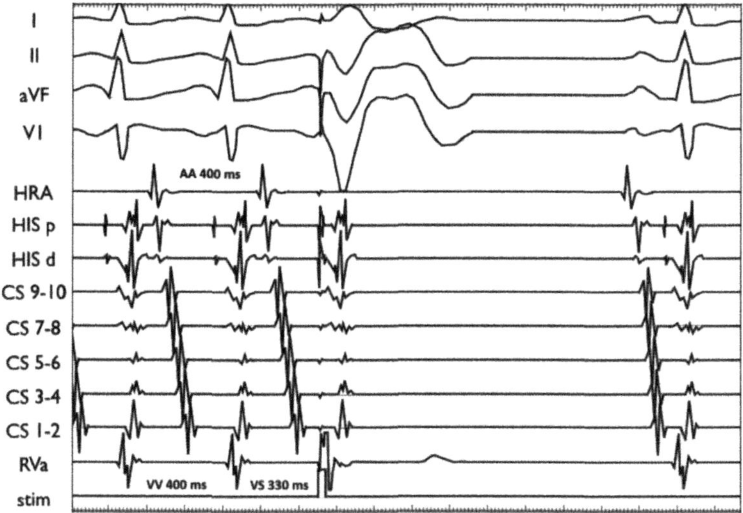

His-synchronous PVC (delivered 70 ms early) terminates the tachycardia without conducting to the atrium. This confirms both the presence of an AP as well as its involvement in the tachycardia (the ventricle is a critical part of the circuit).

- Entrainment via ventricular overdrive pacing
  - Used to distinguish AVRT using a paraseptal AP from AVNRT or AT
  - VA activation should be similar during pacing and tachycardia.
  - With termination of pacing:
    - A **VAV** (AHV) response is observed.
    - The return CL has baseline VA timing intervals (fixed coupling).
    - **PPI – TCL** for AVRT using a septal AP (Stim to V EGM) <115 ms.
    - Corrected post-pacing interval (cPPI) = (PPI – TCL) – (AH_{RVP} – AH_{SVT}) <110 ms
    - **Stim-A_{RVP} – VA_{SVT}** < 85 ms

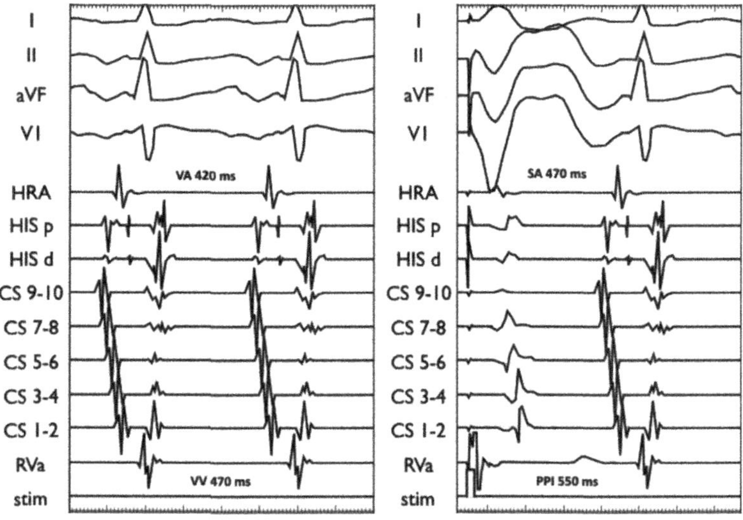

SVT entrainment via RV pacing at 440 ms (TCL 470 ms with a VA time of 420 ms: **left panel**). The Stim-A_{RVP} – VA_{SVT} interval is 50 ms, and the PPI – TCL is 80 ms consistent with an ORT using a right posteroseptal AP.

VAV (AHV) Nodal Response (AVNRT, AVRT)

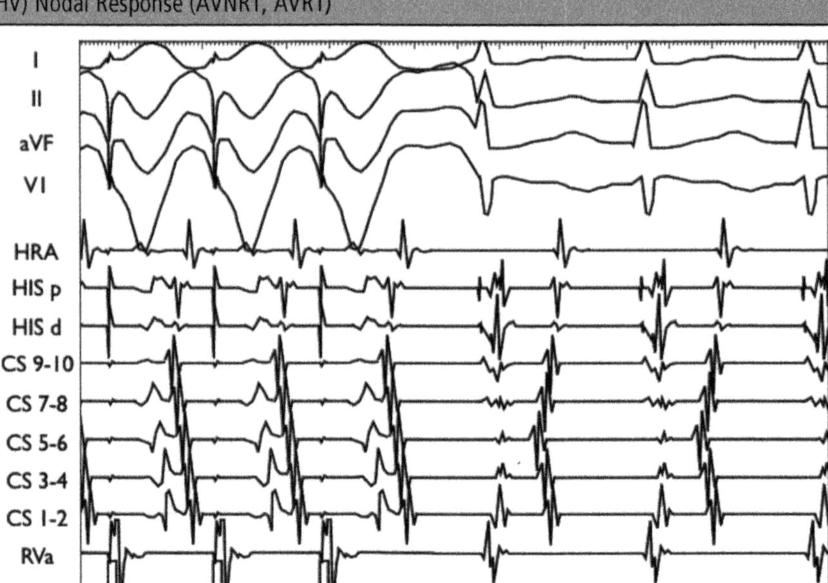

Ventricular entrainment during typical AVNRT results in 1:1 VA conduction. Post cessation of ventricular pacing, the EGM response is atrioventricular (AV).

- Entrainment via atrial overdrive pacing
  - Used to differentiate AVRT from AT.
  - With termination of pacing:
    - The VA of the first return beat should demonstrate a fixed VA timing (<10 ms of tachycardia VA) in AVNRT and orthodromic AVRT (effectively excludes atrial or junctional tachycardia).
    - Post-pacing sequence should be **AHA** in AVRT.
- Differential RV entrainment
  - Entrainment at the RVa and RV base is often used to differentiate AVRT using a paraseptal decremental AP from atypical AVNRT.
  - Interpretation:
    - A [PPI – TCL (base) – PPI – TCL (apex)] <30 ms supports AVRT
    - A [Stim-A_{RVP} – VA_{SVT} (apex) – Stim-A_{RVP} – VA_{SVT} (base)] >0 ms supports AVRT
- Parahisian entrainment
  - Entrainment with and without His capture is often used to differentiate AVRT using a paraseptal decremental AP from atypical AVNRT.
  - Delta SA (His loss – His capture) <40 ms: AVRT
  - Without His capture
    - PPI – TCL (Stim to local V EGM) <100 ms: AVRT
    - Stim-A_{RVP} – VA_{SVT} <75 ms: AVRT

Parahisian Entrainment in Tachycardia: ORT via Posteroseptal AP

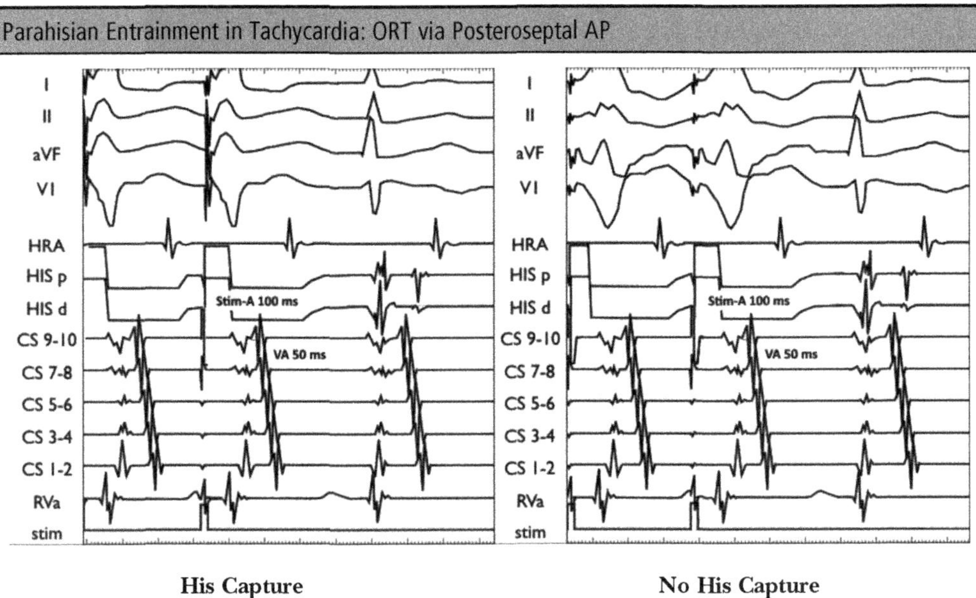

Narrow-complex tachycardia with a long VA time and earliest atrial activation in the proximal CS (CL 295 ms). Shown in the two panels are two separate entrainment maneuvers performed at 250 ms. In the **left panel**, there is His capture; on the **right panel**, there is loss of His capture. The delta Stim-A with loss of His capture was 0 ms, consistent with AVRT (posteroseptal AP).

Maneuvers in Sinus Rhythm

- Parahisian pacing
  - Useful to differentiate an anteroseptal pathway from an anterior AVN exit site.
  - Interpretation – **Extranodal response**:
    - Retrograde atrial activation sequence
      - Changes in the presence of both retrograde AP and retrograde AVN conduction
      - Does not change in the presence of exclusive retrograde AP conduction
    - The Stim-A interval usually decreases or does not change
      - Rarely, the Stim-A interval increases (<40 ms).
    - The His bundle-atrial interval usually decreases (but it may remain stable).

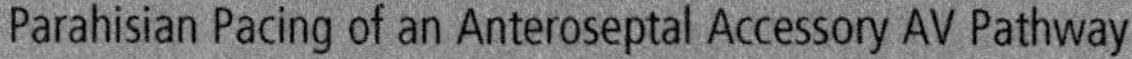

Parahisian Pacing of an Anteroseptal Accessory AV Pathway

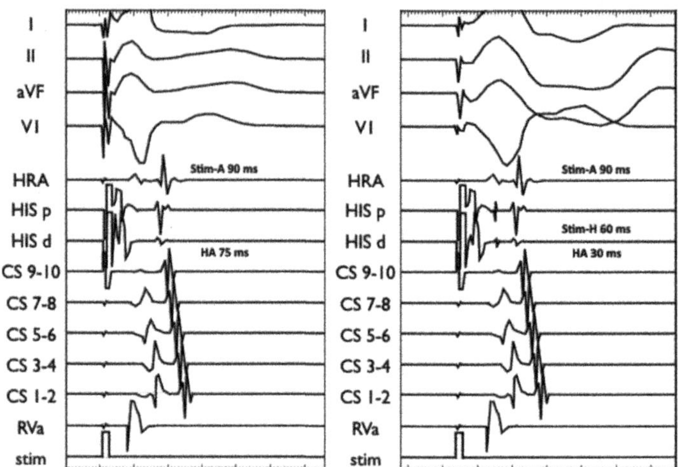

Left panel: Ventricular and HB-RB capture, producing a relatively narrow QRS complex and early activation of the His bundle (buried within the V EGM on the His catheter).
Right panel: Loss of HB-RB capture resulting in widening of the QRS complex, a 45 ms increase in the S-H interval (from 15 to 60 ms), but no change in the Stim-A interval (constant at 90 ms).

The stable **Stim-A** interval (90 ms) indicates that retrograde conduction was dependent on the timing of ventricular activation and not on the timing of the His bundle.

The earliest atrial activation occurs on the His suggesting retrograde conduction occurs over an anteroseptal accessory AV pathway.

- Differential Pacing from the RVa and RV Base/RVOT
  - Useful to differentiate a septal AP from an anterior or posterior AVN exit site
  - In the presence of a right-sided AP, the stimulus can reach the atrium directly (e.g., without traveling to the apex to invade the His-Purkinje system).
    - This results in no change in the Stim-A time from the RV base than the right ventricular apex (RVa).
    - Retrograde atrial activation sequence may change.
    - The septal HA interval increases slightly (<20–30 ms) or becomes negative.

Differential Pacing from the RVa and RV Base

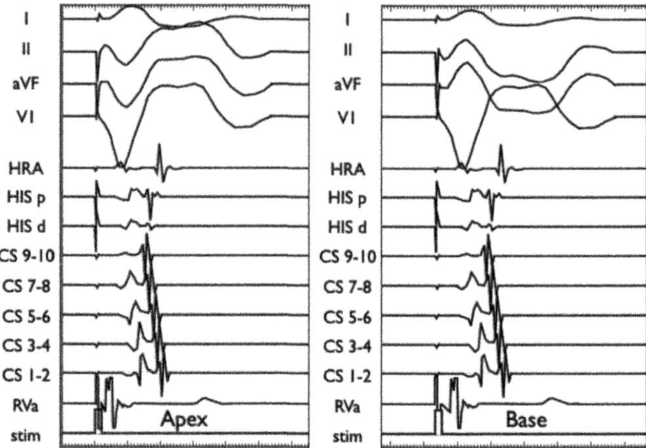

No change in VA time with basal pacing suggests posteroseptal AP.

- Differential atrial pacing
  - Right-sided pathways:
    - Pacing along TVA can identify the shortest stimulus–delta wave interval.
  - Left-sided pathways:
    - Pacing via distal CS will facilitate arrival of the impulse at the AP earlier than AVN; it pre-excites and leads to a shorter stimulus–delta wave interval.

Table 6.4 Concurrent and Countercurrent Pacing

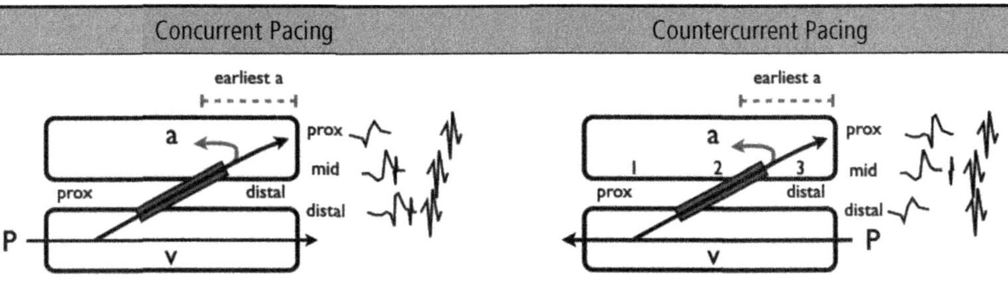

Concurrent Pacing	Countercurrent Pacing
Myocardial and AP activation occur in parallel • Produces overlapping A and V potentials ■ Artificially shortens the local AV/VA interval ■ Masks the AP potential and the site of early activation • Note: The shortest local interval is often recorded beyond the distal end of the AP. ■ That is, a site where ablation is unlikely to be successful.	Reversing the direction of the wavefront activates the local myocardium before activating the AP: • Separates the V and A activation from AP ■ Increases the local AV/VA interval exposing the AP potential and activation sequence

- Atrial pacing at TCL:
  - Interpretation: AH time in pacing is similar to tachycardia (<20 ms longer than tachycardia).

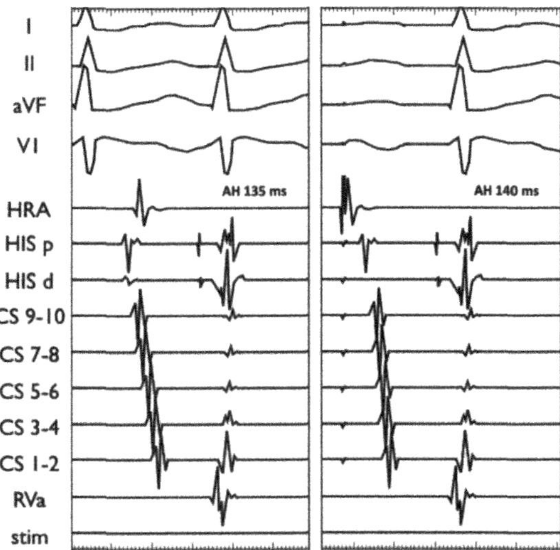

A comparison of AH intervals during orthodromic AV reentrant tachycardia (**left panel**) and high right atrial (HRA) pacing at the TCL (**right panel**). The AH interval is 95 ms during tachycardia (**left panel**) and during atrial pacing (**right panel**) leading to a ΔAH of 0 ms.

- Ventricular pacing at TCL:
  - Interpretation: VA time in pacing is similar to tachycardia (<85 ms longer than tachycardia).
- Induction of retrograde RBBB:
  - Increase in VA timing or TCL ≥ 20 ms
  - Increase in VH > Increase in VA

Conduction Over an AP with Induction of Retrograde RBBB

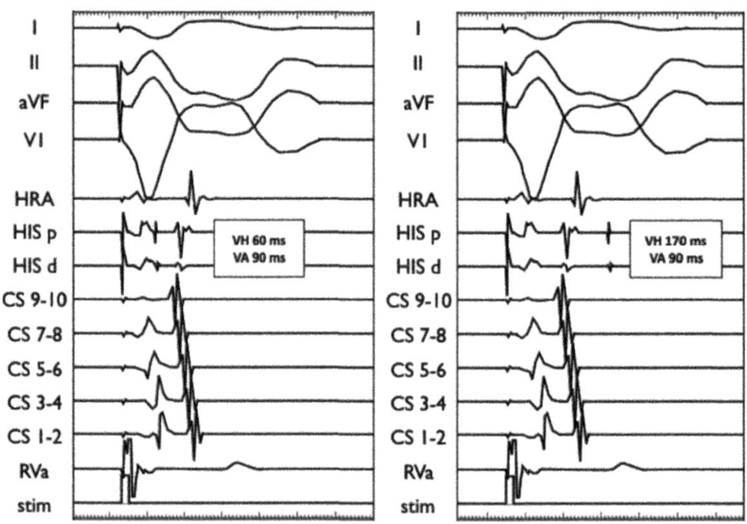

RV apical pacing at 600 ms with an S1-S2 coupling interval of 360 ms results in a retrograde His 60 ms after the QRS with a VA interval of 90 ms. When the coupling interval is decreased to 350 ms retrograde, RBBB is induced without altering VA timing (90 ms): His occurs after atrial activation (~170 ms after QRS onset). Thus, the delta VA is 0 ms with a delta VH of 110 ms.

SPECIAL CIRCUMSTANCES

Antidromic AVRT

Antidromic AVRT is more likely to occur with lateral or right free-wall APs, which allow more conduction time between the AVN and the AP, as well as the AP and His.

- Features
  - A 1:1 VA relationship is present.
  - QRS morphology is consistent with maximal pre-excitation.
  - Changes in VH interval precede changes in TCL.
  - The HA time in tachycardia is >70 ms.
  - Ventricular activation can be advanced by PACs near the atrial insertion and when the atrial septum is refractory.
  - VH time in tachycardia = VH time during pacing at ventricular insertion.

CATHETER ABLATION OF ATRIOVENTRICULAR RECIPROCATING TACHYCARDIA (AVRT)

Indications

- AVRT that is symptomatic, recurrent, or refractory to medical therapy
- Atrial fibrillation with rapid ventricular response

Anticipated Success

- >95%–98% acute success rate
  - Left lateral, 95% (more stable catheter position)
  - Right lateral, 90% (lower catheter stability)
  - Posteroseptal, 90%–95% (may lie deep in the septum or near the conduction system, or RCA)
  - Mid/anteroseptal, 95%
- ~5%–10% 1-year recurrence of conduction
  - Anteroseptal (15% recurrence)
  - Posteroseptal (10% recurrence)
  - Free wall (2%–3% recurrence)

Anticipated Complications

- 2%–4% overall
  - Coronary artery injury/dissection (RCA or LCX)
  - Aorta or aortic valve damage (transaortic approach)
  - Stroke or embolic MI (left-sided pathway)
  - Complete heart block occurs in 0.17%–1% (higher for septal/peri-nodal pathways)

Patient Preparation

- Stop all AADs for 3–5 half-lives before the procedure.
- Conscious sedation is preferred to GA due to the risk of rendering the arrhythmia non-inducible.

Set-Up

- The general set-up is similar to SVT.
- Ablation catheter ± guiding sheath:
  - **Left free wall**: B-curve (small/red) preferred to D-curve (medium/blue) (via transseptal or transaortic)
  - **Right free wall**: B-curve (small/red) to D-curve (medium/blue) curve with aid of a sheath (RAMP or deflectable)
  - **Left septal**: B-curve (small/red) preferred to D-curve (medium/blue) (trans-aortic preferred to transseptal)
  - **Right septal**: B-curve (small/red) to D-curve (medium/blue)

Mapping (Activation Mapping)

- Unipolar vs. bipolar recording
  - Unipolar recording:
    - May be more precise: Bipolar configuration has a larger recording area (decreases accuracy)
    - Can indicate insertion: Unipolar QS unipolar complex (endocardial); RS complex (epicardial)

- Bipolar recording:
  - More accurately indicates timing
  - Can better demonstrate pathway potentials
- AP electrograms
  - The local V and A EGMs should be balanced (1:1 A:V ratio), usually <40–60 ms apart.
    - The exception is a mid/anteroseptal AP, where V should dominate because of the risk of AV nodal damage resulting in complete heart block.
  - There may be continuous electrical activity without an isoelectric interval ± pathway potential.
- AP potentials
  - Low amplitude, high-frequency potentials are detected between the A and V EGM.
    - Represent direct recording of AP activation (analogous to His potentials)
    - Note: An isolated AP potential is usually only apparent with an oblique pathway.
      - In non-oblique pathways, the potential is fused with the atrial or ventricular potential.
  - Accessory pathway potentials can be differentiated from fractionated local potentials by the response to extrastimuli.
    - **Anterograde AP potential**: Verified by ventricular extrastimuli
      - **Late ventricular** extrastimulus **advances the local V** potential **without** advancing the **AP** potential (differentiating the AP potential from local ventricular activation).
      - **Earlier ventricular** extrastimulus **advances the AP** potential **without** advancing the local **atrial** potential (differentiating the AP potential from local atrial activation).
    - **Retrograde AP potential** is verified by atrial extrastimuli.
      - **Late atrial** extrastimulus **advances the local A** potential **without** advancing the **AP** potential (differentiating the AP potential from local atrial activation).
      - **Earlier atrial** extrastimulus **advances the AP** potential **without** advancing the local **ventricular** potential (differentiating the AP potential from local ventricular activation).
- Anterograde conduction time targets the ventricular insertion of manifest pathways only.
  - The earliest local ventricular activation relative to QRS onset is sought along the tricuspid valve annulus (TVA; right-sided pathways) or mitral valve annulus (MVA; left-sided pathways) during sinus rhythm or atrial overdrive pacing.
    - Right-sided AP: Rapid pacing from the high right atrial (HRA) of proximal coronary sinus (pCS)
    - Left-sided AP: Rapid pacing from the distal coronary sinus (dCS)
  - Activation timing is measured to the peak of the first major (sharp) deflection of the bipolar V EGM, or the onset of the monophasic unipolar QS complex.
  - It should have activation that is simultaneous or preceding the onset of the surface QRS.

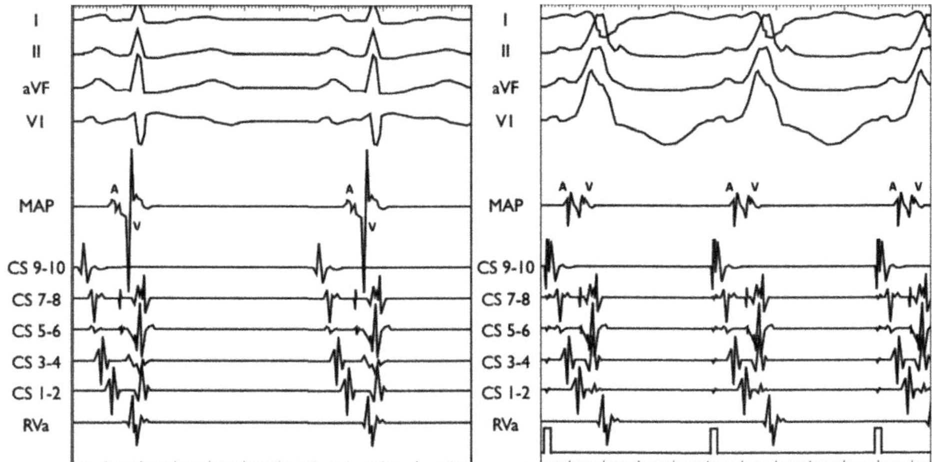

Anterograde mapping during sinus rhythm (**left panel**) and during atrial overdrive pacing (**right panel**). The map catheter is positioned along the lateral MVA. Continuous electrical activity with a large V EGM simultaneous to QRS onset (**left panel**) is observed, suggesting a slightly suboptimal (distal) ablation site. In the **right panel**, a fused, but more balanced A and V EGM is observed, with the local V EGM preceding the delta wave by 10 ms.

- Retrograde conduction timing targets the atrial insertion of retrogradely conducting manifest or concealed APs.
  - The earliest local atrial activation relative to QRS onset is sought along the tricuspid (right-sided pathways) or mitral (left-sided pathways) annulus during orthodromic tachycardia or ventricular pacing.
    - Note: The pacing must be at a rapid rate and ideally close to the presumed AP site in order to avoid retrograde mapping and ablation of the AVN.
  - The onset is measured in reference to QRS onset or pacing stimulus but should precede the retrograde P wave.
  - Note: Mapping during tachycardia is preferred for septal APs to avoid inadvertant AVN ablation.

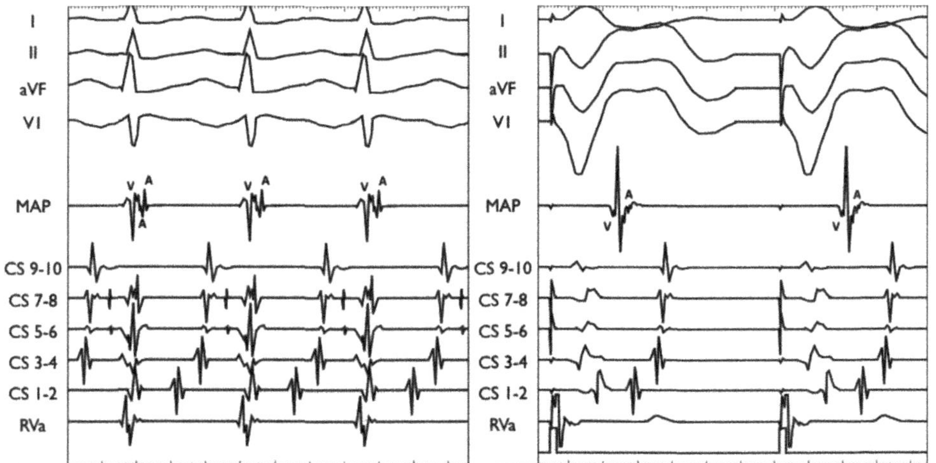

Retrograde mapping during AVRT (**left panel**) and during ventricular overdrive pacing (**right panel**). The mapping catheter is positioned along the lateral MVA. Continuous electrical activity with a relatively large V EGM followed by a small A EGM is demonstrated.

Ablation

- The ideal site of RF application is the location where an AP potential is recorded.
  - In the absence of an AP potential, ablation should be targeted at the site of earliest retrograde atrial activation or earliest anterograde ventricular activation
- Radiofrequency (RF) application:
  - Non-irrigated RF: 50 Watts for 30–60 seconds (target temperature 60–65°C)
    - Irrigated RF may be needed if deep-seated or epicardial pathways are present.
  - At most successful sites, the AP function is eliminated within 5 seconds after the RF current onset.
    - If the pathway function persists after 10–15 seconds of current, then terminate RF because of the risk of edema or clot.
- Note: General anesthesia with a paralytic agent allows 1- to 2-minute periods of apnea to help stabilize the catheter position during mapping and ablation.
  - This is especially useful for right free wall, anteroseptal, and mid-septal APs.

Determinants of Success

- Manifest anterograde conducting pathways:
  - Termination of pre-excitation, ideally within 6 seconds is considered successful.
- Concealed retrograde conducting pathways:
  - Loss of VA conduction in the AP
  - Altered atrial activation (from eccentric to concentric) with a significant increase in the VA block CL during ventricular pacing, ideally within 6 seconds, is considered successful.
- Observation and testing:
  - A minimum 30-minute waiting period should be observed after a successful ablation.
  - Adenosine testing (IV 12–18 mg) can be used to test for recurrent AP conduction.

Catheter Ablation of Specific Anatomic AP Locations

Left Free Wall APs

- Access
  - Transseptal puncture or transaortic approach
- Techniques
  - Attempt to manipulate the CS catheter into a position where it "brackets" the earliest activation.
  - Access via transseptal approach allows for the use of guiding sheaths, which facilitates catheter stability.
- Catheter and power
  - B-curve (small/red) or D-curve (medium/blue) catheter
  - Non-irrigated RF: 50 Watts for 30–60 seconds (target temperature 60–65°C)
  - Irrigated RF 25–35 Watts (target temperature 43°C)

- Troubleshooting
  - No early signals
    - Inability to access target site: Change the approach (transseptal or transaortic) or use a sheath.
    - Epicardial AP: Map within the CS or left atrial appendage (LAA), and perform epicardial ablation via a pericardial access.
    - Ligament of Marshall connection: Map the LA anterior to the left superior pulmonary vein (LPSV) along the ridge.
  - Recurrent AF
    - AVRT degeneration or recurrent PACs: IV flecainide (10 mg increments up to 50 mg), IV procainamide, or IV amiodarone
  - Unsuccessful energy delivery
    - Poor catheter stability: Change approach (transseptal or transaortic); use a sheath
    - Low power delivery: Use an irrigated RF or cryoablation.

Right Free Wall APs

- Access
  - Right femoral is the preferred initial approach.
  - If unsuccessful, try through the subclavian or internal jugular.
- Catheter and power
  - D-curve (mdedium/blue) or F-curve (large/orange) catheter (may require larger catheters to provide extra reach along the TVA)
  - Non-irrigated RF: 50 Watts for 30–60 seconds (target temperature 60–65°C)
  - Irrigated RF 25–35 Watts (target temperature 43°C)
- Troubleshooting
  - No early signals
    - Inability to access target site: Change the approach (inferior/superior), or use a long sheath (SR0-4), or deflectable sheath.
    - Difficulty identifying annulus: Use a multi-electrode catheter or wire within the right coronary artery (RCA).
    - Epicardial AP: Map within the RAA, and consider an epicardial ablation
  - Poor catheter stability
    - Change the approach (inferior/superior).
    - Use a long sheath (SR0-4), deflectable sheath, or cryoablation.
  - Low power delivery
    - Use an irrigated RF or cryoablation.
  - Mechanical block due to a superficial AP location
    - Wait for the recurrent AP conduction without moving the catheter, and visualize with 3D mapping.

Mid-/Anteroseptal APs

- Access
  - Right femoral is the preferred initial approach.
  - If that is unsuccessful, try the subclavian or internal jugular.
- Techniques
  - Risk of an AV block is high for APs at the site recording a sharp His potential (**right anteroseptal AP**), posterior to the His and anterior to the CS (**right midseptal AP**), as well as with **left anteroseptal APs** (even with a retrograde transaortic approach and apnea).
  - Strategies to reduce the risk of compact AVN damage:
    - Ideal site
      - Position the catheter in a relatively ventricular position (large V EGM) compared to other AP ablation sites
      - Unipolar tip EGM: Sharp AP potential with little or no atrial potential
      - Note: A small (<0.15 mV) His may be seen at successful sites.
    - Approach the AP from the ventricular side of the tricuspid valve annulus (TVA) as placement of the ablation catheter under the TV leaflet provides a stable catheter position during ablation of anteroseptal and mid-septal AP (low risk of AV block).
      - Underneath the anterior leaflet (right subclavian venous approach)
      - Underneath the septal leaflet (femoral venous approach)
    - Perform ablation in sinus rhythm (improved catheter stability)
    - Cryoablation: Ability to perform cryomapping (to reduce AVN damage) and improved catheter stability
  - Note: Mid-/anteroseptal APs tend to be superficial leading to mechanical AP block in up to 40% of cases.
- Catheter and power
  - Non-irrigated RF: Start at 10 Watts and increase to 20 Watts after 10s (target temperature 60–65°C)
    - If AP block occurs, continue ablation for 45 seconds.
    - If junctional beats occur, stop the ablation and reposition the catheter in a more ventricular position.
    - If progressive pre-excitation occurs, stop the ablation (AVN ablation is occurring).
    - If no response is shown at 20 Watts after 10 seconds, stop the ablation and reposition the catheter.
  - Post ablation, move the catheter away from the septum to avoid a mechanical AP block.
- Troubleshooting
  - Large His at site of earliest signal
    - **Parahisian AP:** Use incremental RF power or cryoablation.
  - RBBB during RF
    - **Lesion is too distal:** Stop the RF and reposition the catheter.
  - Mechanical AP block
    - **Superficial AP:** Wait for a recurrent AP conduction without moving the catheter; 3D mapping.

Left Mid-Septal APs

- Hallmarks
  - It is the "earliest" retrograde atrial activation recorded nearly simultaneously in His and proximal CS.
    - Activation originates at a site equally distant from the HB and proximal CS.
- Access
  - Transseptal puncture or transaortic approach
- Technique
  - A far-field AP preceding atrial activation may be detected when the mapping catheter is directed vertically into the roof of the CS ostium.
  - Ablation with vertical pressure in the roof of the CS ostium (close to the atrial side of the mid-septal mitral annulus) usually fails to eliminate AP conduction and is associated with an AV block.
- Management
  - Ablation along the mitral annulus (posterior to the His and anterior to the CS) at the site that recorded a large, sharp AP potential eliminates AP conduction without an AV block.

Posteroseptal APs

- Access: Right atrial ablation is the preferred initial approach.
  - Before performing a transseptal puncture, it may useful to extensively map in the CS (and venous branches), because the AP sometimes can be accessed from the right venous structures.

Table 6.5 Characteristics Favoring a Right- or Left-Sided Approach for Posteroseptal AP Ablation

Right-Sided Ablation Preferred	Left-Sided Ablation Preferred
• Negative delta wave in V1 with R > S transition in V2 or V3 • Earliest atrial activation during ORT at proximal CS • Difference between His and shortest CS VA interval <25 ms (short distance between right AP insertion and His)	• R > S in V1 • Earliest atrial activation during ORT at mid-CS • Difference between His and shortest CS VA interval >25 ms (greater distance between left insertion and RA signal)

- Catheter and power
  - D-curve (medium/blue) catheter
  - Non-irrigated RF: 30–50 Watts for 30–60 seconds (target temperature 60–65°C)
  - Irrigated RF: 25–35 Watts (target temperature 43°C) is required in 25% of cases due to a deep location.

- Troubleshooting
  - No early signals:
    - Incomplete mapping or epicardial AP: Map proximal CS, branches, and left atrium.
    - Slow and/or decremental anterograde conduction: Map the AP potentials, shortest AV interval in atrial pacing, or unipolar site of EGM reversal (QS to RS).
  - Low-power delivery:
    - Low blood flow or ablating within the CS: Use irrigated an RF or cryoablation.
  - Epicardial connection near the RCA or LCX artery (AP in the proximal CS)
    - Use cryoablation.

Right Atriofascicular APs

- Right atriofascicular APs are a duplication of the normal AV conduction system.
  - An accessory AVN/His (located along the anterolateral to posterolateral TVA at approximately 8 to 9 o'clock) connects to an isolated bundle of Purkinje fibers that extend to the apical RV free wall (near the moderator band).
- ECG
  - Baseline
    - Pre-excitation may not be evident (slow, decremental, anterograde conduction).
    - A subtle, LBBB-like appearance may manifest (no septal Q in I, aVL, V5 and V6).
  - Antidromic AVRT (CL of 220–450 ms)
    - LBBB-type QRS complex (~RV insertion): R wave in lead I, rS wave in V1
    - Tachycardia QRS duration is usually <150 ms
    - Axis of 0 to −75°
    - QRS transition >V4
- EPS properties
  - Findings at baseline:
    - AP has a long conduction time (no baseline pre-excitation during sinus rhythm).
    - Atrial pacing produces pre-excitation with a relatively long AV interval.
      - Right atrial pacing produces more pre-excitation than left atrial pacing.
    - An AP ("M") potential may be found around the TVA.
    - Decremental anterograde conduction is proximal to the AP potential (fixed AP-to-V interval).
    - Ventricular activation is **earlier at RVa than RV base** (TVA or His catheter) when maximally pre-excited due to the relatively apical AP insertion (into or near the fascicles).
    - No retrograde AP conduction is present.

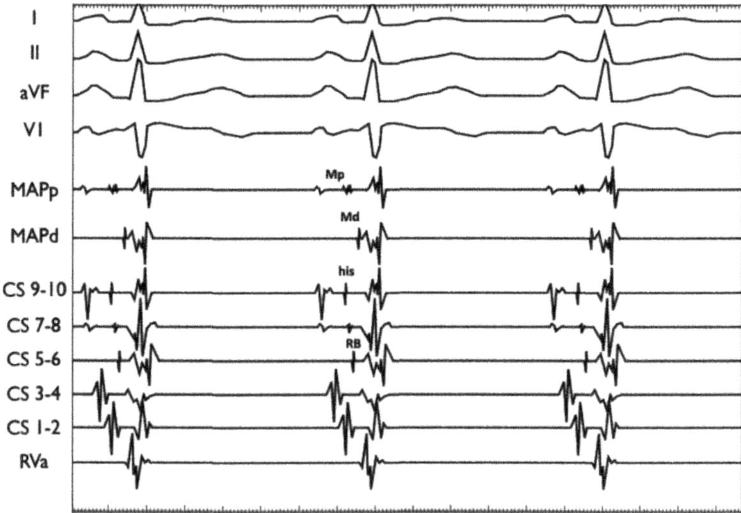

Mapping during sinus rhythm. Ventricular activation is predominantly via the AVN (AH is shorter than the A-Mahaim potential interval; and His bundle depolarization precedes the right bundle [RB] activation).

- Findings during tachycardia:
  - Antidromic AVRT with anterograde conduction via AP and retrograde conduction via:
    - The AVN (antidromic AVRT; 90% to 95% of patients)
    - A concealed AP for retrograde conduction (5% to 10%)
  - QRS complex:
    - LBBB-pattern with a QRS duration <145 ms
    - Rapid QRS onset in I and/or V1 is due to utilization of the right bundle.
  - The anterograde ventricular activation is earlier at the RVa than the RV base.
  - There is an early retrograde activation of the right bundle.
    - This activation results in recording the retrograde right bundle potential and then the His bundle potential within 30 ms of the QRS onset.
  - The tachycardia VH interval is <50 ms (frequently <20 ms).
    - V onset is at the fascicular AP insertion; subsequently, a retrograde His activation occurs rapidly via the normal conduction system.
  - There is an increase in the VA and VH intervals, and TCL with RBBB without a change in pre-excitation.
    - This reflects the participation of the RBB in the retrograde limb of the tachycardia.
  - The HA in tachycardia = HA in RV pacing (VA conduction via the AVN).
    - If the tachycardia is AVNRT with a bystander AP, supraventricular tachycardia (SVT) HA < HA with RV pacing.
  - VH in tachycardia < VH with RV pacing
    - This is because insertion of the AP directly into the fascicle results in a rapid retrograde His activation.
    - Compared to RV pacing of retrograde His activation from a site distant to the fascicle, there is a longer interval.
  - His-synchronous PACs (delivered when the septum is refractory) advance the V and subsequent A.

Antidromic AVRT Over a Right Atriofascicular AP

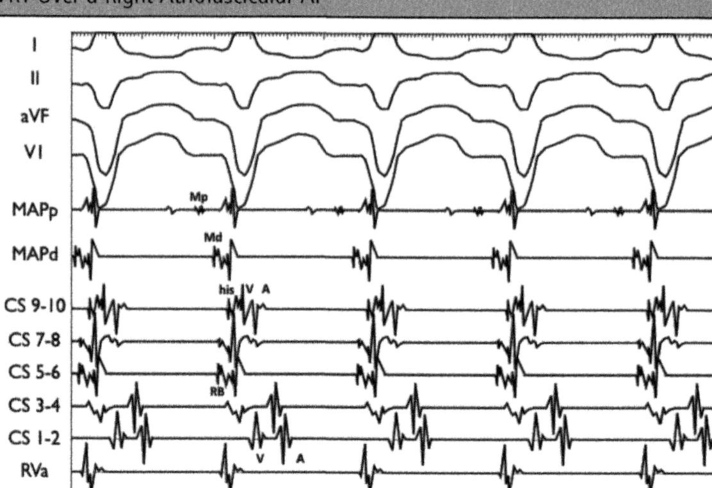

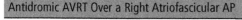

The activation proceeds from proximal to distal "M" potential, followed by retrograde activation from right bundle to His to AVN.

- Management
  - Mapping
    - Look for the discrete AP ("Mahaim" or "M") potential at 8–9 o'clock on TVA
    - Pace the atrium near the atrial insertion of the AP at a relatively rapid rate (maximal pre-excitation), and look for earliest delta wave (the stimulus-delta wave interval).
  - Ablation
    - The optimal ablation site is along the TVA at the AP "M" potential
    - Non-irrigated RF: 50 Watts for 30–60 seconds (target temperature 60–65°C)
    - Irrigated: 25-30 Watts for 30–60 seconds (target temperature 43°C)
    - During ablation a non-sustained pre-excited rhythm may be observed.
  - Advanced techniques
    - If the catheter cannot be stabilized at the TVA, ablation can be performed along the basal or mid RV free wall, where a high-frequency right atriofascicular (RAF) potential (similar to the RBB potential) is recorded.
    - Note: Locations close to the apex should be avoided to prevent ablation of the distal RBB (proximal to the RAF) because this increases antidromic AVRT CL, occasionally producing incessant tachycardia.

Fasciculoventricular APs

- Fasciculoventricular APs arise from the His bundle and insert into the RV myocardium.
- ECG
  - Atrial extrasystoles and atrial fibrillation do not alter the degree of pre-excitation.
  - Junctional ectopy is pre-excited despite no atrial activation.

- EPS
  - Incremental atrial pacing results in:
    - Prolongation of the AH interval without changes in the HV interval
    - A constant degree of pre-excitation
  - Junctional extrasystoles demonstrate the same degree of pre-excitation and short HV interval.
  - No retrograde AP conduction
  - His bundle pacing produces an identical QRS as observed during sinus rhythm.
  - The adenosine challenge induces an AV block without eliciting a greater degree of pre-excitation.
  - Ajmaline or procainamide challenge results in loss of pre-excitation.

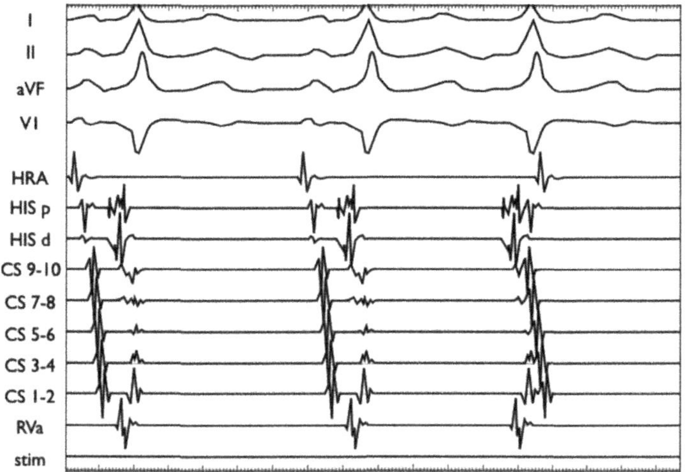

Pre-excited junctional premature arterial contraction (PAC).

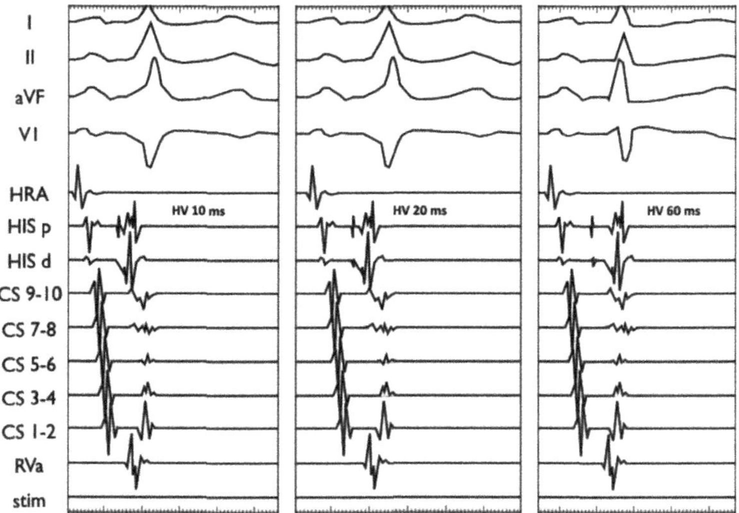

HV prolongation and loss of pre-excitation during Ajmaline infusion: 0 mg (**left panel**); 40 mg (**middle panel**); 60 mg (**right panel**).

- Ablation
  - Not necessary as fasciculoventricular pathways do not participate in tachycardia.

Nodoventricular or Nodofascicular Connections

- Nodoventricular or nodofasicular connections are APs arising from the AVN and inserting into the RV myocardium or right bundle.
- They may result in narrow or broad complex SVT.
  - Antidromic tachycardia: VH interval
    - <50 ms for nodofascicular APs
    - 50–80 ms for nodoventricular APs
  - AV dissociation may occur as the upper turn around is located within the AVN itself.
    - VA block can occur during tachycardia as the atrial myocardium is not part of the circuit.
  - His-synchronous PACs (delivered when the septum is refractory) do not advance.
  - His-synchronous PVCs advance the subsequent His/V or terminates SVT.
  - BBB ipsilateral to AP prolongs the VA interval or TCL.
  - May have a discrete pathway potential in sinus rhythm.

Unusual and Unexpected AP Locations

Coronary Sinus (CS) "Epicardial" AP

- The most common form of epicardial posteroseptal AP results from a connection between the LV epicardium and an extension of the CS myocardial coat.
  - In most cases it extends to the great cardiac vein, thus providing electrical continuity.
  - In <5%, muscular sleeves may cover the terminal part of the middle and posterior cardiac veins.
  - A CS diverticula with associated AP can be found in 20%.
- ECG
  - Steep negative delta wave in lead II: Specificity 80%
  - Steep positive delta wave in aVR: Specificity 98%
  - Deep S wave in V6 ($R \le S$): Specificity 90%
- Mapping
  - Anterograde conduction
    - The earliest endocardial ventricular activation is recorded 25 ms after far-field EGM onset.
      - Nearly simultaneously on the right and left sides of the interventricular septum
      - Approximately 1 to 3 cm apical to the tricuspid and mitral annuli
    - The earliest "epicardial" ventricular activation is recorded 15 ms after the onset of far-field activation from the middle cardiac vein (or other coronary vein or CS diverticulum).
      - Anterograde conduction is preceded by distinct potential from anterograde activation of CS myocardial extension.

- Retrograde conduction characteristically has three distinct potentials that can be recorded from the coronary venous system:
  - **First potential**: Recorded in the coronary vein and generated by retrograde activation of the CS myocardial extension
  - **Second potential**: Recorded along the floor of the proximal CS and generated by leftward activation of the CS musculature
    - Because of fiber orientation, the CS myocardium activates the LA at a location 2–4 cm left of the orifice of the middle cardiac vein.
    - This results in a rapid LA activation in the leftward direction.
    - The left atrial activation in the rightward (septal) direction is delayed as a result of slowing of conduction during the reversal in direction of activation.
  - **Third potential**: Recorded near the orifice of middle cardiac vein and generated by the late LA activation near the orifice of middle cardiac vein
- Ablation
  - The optimal ablation site is within the coronary vein at the site recording the largest, sharpest unipolar potential generated by the CS myocardial extension.
    - Due to extensive connections between the CS myocardium and left atrium
    - Begin at 10–15 Watts and increase power as required up 25–30 Watts.
      - Use an irrigated catheter if poor blood flow limits power.
    - Note: Terminate the RF application as quickly as possible when the impedance rise occurs (3–5 above the lowest value) to prevent adherence of the electrode to the vein.
  - When the optimal ablation site in the vein is located within 4–5 mm of a significant coronary artery, cryoablation is recommended because the risk of coronary artery stenosis is low.
    - A large number of cryoapplications may be required.
    - A frequent, transient AP conduction block lasting up to 60 minutes may be observed.

Epicardial Anteroseptal APs

- Hallmarks
  - Endocardial recordings exhibit far-field early anterograde ventricular and retrograde atrial activation.
  - Unipolar recordings along the TVA show local activation (rapid downstroke) beginning ≥20 ms after the onset of the far-field potential ± tiny far-field AP potential.
- Technique
  - Mapping within the non-coronary cusp demonstrates a sharp unipolar AP potential.
    - Located just opposite the anteroseptal and anterior paraseptal TVA
    - Ablation at this location generally eliminates AP conduction.
  - Note: The risk of AV block for ablation in the non-coronary cusp appears low.

Right and Left Atrial Appendage Connection

- Occurs in <0.5%
- AP conduction can be produced by a band-like muscular epicardial connection between the right (RAA) or left atrial appendage (LAA) and the underlying ventricle (approximately 1 cm apical to the TVA or MVA).
- ECG
  - Pre-excitation similar to anterior or anterolateral APs
- Mapping
  - Relatively long tachycardia VA timing (longer epicardial course)
  - **Earliest retrograde atrial activation**
    - Mapping along the annulus records the local activation (rapid downstroke of the unfiltered unipolar EGM) 30–40 ms after the onset of the far-field potential.
    - Continued mapping along the atrial wall, close to the orifice of the appendage, is earlier but still long after the onset of far-field activation.
  - **Earliest anterograde ventricular activation**
    - Recorded earlier at sites 1–3 cm apical of the annulus but also long after the onset of far-field activation.
  - **Mapping inside the atrial appendage**
    - Locates earliest endocardial activation, which is usually <10 ms from onset of far-field retrograde atrial/anterograde ventricular activation
  - Note: AP potential is not recorded because these pathways result from a direct connection between the atrial appendage and the ventricular myocardium.
  - 3D mapping may be beneficial for localization.
- Ablation
  - Ablation is within the RAA (irrigated catheter; limit power to 15–25 W).
    - High-energy delivery may be needed in the appendage for success.
    - Segmental isolation of the appendage surrounding the ventricular attachment may be required.
  - A percutaneous epicardial approach may prove useful for catheter ablation of these connections.

Multiple APs

- Definition: Multiple (usually 2) APs are separated by at least 1–3 cm along the annulus.
- Incidence: 3%–15% (possibly higher with right free wall or posterior AP)
  - More often seen with Ebstein's anomaly or a history of antidromic AVRT
- Mapping
  - >1 pattern of ventricular pre-excitation during atrial pacing or AF
  - >1 pattern of atrial activation during RV pacing or AVRT
  - Pathway-to-pathway tachycardia
    - Especially if BBB during tachycardia does not affect the TCL
  - Mismatch (>1 cm) between anterograde and retrograde limbs of the tachycardia circuit
  - A switch from orthodromic to antidromic AVRT (and vice versa)

- Ablation
  - Recognition of >1 AP is essential to avoid primary ablation failure.
  - A completed RF application at target sites should be undertaken before remapping.
  - Close observation of the surface ECG for changes in the pre-excitation pattern during RF application is essential to avoid multiple, incomplete RF applications.
  - Multipolar mapping catheters (CS or Halo catheters for left- and right-sided APs, respectively) are useful to identify subtle changes in the intracardiac activation sequence.
- Success
  - Acute success rate: 86%–98%
  - Recurrence rate: 8%–12%

Permanent Junctional Reciprocating Tachycardia (Atypical Chronic Orthodromic Tachycardia)

- Slowly conducting, concealed, right posterosepal AP results in incessant SVT.
  - Anterograde conduction down the AVN and the bundle of His
  - Atria are activated retrograde by the slowly conducting AP usually from the right posterior septum.
- Clinical features
  - Classically seen in children and adolescents
  - If not corrected, it may lead to a dilated cardiomyopathy.
- ECG diagnosis
  - Incessant SVT
  - Tachycardia initiates with a sinus beat.
  - Normal QRS width (no pre-excitation at baseline)
  - Negative P waves in inferior leads and V3–V6
  - Long RP interval

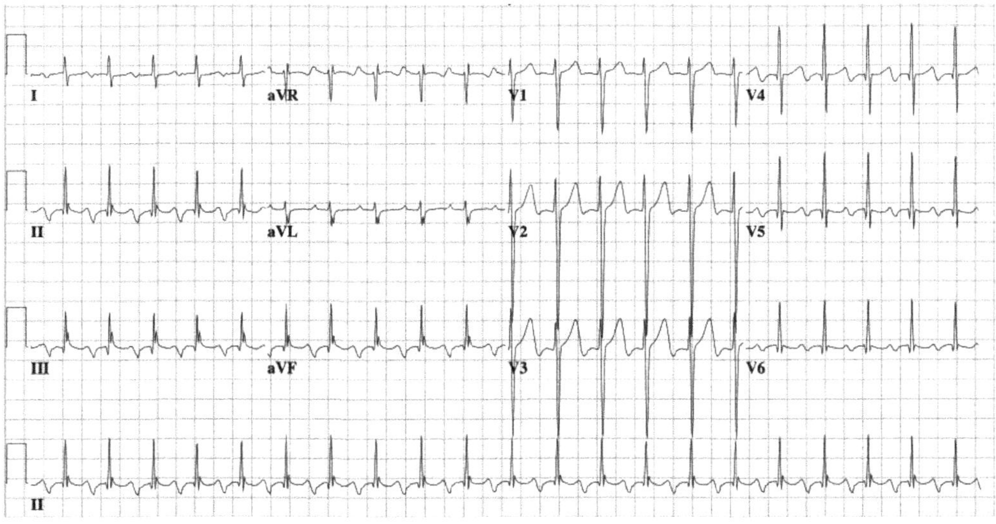

- Mapping
  - Decremental, retrograde only conducting right posteroseptal AP
  - Atrial insertion is usually near the CS os.
  - Initiation with a VPB during sinus rhythm when the His is refractory
  - During entrainment, the VA interval prolongs due to the decremental properties of the AP.
  - During tachycardia, the A may be advanced with a His-synchronous VPB.
    - Decremental AP properties may mean result in A delay.
  - During tachycardia, the VA interval increases with ipsilateral BBB.
- Ablation
  - Target the site of earliest atrial activation (with reference to P wave onset or CS activation).
- Prognosis
  - Cardiomyopathy typically resolves within 6 months of AP ablation.

Key References for Further Reading

- Delacrétaz E. Supraventricular tachycardia. *N Engl J Med.* 2006;354:1039–1051.
- Gonzalez-Torrecilla E, Almendral J, Arenal A, Atienza F, Atea LF, del Castillo S, et al. Combined evaluation of bedside clinical variables and the electrocardiogram for the differential diagnosis of paroxysmal atrioventricular reciprocating tachycardias in patients without pre-excitation. *J Am Coll Cardiol.* 2009;53:2353–2358.
- Veenhuyzen GD, Quinn FR, Wilton SB, Clegg R, Mitchell LB. Diagnostic pacing maneuvers for supraventricular tachycardia: Part 1. *PACE.* 2011;34:767–782.
- Knight BP, Ebinger M, Oral H, Kim MH, Sticherling C, Pelosi F, et al. Diagnostic value of tachycardia features and pacing maneuvers during paroxysmal supraventricular tachycardia. *J Am Coll Cardiol.* 2000;36:574–582.
- Nakagawa H, Jackman WM. Catheter ablation of paroxysmal supraventricular tachycardia. *Circulation.* 2007;116:2465-2478.

CHAPTER

7

Focal Atrial Tachyarrhythmia

UNDERSTANDING AND MANAGING FOCAL ATRIAL TACHYCARDIA

Epidemiology and Clinical Features

Focal atrial tachyarrhythmia (FAT) is observed in 0.3-0.4% of the asymptomatic population and 0.4-0.5% of the symptomatic population. It can present as:

- Paroxysmal tachycardia
- Persistent tachycardia with palpitations, chest pain, fatigue, dyspnea, or effort intolerance
  - If rapid rates persist, then heart failure may result (tachycardia-induced cardiomyopathy).
- Syncope is rare, but it can occur with rapid tachycardia and 1:1 conduction.
- "Silent" atrial tachycardia is detected in asymptomatic patients on electrocardiogram (ECG), Holter, or implantable devices.

Anatomy and Pathophysiology (Mechanism)

- Basic mechanism is an impulse originating from a right (80%; crista terminalis; superior vena cava [SVC]; inferior vena cava [IVC]) or left (20%; pulmonary vein, atrial septum, mitral annulus) atrial focus.
- Sub-classified based on mechanism
  - **Abnormal automaticity** (i.e., automatic ectopic atrial tachycardia [AEAT])
  - **Triggered activity** (i.e., non-automatic focal atrial tachycardia [NAFAT])
  - **Localized (micro) reentry**

Etiology

- Pulmonary disease: Chronic obstructive pulmonary disease (COPD), pulmonary hypertension, or chronic hypoxia
- Hyper-adrenergic states: Myocardial ischemia or infarction
- Metabolic or electrolyte: Hypokalemia/hypomagnesemia
- Drugs: Digoxin, theophylline
- Cardiothoracic surgery (especially for congenital heart disease)

The Clinical Cardiac Electrophysiology Handbook © 2016 Jason Andrade.
Cardiotext Publishing, ISBN: 978-1-942909-00-2.

Classification

- **Benign atrial tachyarrhythmia**
  - Paroxysmal, regular, narrow-complex tachyarrhythmia at 80–140 bpm
- **Incessant atrial tachyarrhythmia**
  - Persistent/permanent, regular, narrow-complex tachyarrhythmia at 100–160 bpm
- **Focal atrial tachycardia with an AV block**
  - Regular atrial tachyarrhythmia with variable ventricular rate
  - Typically this is seen with digoxin toxicity, which has parasympathetic (inhibitory) effects on sinoatrial (SA node) and atrialventricular nodes (AVN) but sympathetic (stimulatory) effects on pacemaker cells (increased automaticity).
- **Multifocal atrial tachycardia**
  - Irregular tachyarrhythmia (100–250 bpm) because of simultaneous activation of multiple (>3) foci
    - Most often enhanced automaticity is seen during an acute medical illness (typically pulmonary disease).
  - **A wandering atrial pacemaker** is similar to multifocal atrial tachycardia except for the heart rate <100.
- **Junctional tachycardia (JT)**
  - Persistent/permanent tachyarrhythmia because of enhanced automaticity or triggered activity originating at the junction between AVN and His bundle
  - Classification
    - **Focal junctional tachycardia**: A heart rate of 110–250 bpm is usually due to trauma, infiltrative hemorrhage, inflammation, or pediatrics.
    - **Non-paroxysmal junctional tachycardia**: The heart rate of 70–120 bpm is usually a marker for significant pathology (e.g., digitalis toxicity, ischemia, myocarditis).

12-Lead ECG

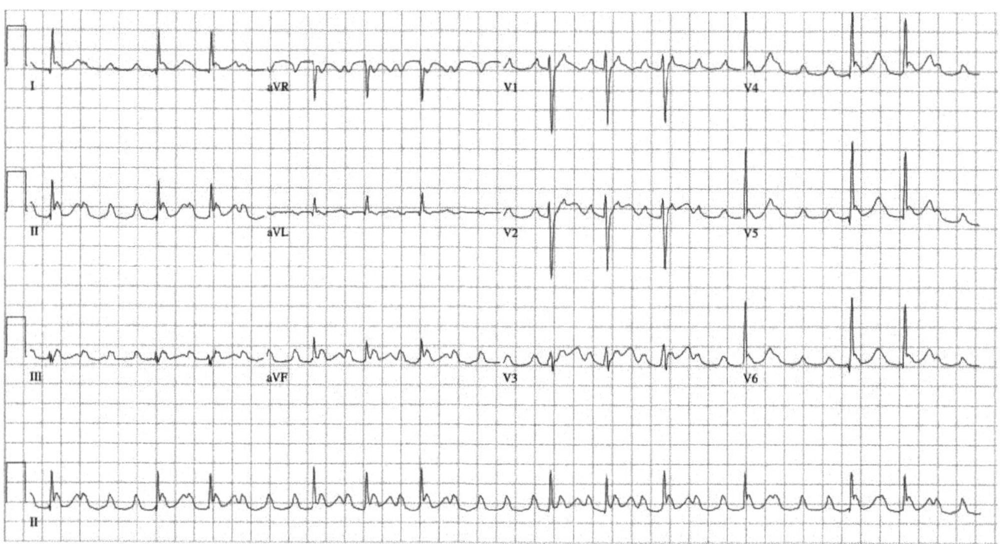

- **Rate**: Atrial rate of 100–250 bpm
- **Rhythm**: Ventricular conduction is variable:
  - **Regular** (constant ventricular conduction): Usually 1:1, 2:1, or 4:1 AV association
    - Odd conduction ratios (e.g., 3:1) are rare.
  - **Regularly irregular** (dual-level AV block; i.e., 6:2)
  - **Irregularly irregular** (variable AV conduction)
    - Variable AV block may be confused with irregular ventricular rhythm for atrial fibrillation.
- **P wave**: Ectopic, unifocal P′ waves differ from the sinus node P wave.
  - **FAT**: Discrete P waves separated by isoelectric baseline in all leads
  - **MAT**: Multiple (≥3) different discrete P-wave morphologies with no dominant pacemaker

Table 7.1 ECG Features to Localize the Site of Origin of an Atrial Tachycardia

	Right Atrium V1: Negative P wave (Spec 100%) aVL: Positive or biphasic (Spec 76%)	Left Atrium V1: Positive (Spec 90%) aVL: Negative P wave (usually)
High II, III, aVF – positive	**SVC** • Large P wave mimicking P pulmonale **Crista Terminalis** • P wave resembles sinus • P is negative in aVR (Spec. 93%)	**Superior PVs** • Amplitude in lead II is ≥0.1 mV (Sp. 74%) • P wave is larger in ectopy than sinus (lead II; Sp. 85%) **Left-sided PVs** • Notching in lead II (only during ectopy; Spec. 95%) • P-wave ratio in lead III:II ≥0.8 (Spec. 75%) • V1 positive phase ≥80 ms (Spec. 73%) **Right-sided PVs** • Positive P wave in aVL (Spec. 100%) • P-wave amplitude in lead I ≥50 mcV (Spec. 99%)
Low II, III, aVF – negative	**Inferolateral** • **Positive** P wave in V5–V6 **Inferomedial** • **Negative** P wave in V5–V6 **Apex of Triangle of Koch or Septal** • P-wave duration is shorter than sinus	

- **PR interval**: Isoelectric PR interval with long RP (period of absent atrial activation)
- **QRS**: Narrow complex unless it is an aberrancy or bundle branch block (BBB)
- **Onset/termination**: Paroxysmal or non-paroxysmal
  - May exhibit a rate increase ("warm-up") at onset or a decrease ("cool down") at termination
- **Maneuvers**: Carotid sinus massage or adenosine usually increases the degree of AV block and facilitates the identification of P waves. Adenosine may rarely terminate the tachycardia.

Other Investigations

- **Laboratory investigations**
  - Investigations into underlying cause (see Etiology)
- **24-hour Holter monitor**
  - Useful for diagnosis with episodes occurring more frequent than weekly
- **Event recorder**
  - Useful for diagnosis with symptomatic episodes occurring weekly to monthly
- **Echocardiogram**
  - Assessment of LV function and to exclude structural or congenital heart disease
- **Electrophysiology study (EPS)**
  - See below.

Management

Acute Management

- Cardioversion
  - Effectiveness depends on the mechanism.
  - Automatic FAT is usually unresponsive to attempts at electrical cardioversion.
  - Options
    - DC Cardioversion (class I)
    - Adenosine, β-blockers, ND-CCB (class IIa)
    - Antiarrhythmics (class IIa): Procainamide, flecainide, propafenone, amiodarone, and sotalol aim to directly suppress the focus.
- Rate control
  - β-blockers, ND-CCB (class I)
  - Digoxin (class IIb)

Chronic Management

Table 7.2 Management of Focal Atrial Tachyarrhythmia

	Recurrent Symptomatic	Incessant SVT	Non-sustained Asymptomatic
Nothing	—	—	—
BB/ND-CCB	I	—	—
Disopyramide	IIa	—	—
Flecainide/propafenone	IIa	—	—
Sotalol/amiodarone	IIa	—	—
Ablation	I	I	III

I: Should be performed; IIa: May be considered; IIb: Reasonable alternative; III: Not indicated.

- Non-pharmacologic therapy
  - Treat the underlying cause (i.e., for MAT, use ipratropium instead of salbutamol for COPD/asthma.
- Pharmacologic therapy
  - β-blockers, flecainide, propafenone, sotalol, and amiodarone are variably successful.
- Invasive therapy
  - Catheter ablation is preferred in most cases of recurrent atrial tachycardia.

Electrophysiology Study

Anterograde Conduction

- Usually normal decremental AVN conduction

Retrograde Conduction

- If present will be decremental and concentric.

Tachycardia Induction

- Programmed stimulation (atrial extrastimuli or burst atrial pacing) with or without isoproterenol infusion
  - Tachycardia is almost never induced with ventricular pacing.
- Non-inducibility or induction of a non-clinical arrhythmia are common reasons for procedural failure.

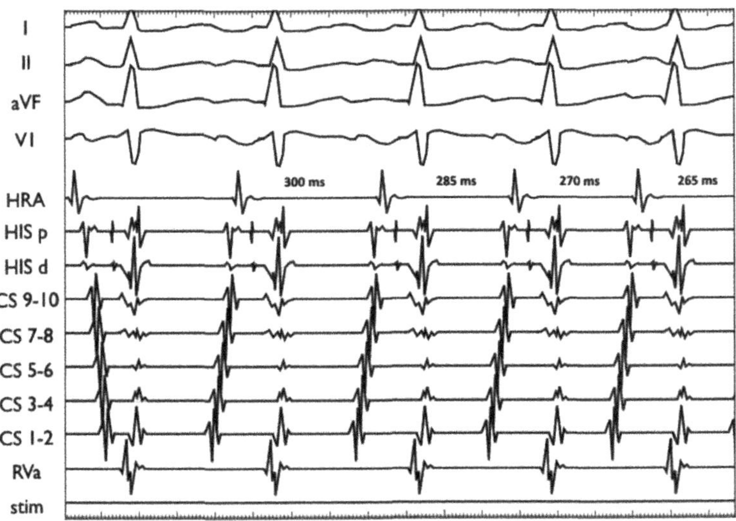

Arrhythmia onset is preceded by an atrial extrasystole (altered P-wave morphology and atrial activation). Thereafter, an atrial tachycardia (AT) is initiated. Note the gradual increase in tachycardia at arrhythmia onset.

Observations During Tachycardia

- The AV relationship is usually 1:1 or ≥2:1.
  - An uninterrupted tachycardia during an AV block is typical of AT because the AVN is **not** critical to the circuit.
  - The A:V ratio ≥2:1 excludes AVRT and makes AVNRT less likely.
- Change in the AA interval precedes a change in the HH and VV intervals as the AVN is not a critical part of the circuit.
- The VA interval is variable.
- BBB has no effect on the tachycardia cycle or VA timing.
- **Tachycardia CL variability**
  - [(longest CL – shortest CL) / mean TCL] over 1 minute
    - >15% variability: Suggests focal origin
    - <15% variability: Suggests macroreentrant or focal origin
- CS activation sequence

Table 7.3 Activation Sequence in the CS

	Right Atrium	Left Atrium	
		FAT	MRAT
Proximal to distal	**FAT** – any **MRAT** – any	PV tachycardia (RSPV, RIPV) FAT: Interatrial septum or right-sided LA FAT with previous mitral isthmus line	Counterclockwise peri-mitral AFL Right-sided roof-dependent AFL
Distal to proximal	—	PV tachycardia (LSPV, LIPV) FAT (left-sided LA)	Clockwise peri-mitral AFL Left-sided roof-dependent AFL
Flat	—	FAT (roof or posterior wall)	Roof-dependent AFL

AFL: atrial flutter; LIPV: left inferior pulmonary vein; LSPV: left superior pulmonary vein; MRAT: macroreentrant atrial tachycardia; PV: pulmonary vein; RIPV: right inferior pulmonary vein; RSPV: right superior pulmonary vein.

Maneuvers During Tachycardia

- Ventricular overdrive pacing
  - This maneuver is used to distinguish AT from nodal reciprocating tachycardias (AVNRT or AVRT).
  - It should not entrain the tachycardia.
  - The retrograde atrial activation sequence should differ from tachycardia.
  - VA dissociation will not terminate tachycardia.
  - With termination of pacing:
    - The return CL differs from the baseline VA timing (variable coupling).
    - Post-pacing sequence is VAAV or AAHV

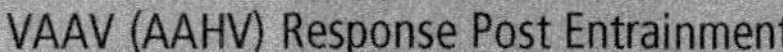

VAAV (AAHV) Response Post Entrainment

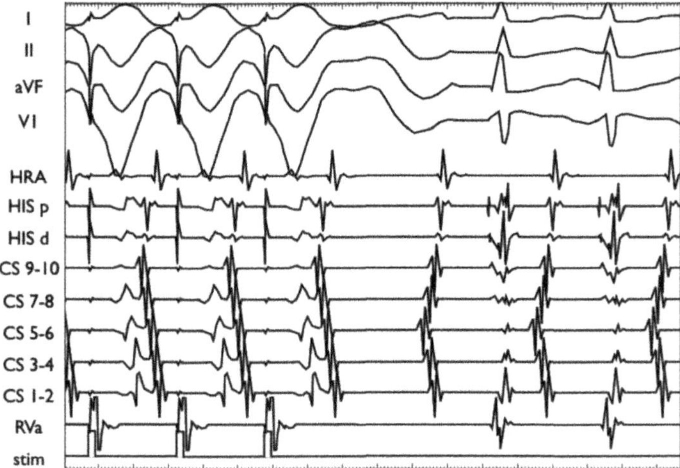

Ventricular entrainment during atrial tachycardia results in 1:1 VA conduction. Post cessation of ventricular pacing, the EGM response is atrial-atrial-ventricular (AAV).

No VA Linking Post Entrainment

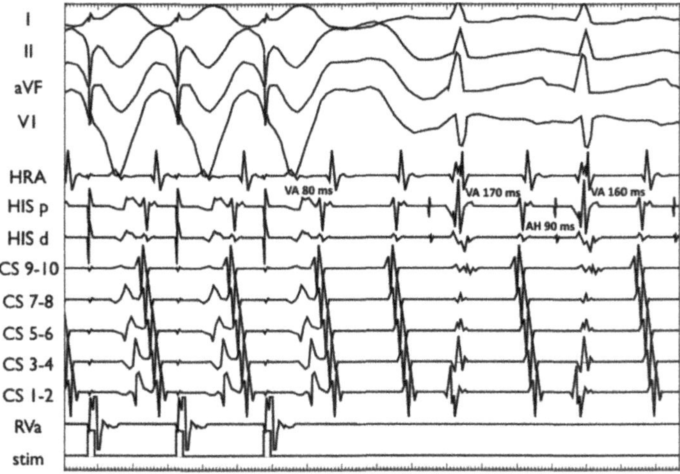

Entrainment of a septal AT via RV pacing. The VA interval on the first post-paced ventricular beat is >10 ms different from the tachycardia VA interval, thus demonstrating no VA linking. Note: Despite variable VA timing, the AH and HV intervals are stable.

- Entrainment via atrial overdrive pacing
  - Used to differentiate AT from nodal reciprocating tachycardia (AVNRT or AVRT)
  - With the termination of pacing:
    - The VA of first return beat should demonstrate variable VA timing (>10 ms of tachycardia VA).
    - Post-pacing sequence: AHHA or AHV

Entrainment of Junctional Ectopic Tachycardia (JET)

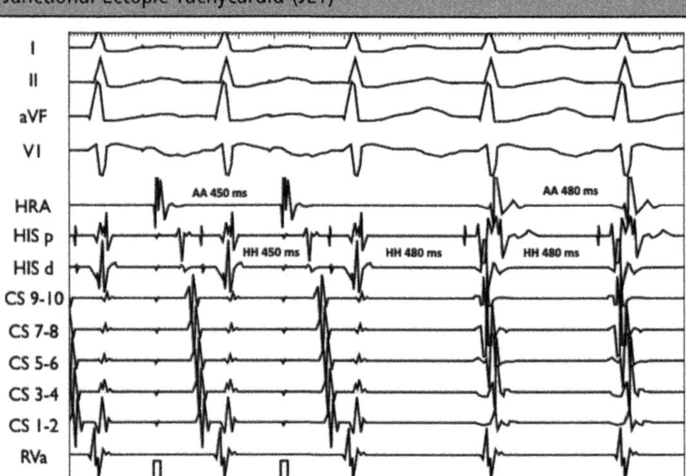

Entrainment is performed via HRA pacing at 450 ms (TCL 480 ms). After pacing, an AHHA response is observed.

Maneuvers in Sinus Rhythm

- Atrial pacing at TCL
  - Interpretation: AH time with pacing – AH interval during tachycardia is <10 ms

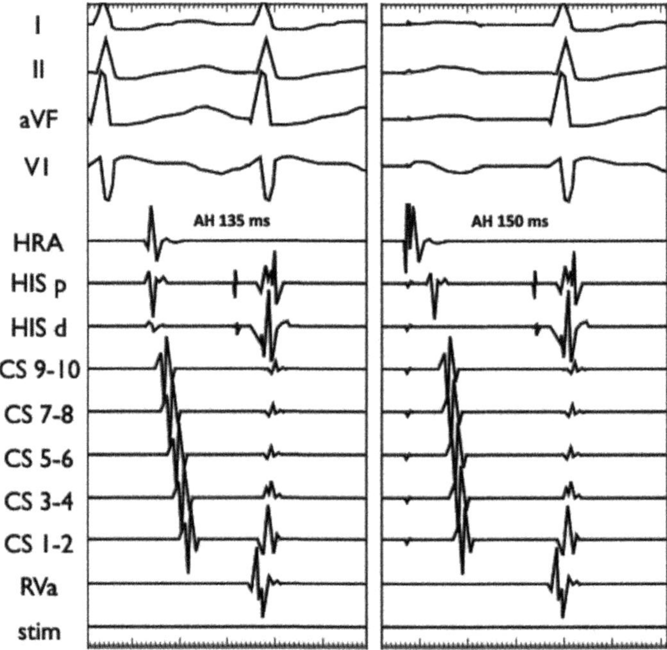

A comparison of AH intervals during atrial tachycardia (**left panel**) and HRA pacing at the TCL (**right panel**). The AH interval is 135 ms during tachycardia (**left panel**) and 150 ms during atrial pacing (**right panel**), leading to a delta AH of 15 ms.

CATHETER ABLATION OF ATRIAL TACHYARRHYTHMIA (AT)

Indication

- For treatment of AT that is symptomatic, recurrent, or refractory to medical therapy

Anticipated Success

- 85% acute success rate
  - Non-inducibility or induction of a non-clinical arrhythmia are common reasons for procedural failure.
- 8% recurrence

Anticipated Complications

- Similar to all invasive ablation procedures
- Specific risks are dependent of specific location of tachycardia.
  - Stroke risk is higher with left atrial origin.
  - The AV block risk is higher with peri-nodal origin.

Patient Preparation

- Stop all AAD for 3–5 half-lives before the procedure.
- Conscious sedation is preferred to GA due to the risk of rendering the arrhythmia non-inducible.

Set-Up

- 3D mapping system
- Irrigated RF ± sheath (stability and facilitates catheter orientation)
- Multipolar catheter in the CS
- Consider quadripolar catheter: HRA, RVa, and His

Mapping

- Activation mapping
  - Centrifugal spread from a fixed point: FAT
    - Once a "hot spot" is located, then a concentration of points should be taken to ensure there is centrifugal spread from a single origin.
    - Note: If the hot spot is septal and non-discrete, consider a breakthrough from opposite atria (Bachman's bundle, mid-septum, or CS)
  - Full range of cycle length with "early-meets-late": Reentry
    - Note: Focal AT located in the vicinity of a complete ablation line or associated with interatrial delay may lead to the activation propagating around the atrium in a fashion simulating the activation observed during macroreentry. Entrainment/resetting will discriminate between a macroreentrant and a focal AT.

- Overdrive pacing/entrainment mapping
  - Assessment
    - Pace a single atrial site at 10, 20, and 30 ms below the TCL.
  - Interpretation
    - Inconsistent PPIs (PPI variability >30 ms): FAT
    - Consistent PPIs (PPI variability <10 ms): Reentry (micro or macro)
    - Concealed entrainment with PPI = TCL: In circuit response
      - Entrainment with fusion and PPI > TCL: Out of circuit response
      - Concealed entrainment with PPI > TCL: Bystander location
  - Repeat the pacing maneuver at 2–3 distant sites.
    - If the maneuver is within the circuit, then the PPI should remain ≤20 ms.
- Special circumstances
  - Multiple unstable focal ATs firing sequentially
    - Ablation of the most frequent AT usually results in the organization of the atria and allows for mapping and ablation of other ATs.

Ablation Target

- Activation time >30 ms in advance of the surface P wave onset with centrifugal spread
- **FAT**: Unipolar recording usually shows a sharp negative QS deflection ± diastolic potentials
- **Microreentry**: Fractionated low-voltage EGMs spanning the entire AT cycle length within a surface of less than 2 cm of diameter

Activation Mapping of a HRA Tachycardia

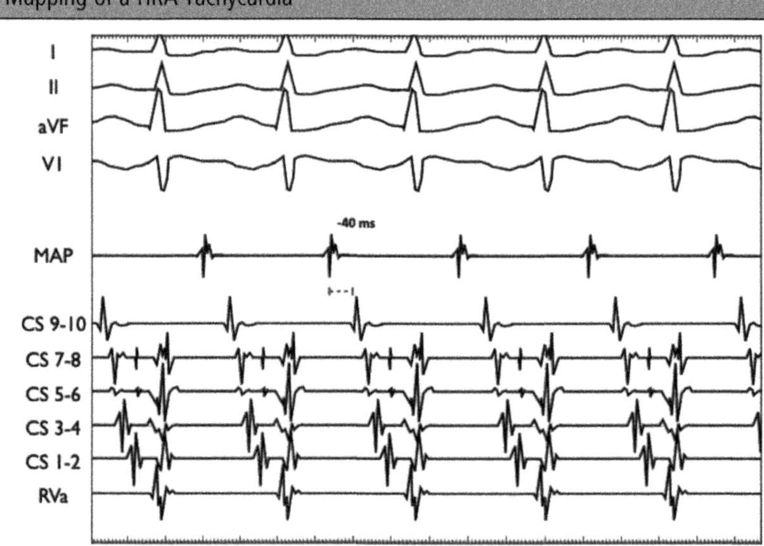

An ideal ablation site displays a local atrial EGM preceding the reference (HRA) by 40 ms.

RF Application

- Non-irrigated: 40–60 Watts (temperature limit of 60°C) for 45–60 seconds per lesion
- Irrigated: 25–35 Watts (temperature limit of 43°C) for 45–60 seconds per lesion

Determinants of Success

- Termination of the tachycardia during RF application:
  - Arrhythmia may transiently accelerate before terminating (automatic).
    - Transient acceleration without termination suggests a proximity to the focus.
  - Arrhythmia may slow before terminating (especially if it is microreentrant).
- Elimination of inducible tachycardia (rest and with isoproterenol stimulation) predicts long-term success.

Ablation of Specific AT Substrates

PV Tachycardia

- PV tachycardia may occur as an isolated AT in younger patients with normal hearts.
- Activation mapping localizes the tachycardia to within the PV ostia.
- Ablation should be performed at an antral or ostial level (i.e., outside the vein) as per standard pulmonary vein isolation (PVI; see Chapter 9).

Peri-nodal AT

- Requires careful differentiation from typical and atypical AVNRT
- 3D mapping may be beneficial to delineate the normal conduction system
- If ablation is to be performed:
  - Cryoablation is preferred given the proximity to the normal conduction system.
  - Otherwise, use RF with stepwise energy titration (10 W →15 W → 20 W → 25 W) until the tachycardia is suppressed.
    - Pay careful attention to the induction of junctional rhythm. If present, halt the ablation.

Key References for Further Reading

- Roberts-Thomson KC, Kistler PM, Kalman JM. Focal atrial tachycardia I: Clinical features, diagnosis, mechanisms, and anatomic location. *PACE.* 2006;29:643–652.
- Roberts-Thomson KC, Kistler PM, Kalman JM. Focal atrial tachycardia II: Management. *PACE.* 2006;29:769–778.
- Rosso R, Kistler PM. Focal atrial tachycardia. *Heart.* 2010;96:181–185.
- Chen SA, Chiang CE, Yang CY, Cheng CC, Wu TJ, Wang SP, et al. Sustained atrial tachycardia in adult patients. Electrophysiological characteristics, pharmacological response, possible mechanisms, and effects of radiofrequency ablation. *Circulation.* 1994;90;1262–1278.
- Kistler PM, Roberts-Thomson KC, Haqqani HM, Fynn SP, Singarayar S, Vohra JK, et al. P-wave morphology in focal atrial tachycardia: Development of an algorithm to predict the anatomic site of origin. *J Am Coll Cardiol.* 2006;48:1010–1017.
- Miyazaki H, Stevenson WG, Stephenson K, Soejima K, Epstein LM. Entrainment mapping for rapid distinction of left and right atrial tachycardias. *Heart Rhythm.* 2006;3:516–523.

CHAPTER

8

Atrial Flutter and Macroreentrant Atrial Tachycardia

ATRIAL FLUTTER (AFL)

General Information

- Regular, narrow-complex tachyarrhythmia due to a macroreentrant loop in the atria
  - Due to activation encircling a large central anatomic (valves, veins, scar) or functional obstacle
    - No single point of origin
    - Activation can be recorded throughout the entire cycle length (CL).

Epidemiology and Clinical Features

- Paroxysmal or persistent tachycardia with palpitations, chest pain, fatigue, dyspnea, or effort intolerance
  - Note: If persistent rapid rates are present, then heart failure may result (tachycardia induced cardiomyopathy).
- Syncope is rare but can occur with rapid 1:1 conduction.
- "Silent" atrial tachycardia: Detected in asymptomatic patients on electrocardiogram (ECG), Holter, or implantable devices

Classification of Macroreentrant Atrial Tachycardia (MRAT)

Cavotricuspid Isthmus-Dependent MRAT

- Macroreentrant circuit confined to the right atrium (passive LA activation)
  - Encircles the tricuspid valve (TV) with a posterior boundary (superior vena cava [SVC], inferior vena cava [IVC], and crista terminalis)

The Clinical Cardiac Electrophysiology Handbook © 2016 Jason Andrade.
Cardiotext Publishing, ISBN: 978-1-942909-00-2.

- Can be subdivided into:
  - **Typical AFL**: Counterclockwise activation
  - **Reverse-typical AFL**: Clockwise activation
  - **Double-wave reentry**: Two waves in the typical pathway
    - Usually unstable; self-terminates or degrades into atrial fibrillation (AF)
  - **Lower loop reentry**: MRAT encircling inferior vena cava with an upper turn around point is located in the posterior RA via a conduction gap in the crista terminalis.

Non-cavotricuspid Isthmus-Dependent MRAT

- Right atrial MRAT
  - **Upper loop reentry**: MRAT encircling the SVC with a lower turn-around point is located at a conduction gap in the crista terminalis.
    - Counterclockwise: Descending activation sequence in the free wall anterior to the crista
    - Clockwise: Ascending activation sequence in the free wall anterior to the crista
  - **RA free wall flutter**: MRAT encircling a low-voltage zone in the anterior free wall
  - **RA "figure-of-eight" reentry**
    - **Type 1:** Simultaneous upper and lower loop reentry share a common pathway through conduction gap in the crista terminalis. The two separate obstacles are the SVC combined with upper crista and the IVC combined with lower crista.
    - **Type 2**: Simultaneous upper loop reentry and free wall reentry share a common pathway between the crista terminalis and the low-voltage zone. The two separate central obstacles are the SVC with upper crista and a part of the low-voltage zone.
- Left atrial MRAT
  - **Peri-mitral flutter**: MRAT encircling the mitral annulus; isthmus between the mitral annulus and left inferior pulmonary vein (LIPV)
  - **Peri-venous flutter**: MRAT encircling the ipsilateral pulmonary veins (PVs) via a gap between the superior PVs
  - **"Small loop" reentry**: MRAT confined to a region of <3 cm; usually across two gaps in an ablation line (i.e., circumferential PV isolation)
  - **Coronary sinus (CS) macroreentry**: MRAT involving the coronary sinus (CS) musculature and atrial septum
- "Lesion-related MRAT" (scar-related flutter)
  - Post cardiac surgery: Right atriotomy, suture line, or prosthetic patch;
  - Post surgical MAZE or percutaneous catheter ablation

12-Lead ECG

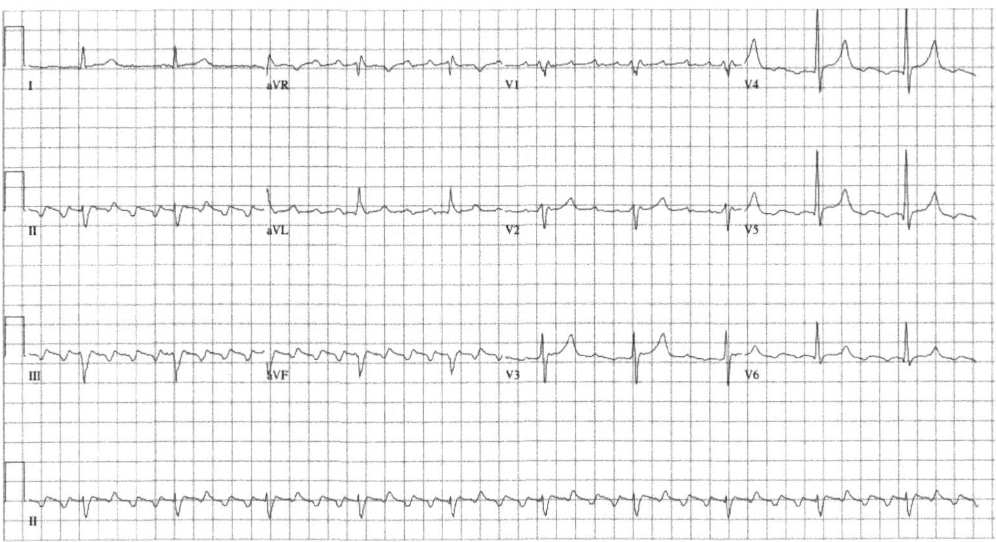

- Rate: The atrial rate is between 250 and 350 bpm.
  - It can be slower in the presence of class 1a, 1c, III antiarrhythmics.
- **Rhythm**: Ventricular conduction is variable:
  - **Regular**: Usually 1:1, 2:1, or 4:1 AV association
    - Odd conduction ratios (e.g., 3:1) are rare.
  - **Regularly irregular**: Dual-level AV block; e.g., 6:2
  - **Irregularly irregular**: Variable AV conduction may be confused with AF.
- Flutter waves
  - Morphology depends on the location of the reentrant loop.
    - **Typical**: Counterclockwise activation along the TV results in:
      - Negative F waves in the inferior leads and V6; positive F wave in V1–V5
    - **Reverse-typical**: Clockwise activation along the TV results in:
      - Positive F waves in inferior, V6; negative F waves in V1–V5
- PR: No isoelectric PR interval
- QRS: Narrow complex unless aberrancy or bundle branch block (BBB)
- Onset/termination can be paroxysmal or non-paroxysmal
- Maneuvers: Carotid sinus massage or adenosine usually increases the degree of AV block and facilitates identification of flutter waves.

Other Investigations

- **Laboratory investigations**
  - Investigations into underlying cause (see Etiology)
- **24-hour Holter monitor**
  - Useful for diagnosis with episodes occurring more frequent than weekly
- **Event recorder**
  - Useful for diagnosis with symptomatic episodes occurring weekly to monthly
- **Echocardiogram**
  - Assessment of LV function and to exclude structural or congenital heart disease
  - **Electrophysiology study (EPS)**: See below.

Management

Acute Management

Table 8.1 Management of AFL or MRAT

	Not Tolerated	Stable – Conversion	Stable – Rate Control
BB/ND-CCB	IIa	—	I
Digoxin	IIb	—	IIb
Ibutilide	—	IIa (38%–76% success)	—
Amiodarone	IIb	IIb	IIb
Class Ic: Flecainide, procainamide **Class Ia: Propafenone** **Class III: Sotalol**	—	IIb (<40% success)	—
DC cardioversion	I	I (>95% success)	—
Pacing (atrial/esophageal)	—	I (80% success)	—

I: Should be performed; IIa: May be considered; IIb: Reasonable alternative; III: Not indicated.
BB, β-blockers; ND-CCB, non-dihydropyridine calcium-channel blockers.

- Rate control
  - Difficult to achieve
  - β-blockers or non-dihydropyridine calcium-channel blockers (ND-CCB) are preferred
  - Digoxin or amiodarone are second line
- Cardioversion
  - **Medical**: Ibutilide, procainamide, sotalol, amiodarone, quinidine
    - A β-blocker or ND-CCB (diltiazem or verapamil) should be given before administering a class I AAD (i.e., procainamide, propafenone, flecainide), because these agents have can potentially slow the atrial rate, resulting in rapid conduction across the AV node (AVN) (e.g., paradoxical increase in the ventricular rate).
  - **Electrical**: DC shock at low synchronized energy levels (30–50 J) terminates the reentrant circuit, inducing uniform refractoriness.
  - **Overdrive pacing:** Pace the atrium from atrial or esophageal leads at a rate > than flutter can terminate the circuit.

Chronic Management

- Anticoagulation
  - See AF section.
- Pharmacologic therapy
  - Rate control: β-blocker, verapamil/diltiazem, digoxin
  - Rhythm control: Dofetilide preferred to other antiarrhythmic drugs (AADs).

Table 8.2 Chronic Management of AFL or MRAT

	First Episode Tolerated	Recurrent Tolerated	Poorly Tolerated	After AAD for AF	Non-CTI Failed AAD
Cardioversion alone	I	–	—	—	—
Dofetilide	—	IIa (>70% 1y success)	—	—	—
Antiarrhythmic drugs - Class III, class Ic, class Ia	—	IIb (~50% 1y success)	—	—	—
Catheter ablation	IIa	I	I	I	IIa

I: Should be performed; IIa: May be considered; IIb: Reasonable alternative; III: Not indicated.

- Invasive therapy
  - Catheter ablation: Preferred over AADs

CATHETER ABLATION OF MACROREENTRANT ATRIAL TACHYCARDIA (MRAT)

Indication

- AFL or MRAT that is symptomatic, recurrent, or refractory to medical therapy (class I indication).

Anticipated Success

- **Cavotricuspid isthmus (CTI)-dependent flutter**: >95% acute success; 5%–10% redo rate
  - 30% will go on to develop AF after AFL ablation (compared to >50% with AFL not undergoing CTI ablation)
- **Non-CTI-dependent flutter**: 50%–88% chronic success rate
- **Co-existing AF and AFL**: Arrhythmia-free survival depends on the dominant rhythm.
  - Predominantly AFL: 60% free of both AF and AFL
  - Predominantly AF: 25–30% free of both AF and AFL

Anticipated Complications

- Similar to all invasive ablation procedures
- <0.5% risk of AV block (particularly with ablation near the septum, due to damage to the AV nodal artery.

Patient Preparation

- Stop all AAD for 3–5 half-lives before the procedure.
- If in continuous flutter for >48 hours or of unknown duration
  - Anticoagulation 3 weeks prior to the procedure or perform a pre-procedure transesophageal echocardiography (TEE) to exclude LAA thrombus
  - Consider performing the procedure on uninterrupted oral anticoagulation.

Set-Up

- Multipolar catheter in the CS
- Ablation catheter: D-curve (medium/blue) or F-curve (large/orange) ± RAMP/ SR0/deflectable sheath
  - An irrigated tip radiofrequency (RF) or non-irrigated RF (8 mm) is preferred, but a cryoablation 8-mm tip is reasonable
- Consider the following:
  - Quadripolar catheter in RV or His
  - HALO catheter (or decapolar ± RAMP sheath) along lateral RA and positioned anterior to the eustachian ridge (ER).
    - **If behind the ER**: With proximal CS pacing, the atrium may be activated counterclockwise posteriorly even though conduction continues medial to lateral within the CTI (pseudoblock along the CTI).
    - **If on the ER**: Double potentials/fragmented signals give the appearance of slow conduction across the isthmus when a block is present (pseudoconduction across the CTI).
  - 3D mapping system

Mapping of MRAT

Tachycardia Induction

- Atrial burst pacing or extrastimuli ± isoproterenol

Observations During Tachycardia

- CS activation:
  - Proximal to distal
    - **Right atrial MRAT**
    - **Left atrial MRAT**: Counterclockwise peri-mitral flutter, right-sided roof flutter
  - Distal to proximal
    - **Left atrial MRAT**: Clockwise peri-mitral flutter, left-sided roof flutter
  - Flat
    - Roof-dependent left atrial MRAT

Activation Mapping

- Activation mapping should be able to demonstrate the entirety of the tachycardia circuit.
  - No single point of origin.
  - Activation can be recorded throughout the entire CL.
    - Consider an alternate mechanism if <50% of TCL is recorded.

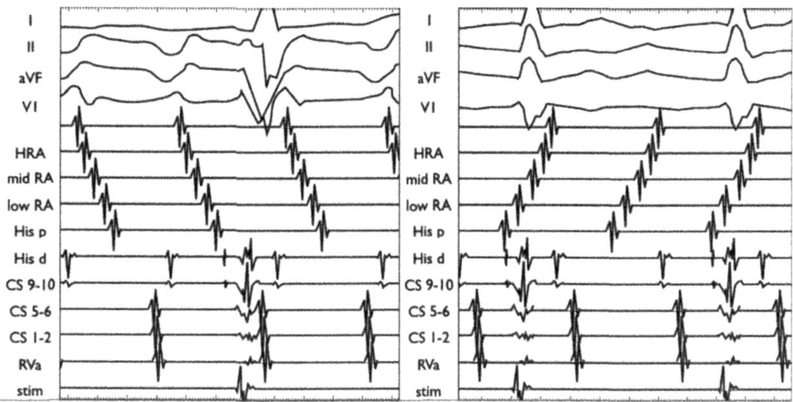

Atrial activation of a typical (counterclockwise) AFL (pCS → His → high lateral RA → low lateral RA)

Atrial activation of a reverse typical (clockwise) AFL (pCS → low lateral RA → high lateral RA → His)

Maneuvers in Tachycardia

- Atrial entrainment from atrial overdrive pacing
  - Consistent PPIs (PPI variability <10 ms) suggest the mechanism is reentry (micro or macro)
- Atrial entrainment (30 ms below the TCL) from ≥3 segments of the chamber of interest (for example cavotricuspid isthmus, lateral RA, and septum for CTI-dependent flutter)
  - Concealed entrainment with PPI – TCL ≤20 ms: In-circuit response
  - Concealed entrainment with PPI – TCL >20 ms: Bystander location
  - Entrainment with fusion and PPI – TCL >20 ms: Out-of-circuit response

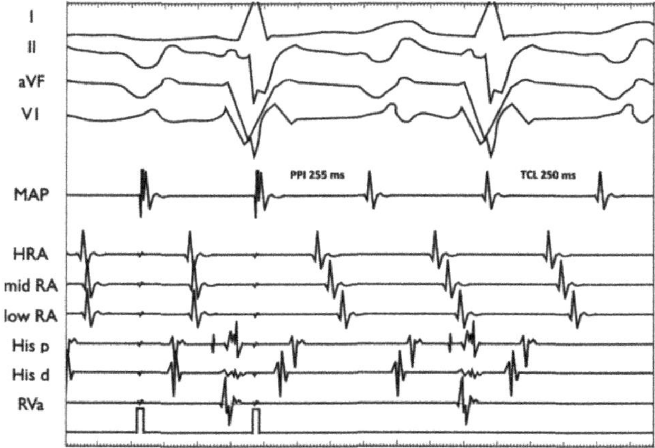

Entrainment mapping from mapping catheter placed within the cavotricuspid isthmus. At cessation of pacing the post-pacing interval (PPI) is 255 ms. The TCL is 250 ms giving a PPI – TCL of 5 ms, indicating the cavotricuspid isthmus is within the tachycardia circuit.

Ablation Target

A linear ablation of the putative isthmus is guided by anatomic landmarks.

- Right atrial MRAT
  - Cavotricuspid isthmus CTI-dependent flutter (typical and reverse typical)
    - Ablation line the joining the IVC to the tricuspid annulus (see below)
  - Lower loop reentry
    - Ablation of the cavotricuspid isthmus (as above)
  - Upper loop reentry
    - Ablation of the conduction gap in the crista terminalis
  - RA free wall flutter (lesion-related or incisional MRAT)
    - Ablation of the channel between the IVC or tricuspid annulus and the central obstacle (i.e., scar or gap in the atriotomy)
  - RA figure-of-eight reentry
    - Type 1 (upper and lower loop reentry): Ablation of the gap in the crista terminalis
    - Type 2 (upper and free wall reentry): The channel between the crista and low-voltage zone
- Left atrial MRAT
  - Roof-dependent flutter
    - Ablation joining the left superior pulmonary vein (LSPV) to the right superior pulmonary vein (RSPV) along mid-anterior portion
  - Peri-mitral flutter
    - Ablation from the joining the left inferior pulmonary vein (LIPV) to the mitral annulus (lateral or mitral isthmus line)
      - May need ablation in the distal CS to complete the line of block
    - Alternatively, linear ablation joining the right inferior pulmonary vein (RIPV) to the mitral annulus (septal line)

RF Application

- **Non-irrigated**: 25–50 Watts (temperature limit of 60°C) for 45–60 seconds per lesion
- **Irrigated**: 25–35 Watts (temperature limit of 43°C) for 45–60 seconds per lesion
  - **Mitral isthmus**: 30–35 Watts near the inferior PV; up to 40 Watts near the mitral valve area (MVA)
  - **Roof**: 30 Watts if catheter tip is perpendicular; 25 Watts if catheter tip is parallel (risk of "popping")
  - **CS**: 15–25 Watts

Determinants of Success

- Slowing and termination of the tachycardia during RF application
- Widely split double potentials along the isthmus
- Confirmation of bidirectional block across the linear lesion (see below)

Advanced Techniques

- Fusion between two simultaneous macroreentrant circuits (e.g., perimitral and a roof-dependent circuit)
  - Suspected when activation is compatible both with perimitral (activation spanning all the AT CL around the mitral annulus) and roof-dependent AT (activation spanning all the CL around the right or left PVs, with inferior activation of either the anterior or posterior wall).

- PPI – TCL <20 ms around the mitral annulus and both anterior and posterior LA near the roof
  - Management: Ablation of one loop will result in transition to the other.
- Double gap present at a linear lesion
  - Two alternating CLs are observed despite identical activation sequence.
  - Management: Ablation of both gaps will complete electrical block.

CATHETER ABLATION OF CAVOTRICUSPID ISTHMUS MACROREENTRANT ATRIAL TACHYCARDIA (MRAT)

Anatomy

- Inferior (cavotricuspid) isthmus
  - The region in the low RA is bordered by the IVC orifice posteriorly and the tricuspid annulus anteriorly.
    - It contains trabecular, membranous, and vestibular components.
    - The length varies from a few millimeters to several cm.
    - It tends to be thinnest in its central portion and thicker more laterally (due to the pectinates).
    - It tends to becomes broader (~6 mm) more inferolaterally than septally.
  - The Eustachian valve and ridge (ER)
    - **Eustachian valve**: Separates the IVC from the right atrium.
    - **Eustachian ridge**: Muscular ridge extending from the CS ostium (os) to the oval fossa.
    - Divides the inferior isthmus into two portions:
      - **The sub-eustachian isthmus** between the TV and the ER
      - **The post-eustachian isthmus** from the crest of the ER downward to the IVC
- Septal isthmus
  - Bounded by the CS posteriorly and the hinge of the TV anteriorly

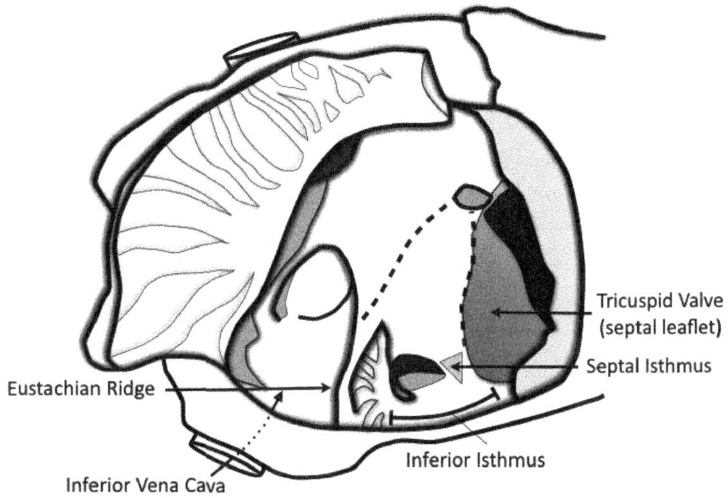

Ablation Target

- The procedure is commenced by advancing the ablation catheter across the TV.
- The catheter is deflected to the RA floor and withdrawn until the bipolar signal exhibits a dominant V with a small A (**distal position**).
  - During sinus rhythm, the ideal catheter orientation is at approximately 6 o'clock when in an LAO angle of 45°.
    - Anterolateral (beyond 7 o'clock) is difficult as the isthmus myocardium is broader, longer and thicker.
    - Septal (beyond 5 o'clock) confers a risk of an AV block (due to AV nodal artery damage) and myocardial infarction (due to inadvertent ablation in the middle cardiac vein).
  - During a counterclockwise flutter, the ideal catheter orientation is where the local activation activates in the middle of the plateau on the surface ECG (i.e., is within the area of slow conduction).
- The RF application for 45–60 seconds is performed until the atrial (A) EGM has diminished.
- The catheter is then slightly withdrawn towards the IVC until a fresh set of EGMs are observed, and ablation is reapplied.
  - Progressive catheter withdrawal results in atrial (A) EGM dominance with the disappearance of ventricular (V) EGM, followed by loss of local EGMs once the IVC is reached.

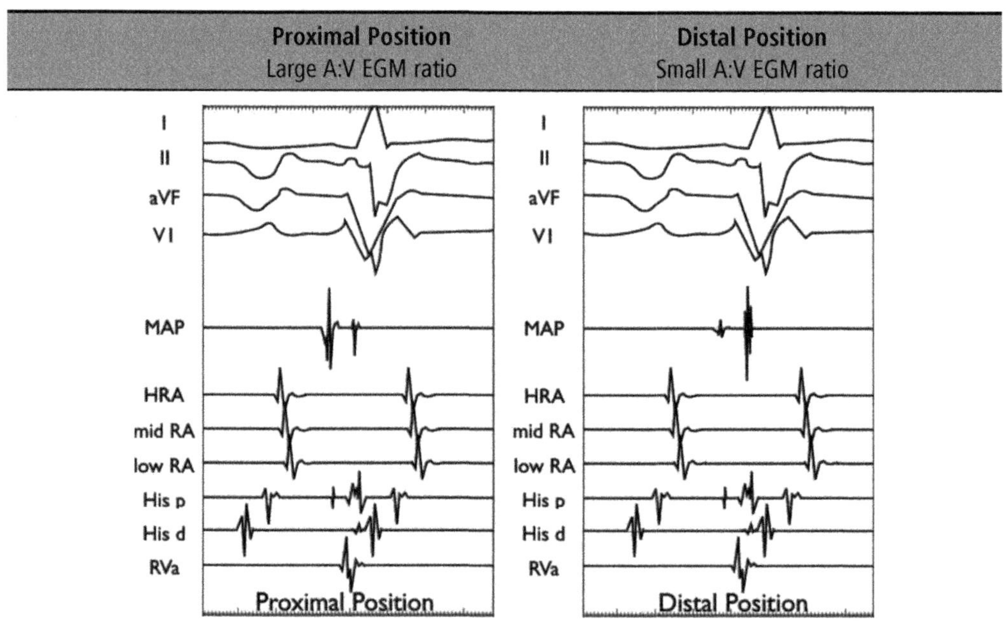

RF Application

- Non-irrigated (8-mm tip): 40–60 Watts (temperature limit of 60°C) for 45–60 seconds per lesion
- Irrigated: 25–35 Watts (temperature limit of 43°C) for 45–60 seconds per lesion

Determinants of Success

- Slowing and termination of the tachycardia during RF application
- Widely split double potentials:
  - The isthmus block is characterized by recording widely split EGMs, separated by an isoelectric baseline (e.g., double potentials separated by >90 ms) along the entire course of the ablation line.
    - The early component represents activation from the ipsilateral side of the line.
    - The late component represents activation around the atrium to the opposite side of the line.
- Bidirectional conduction block
  - This results in a greater long-term success than arrhythmia non-inducibility (<10% recurrence vs. >30%).
  - Assessed via pacing adjacent to the lateral aspect of the line (e.g., low lateral RA via the Halo or ablation catheter), and note the activation sequence at the His and proximal CS catheter.
    - Prior to the conduction block, the activation should be bidirectional, with the activation proceeding from the low lateral RA catheter to the proximal CS and His, with a collision on the septum.
      - The conduction time from pacing stimulus to proximal CS should be <100 ms.
    - After the conduction block, the activation should be clockwise from the low lateral RA to His to proximal CS.
      - A >25 ms increase from baseline in stimulus to proximal CS time should be seen.
      - Note: Isthmus block is likely if the conduction interval is >140 ms (in the absence of AADs); however, residual conduction is likely if the conduction interval is <120 ms.

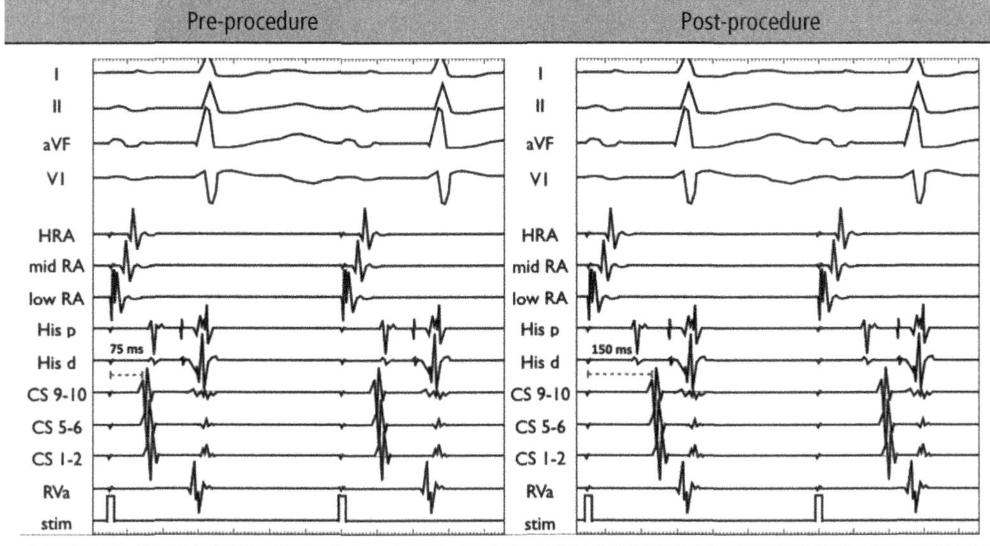

Pacing from the low lateral RA adjacent to the line. Activation from low lateral RA to proximal CS is 75 ms, with pCS activating before His.

Pacing from the low lateral RA adjacent to the line. Activation from low lateral RA to proximal CS is 150 ms, with His activating before pCS.

- Repeat the process for pacing from the medial side of the ablation line (via the proximal CS catheter) and note the activation sequence at the His and low lateral RA catheter.
  - Prior to the conduction block the activation should be bidirectional, with activation proceeding from the proximal CS to the low lateral RA catheter and His, and with the collision in the high lateral RA.
  - After the conduction block, activation should reverse from the proximal CS to His to the low lateral RA
    - A >25 ms increase in the stimulus to lateral RA time should be seen.
    - Note: Isthmus block is likely if conduction interval >140 ms (in the absence of AADs); however, residual conduction is likely if the conduction interval <120 ms.

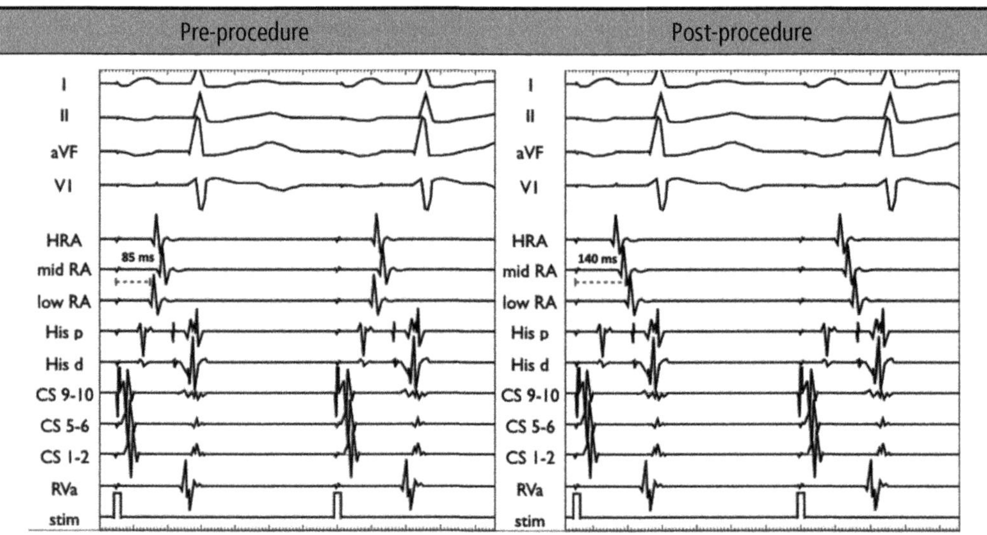

Pacing from the proximal CS (medial to the line). Activation from proximal CS to low lateral RA (85 ms)

Pacing from the proximal CS (medial to the line). Activation from proximal CS to low lateral RA (140 ms)

- Note: Pacing further away from the line results in a shorter conduction time.

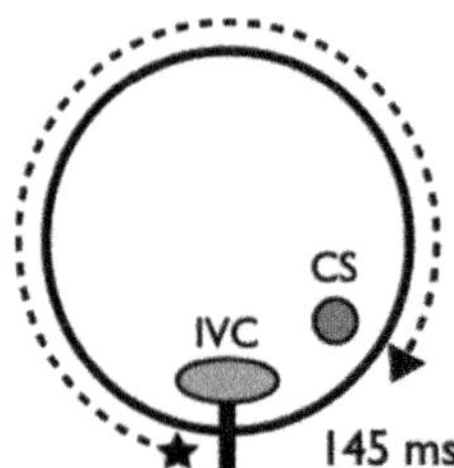

Pacing lateral to the ablation line results in a 145 ms time to activation at the proximal CS.

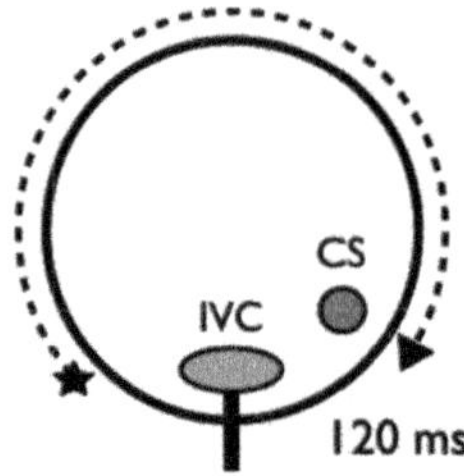

When pacing is performed more lateral from the ablation line, there is a shortening in the activation timing at the proximal CS (120 ms), suggesting that the impulse is travelling clockwise around the valve, and the line has a counterclockwise block.

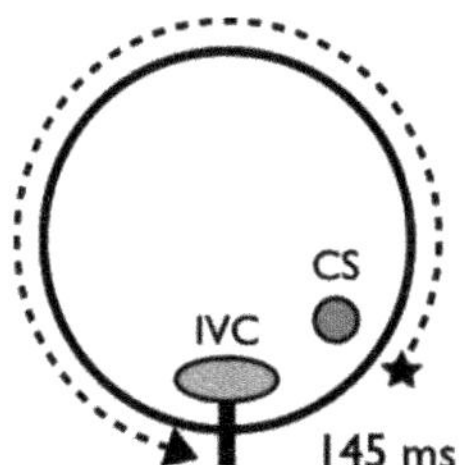

Pacing medial/septal to the ablation line results in a 145 ms time to activation at the lateral aspect of the ablation line.

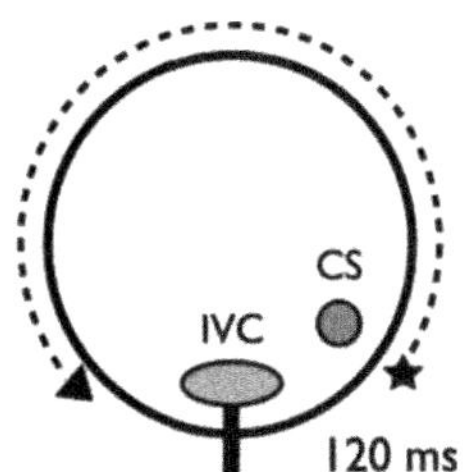

When the mapping catheter is moved more lateral from the ablation line there is a shortening in the activation timing while pacing from the proximal CS (120 ms), suggesting that the impulse is travelling counterclockwise around the valve, and the line has clockwise block.

- Pseudo-block (medial to lateral block) during CS pacing may occur as a result of:
  - **LA activation**: Wavefront proceeds via Bachmann's bundle along the anterior tricuspid annulus to reach the lateral wall, masking a persistent, but extremely slow medial to lateral CTI conduction.
  - **Lower loop conduction**: Wavefront proceeds posteriorly across the lower loop to rapidly reach the lateral aspect of the CTI (apparent medial-lateral CTI block).

Approach to a Difficult Cavotricuspid Isthmus Ablation

Confirm the Diagnosis

- Perform entrainment maneuvers in the medial and lateral isthmus.

If an Isthmus-Dependent Flutter Exists, Consider Anatomic Barriers

- Large sub-eustachian pouch
  - Results in:
    - Inadequate power delivery (due to poor blood flow within the pouch)
    - Inadequate myocardial contact because of the profound depth
  - Solution
    - Use irrigated RF (limits temperature rise and enhances power delivery).
    - Use an appropriate guiding sheath (RAMP/SR0/deflectable sheath).
    - Perform an ablation more laterally (the pouch lies medial) or encircle the pouch and anchor it to the tricuspid annulus as well as to the IVC.
- Large pectinate muscles
  - Results in:
    - An inadequate power delivery (due to poor blood flow between pectinates)
    - Difficulty in creating transmural lesions (due to thick myocardial bundles)
    - Difficulty with catheter manipulation (due to catheter instability)

- Solution
  - Use irrigated RF (limits temperature rise, enhances power delivery).
  - Perform ablation more medially. (The pectinates are more prominent inferolaterally.)
- Prominent Eustachian Ridge (ER)
  - Results in:
    - Difficulty with catheter manipulation (the ER acts as a fulcrum, causing clockwise torque to push the tip of the catheter toward the lateral RA rather than toward the septum)
    - Inadequate myocardial contact (usually on the upslope between the crest and annulus)
  - Solution
    - Use of an appropriate guiding sheath (RAMP/SR0/deflectable sheath)

If an Apparent Adequate Ablation Exists, Consider "Pseudo-Conduction"

- Lower loop conduction
  - A rapid conduction proceeds posteriorly across the lower loop to reach the lateral CTI.
    - This falsely gives the appearance of a continued (possibly) slow conduction across the CTI.
  - Solution
    - Manipulating the catheter posteriorly will demonstrate lower loop activation; however, when the catheter is placed directly on the ablation line there will be demonstration of conduction block.

Table 8.3 Mapping of Focal and Macroreentrant Atrial Tachycardias (MRAT)

RA Tachycardia	Surface ECG	CS Activation	Atrial Activation	Activation Map	Entrainment
CTI-dependent • Counter-clockwise	Positive P V1 Sawtooth inferior	P→D	Asc: Septum Desc: Lateral	Entire CL around TV	Concealed fusion from TV Long PPI from dCS
• Clockwise	Negative/biphasic P V1 Sawtooth inferior		Asc: Lateral Desc: Septum		
Upper loop reentry	Positive P inferior	P→D	descends	Entire CL around SVC	Long PPI from dCS and TV
Lower loop reentry	Negative P inferior	P→D	ascends	Entire CL around IVC	Concealed fusion from TV Long PPI from dCS

(*Continued*)

Table 8.3 (*Continued*)

RA Tachycardia	Surface ECG	CS Activation	Atrial Activation	Activation Map	Entrainment
Post incisional	Variable	P→D	Variable	Entire CL around scar	Concealed fusion around the incision Long PPI from dCS and TV
Focal AT	Variable (see above) isoelectric baseline	P→D	Variable	Centrifugal spread from site of early activation	Variable PPI (auto) Consistent PPI (micro)
LA Tachycardia					
PV tachycardia	Positive P V1–V6	Flat (usual) P→D (R PVs) D→P (L PVs)	Descends	Centrifugal spread from PV or antrum	Variable PPI
Focal AT	Variable isoelectric baseline	Variable	Variable	Centrifugal spread from site of early activation (PV, antrum, CS, roof, septum, or LAA base)	Variable PPI Consistent PPI (micro)
Peri-mitral • Clockwise	Negative P V1 Sawtooth inferior	D→P	ascends	Entire CL around MV	Concealed fusion from MV Short PPI on pCS and dCS Long PPI from roof and RA
• Counter-clockwise	Positive P V1 Sawtooth inferior	P→D	ascends		
Roof-dependent	Discrete P waves	Flat – 40% P→D (right) D→P (left)	Asc: Anterior Desc: Posterior (or opposite)	Entire CL includes roof and one pair of PVs	Concealed fusion from LA roof and either dCS or pCS Long PPI from RA

Asc: ascending; D: distal; dCS: distal coronary sinus; Desc: descending; P: proximal; pCS: proximal coronary sinus.

Key References for Further Reading

- Pérez FJ, Schubert CM, Parvez B, Pathak V, Ellenbogen KA, Wood MA. Long-term outcomes after catheter ablation of cavo-tricuspid isthmus dependent atrial flutter: A meta-analysis. *Circ Arrhythm Electrophysiol.* 2009;2:393–401.
- Asirvatham SJ. Correlative anatomy and electrophysiology for the interventional electrophysiologist: Right atrial flutter. *J Cardiovasc Electrophysiol.* 2009;20(1):113–122.
- Shah D, Haïssaguerre M, Takahashi A, Jaïs P, Hocini M, Clémenty J. Differential pacing for distinguishing block from persistent conduction through an ablation line. *Circulation.* 2000;102:1517–1522.
- Takahashi A, Shah DC, Jaïs P, Haïssaguerre M. How to ablate typical atrial flutter. *Europace.* 1999;1(3):151–155.
- Veenhuyzen GD, Knecht S, O'Neill MD, Phil D, Wright M, Nault I, et al. Tachycardias encountered during and after catheter ablation for atrial fibrillation: Part I: Classification, incidence, management. *Pacing Clin Electrophysiol.* 2009;32(3):393–398.
- Knecht S, Veenhuyzen G, O'Neill MD, Wright M, Nault I, Weerasooriya R, et al. Atrial tachycardias encountered in the context of catheter ablation for atrial fibrillation part ii: mapping and ablation. *Pacing Clin Electrophysiol.* 2009 Apr;32(4):528-38.

CHAPTER

9

Atrial Fibrillation

UNDERSTANDING AND EVALUATING ATRIAL FIBRILLATION (AF)

Anatomy and Pathophysiology (Mechanism)

- Structural (fibrosis, hypertrophy, dilation, etc.) and/or electrophysiologic abnormalities (ion current or connexin changes affecting action potential duration [APD] and/or conduction) promote abnormal impulse formation and/or propagation.
- After the onset of AF, there are immediate (within minutes) and early (hours to days) alterations in the atrial electrophysiological properties (shortening of the atrial APD and ERP, abnormal action potential rate adaptation), followed by later changes in atrial structure (e.g., fibrosis, dilation) and mechanical function.
    - These changes are largely because of the down-regulation of the L-type inward calcium current, impaired intracellular calcium release, up-regulation of inward rectifier potassium current, and alterations of myofibrillary energetics.

Hypotheses Regarding the Initiation and Perpetuation of AF

- Initiation (triggers):
    - Ectopic foci initiate rapid repetitive discharges due to triggered activity (delayed > early afterdepolarization) or enhanced automaticity.
    - The predominant triggers are located in the pulmonary veins (PVs).
        - The PVs contain sleeves of left atrial (LA) myocardium:
            - These sleeves extend ~1.5–2.5 cm beyond the LA–PV junction.
            - These sleeves are thickest in the carina and venoatrial junction (mean 1.1 mm).
            - These sleeves are longer in the superior PVs with the left superior pulmonary vein [LSPV] sleeve being longer than the right superior pulmonary vein [RSPV] sleeve.
        - The sleeves have shorter effective and functional refractory periods compared to LA, with critical zones of conduction delay and non-uniform anisotropy related to abrupt changes in fiber orientation.

  - Non-PV triggers include: the SVC, LA free wall, left atrial appendage (LAA), coronary sinus (CS) ostium, ligament of Marshall, crista terminalis, RA free wall, and the interatrial septum.
- Perpetuation (substrate)
  - **Multiple-wavelet hypothesis**: Postulates that AF results from the continuous annihilation and regeneration of multiple independent coexisting wavelets propagating randomly throughout the atria. It suggests that AF could be indefinitely perpetuated as long as the atrium had a sufficient electrical mass to prevent the simultaneous termination of all of the reentrant activity.
  - **Localized-source hypothesis**: Postulates that AF is perpetuated by discrete, organized and rapid reentrant circuits (e.g., spiral wave reentrant circuits or "rotors"), or focal impulses that disorganize into fibrillatory waves at their periphery (e.g., drivers close to cardiac ganglion plexi with central organized activation and surrounding variable propagation and fractionation).

Classification

- **First detected episode**
- **Paroxysmal**: An AF that terminates spontaneously within 7 days of onset is defined as paroxysmal. According to some definitions, AF terminated by electrical or pharmacological cardioversion within 7 days is also considered paroxysmal.
- **Persistent**: Episodes that last longer than 7 days
- **Longstanding persistent**: Continuous AF of longer than 12 months duration
- **Permanent**: Acceptance of AF (decision to cease further attempts of rhythm control)
- **Lone**: AF in patients <60 years old with no structural heart disease
- **Non-valvular AF**: AF in the absence of rheumatic mitral stenosis or a mechanical heart valve

Epidemiology and Clinical Features

- AF is the most common sustained arrhythmia seen in clinical practice.
  - Prevalence: 1%–2% of the population
    - Increases with age: <1.0% at 50 years, 1%–4% at 65 years, and 6%–15% at 80 years
    - Less common in women: Male sex is associated with a 1.5× increased risk.
    - Lifetime-risk of developing AF for individuals 40–55 years of age is estimated to be 22%–26%.
  - AF accounts for 1.0%–2.7% of total annual healthcare expenditures.
- AF is associated with:
  - Reductions in quality of life, functional status, and cardiac performance
  - Reduced overall survival (RR of death with AF is 1.4–3.0)
  - Increased risk of cardiac thromboembolism
    - Valvular AF (rheumatic mitral stenosis [MS] or mechanical heart valve): Up to 17× increased risk of stroke (vs. sinus rhythm)
    - Non-valvular AF: 3.5× increased risk of stroke (vs. sinus rhythm)
    - Note: AF-related strokes are often recurrent and relatively more severe, causing significantly greater long-term disability, and mortality (25:1 hemispheric to transient ischemic attack [TIA] ratio vs. 2:1 for carotid sources).

- Increased risk of cognitive dysfunction
  - There is a 1.7- to 3.3-fold increased risk of cognitive impairment (vs. sinus rhythm).
  - There is a 2.3-fold increased risk of dementia (vs. sinus rhythm).

Table 9.1 Factors Predisposing Patients to AF

• Hypertension (BP >140/90 mm Hg): RR 1.2–1.5 ■ Pre-hypertension (sBP 130–139 mm Hg): RR 1.3 ■ Increased pulse pressure: RR 1.3 per 20 mm Hg • Valvular heart disease: RR 1.8–3.4 • LV systolic dysfunction: RR 4.5–5.9 ■ Diastolic dysfunction: RR 3.3–5.3 ■ Hypertrophic cardiomyopathy: RR 4–6 • Diabetes: RR 1.4–16 • Thyroid dysfunction: RR 3–6 ■ Subclinical hyperthyroidism: RR 1.4	• Obesity: RR 1.4–2.4 • Alcohol consumption (≥36 g/day): RR ~1.4 • Obstructive sleep apnea: RR 2.8–5.6 • Physical activity (lifetime >1500 h): RR 2.9 • Familial and genetic (AF in ≥1 parent): RR 1.85 • Congenital heart disease • Chronic kidney disease: RR 1.3–3.2 • Inflammation: RR 1.5–1.8 • Pericardial fat: RR 1.3–5.3 • Tobacco use: RR 1.5–2.1

- Clinical evaluation
  - Define the duration and frequency of episodes.
    - Date of first symptomatic attack or AF discovery
    - Onset of current episode
    - Clinical classification (Categorize the patient by the most frequent presentation.)
  - Define the presence and nature of symptoms.
    - Palpitations, dyspnea, fatigue, effort intolerance and pre-syncope predominate, but 21% are asymptomatic.
    - Symptoms are usually secondary to the tachycardia and generally are alleviated with adequate rate control.
  - Identify precipitating factors.
    - Caffeine, exercise, alcohol, sleep deprivation, and emotional stress.
    - Sleep or after a large meal (vagal-mediated AF)
  - Review past evaluations and treatments.
  - Assess the presence of underlying heart disease or other reversible conditions
- Classification of AF-related symptoms
  - Canadian Cardiovascular Society Severity of Atrial Fibrillation (CCS-SAF)
    - **Class 0**: Asymptomatic with respect to AF.
    - **Class 1**: AF has a minimal effect on quality of life (QOL)
      - Minimal or infrequent symptoms.
    - **Class 2**: AF has a minor effect on QOL
      - Mild awareness of symptoms or rare episodes of paroxysmal AF.
    - **Class 3**: AF has a moderate effect on QOL.
      - Awareness of symptoms on most days (persistent)
      - More common episodes (every few months) or more severe symptoms (paroxysmal)
    - **Class 4**: Symptoms of AF have a severe effect on QOL.
      - Unpleasant symptoms (persistent) or frequent/highly symptomatic episodes (paroxysmal)
      - Syncope or heart failure due to AF

- European Heart Rhythm Association (EHRA) score
  - Class I: No symptoms
  - Class II: Mild symptoms – normal daily activity not affected
  - Class III: Severe symptoms – normal daily activity affected
  - Class IV: Disabling symptoms – normal daily activity discontinued

12-Lead ECG

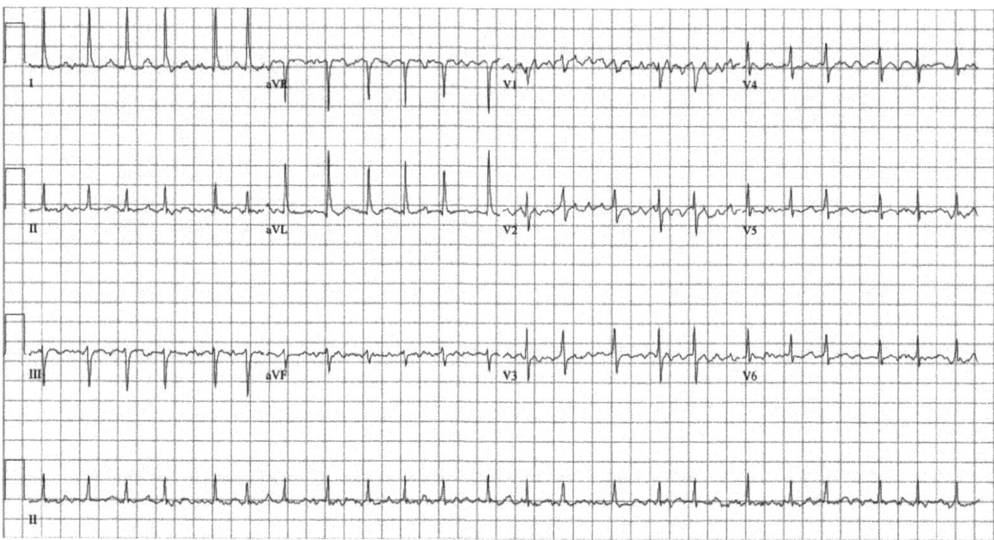

- **Rate**: The atrial rate is usually 350–600 bpm.
  - Due to multiple (~5–6) microreentrant circuits within the atria
- **Rhythm**: The ventricular response is irregularly irregular (usually 100–180 bpm).
  - <60 bpm: Slow ventricular response
    - Due to intrinsic conduction abnormalities, or medications
  - 70–110 bpm: Controlled ventricular response
    - Due to intrinsic conduction abnormalities, or medications
  - >120 bpm: Rapid ventricular response
    - Hyper sympathetic state (generally rates >150 bpm): Drugs, stress, myocardial ischemia, pain, anxiety, infection, hypotension, anemia, thyrotoxicosis, hypoxemia, or hypoglycemia
    - Pre-excitation (especially if rate >200 bpm)
      - The ventricular rate is dependent on the refractory period of the AP.
- **P wave**: There are no distinct P waves, but merely an undulating baseline (fibrillatory waves).
- **QRS**: This is a narrow complex unless an aberrancy or bundle branch block [BBB]
- **Other**: An ST segment shift is common, but only ⅓ have significant coronary disease.

Other Investigations

- Essential investigations
  - Laboratory
    - Complete blood count, electrolytes, renal function, hepatic function, thyroid function
  - Electrocardiogram (ECG)
    - P-wave duration and morphology (if in sinus), chamber hypertrophy, evidence of myocardial infarction
    - R-R, QRS, and QT intervals: Baseline assessment prior to the initiation of antiarrhythmic drugs (AADs)
  - Transthoracic echocardiogram (TTE)
    - Structural heart disease (valvular pathology, cardiomyopathy, congenital heart disease)
    - LA size, LV hypertrophy
- Additional testing
  - 6-minute walk
    - Adequacy of rate control
  - Exercise stress test
    - Exclude active ischemia prior to the initiating class Ic AADs in those at risk of ischemic heart disease.
    - To assess the adequacy of rate control, AF-related symptoms, and to diagnose exercise-induced AF
  - 24-hour Holter monitor or event recorder
    - To confirm the diagnosis of AF
    - To assess the adequacy of rate control

Management

Exclude Reversible Causes

- Myocardial disease: Myocardial infarction, myo-pericarditis
- Pulmonary disease: Embolism, pneumonia, sleep-disordered breathing
- Thyroid disease: 5.4% have subclinical hyperthyroidism; 1% have overt hyperthyroidism
- Acute alcohol and substance use
- Surgery: Cardiac (40%), thoracic (25%), orthopedic (15%), esophageal (5–10%)
  - Peak incidence on day 2 (usually within 5 days)
  - **Prophylaxis**: Oral β-blocker (class I) or amiodarone in high-risk patients (class IIa)
    - Consider amiodarone for patients who are older, have peripheral vascular disease, valvular disease, chronic lung disease, or a large LA

Prevention of Thromboembolism

- Antithrombotic therapy is generally recommended for patients with AF unless contraindicated (see Table 9.2).

Table 9.2 Antithrombotic Therapy Recommendations for Patients with AF

	Recommended Therapy
Valvular AF • Mitral stenosis, mechanical prosthesis	Oral anticoagulation
Hypertrophic cardiomyopathy	Oral anticoagulation
Hyperthyroidism • Until a euthyroid state has been restored	Oral anticoagulation
Non-valvular AF (estimate based on the CHADSVASc score)	
0–1 point	ASA 81–325 mg or nothing
≥2 points	Oral anticoagulation

- Review the stroke risk scores for non-valvular AF (see Table 9.3).

Table 9.3 Stroke Risk for Patients with Non-Valvular AF

			Yearly Risk of Stroke		
	CHADS	CHADSVASc	Score	CHADS	CHADSVASc
Clinical HF or LVEF <40%	1 point	1 points	0	1.9%	0%
Hypertension	1 point	1 points	1	2.8%	1.3%
Age ≥75	1 point	2 points	2	4%	2.2%
Diabetes	1 point	1 points	3	5.9%	3.2%
Stroke/TIA/ thromboembolism	2 points	2 points	4	8.5%	4%
Vascular disease (MI, PVD)	—	1 points	5	12.5%	6.7%
Age 65–74	—	1 points	6	18.2%	9.8%
Sex (female)	—	1 points	7		9.6%
			8		6.7%
			9		15.2%

HF: heart failure; LVEF: left ventricualr ejection fraction; MI: myocardial infarction; PVD: peripheral vascular disease; TIA: transient ischemic attack.

- Consider the risk of bleeding with warfarin therapy (see Table 9.4).

Table 9.4 Risk of Bleeding with Anticoagulation

HASBLED Score		Outpatient Bleeding Risk Index	
Criteria		**Criteria**	
• Hypertension (sBP >160 mm Hg)	1 point	• Age ≥65y	1 point
• Abnormal renal function (Cr >200 µmol/L)	1 point	• History of stroke	1 point
• Abnormal liver function	1 point	• History of GI bleed	1 point
• Stroke	1 point	• Comorbidity	1 point
• Bleeding	1 point	▪ Recent myocardial infarction	
• Labile INR	1 point	▪ Hct <30%	
• Elderly (age >65 years)	1 point	▪ Cr >1.5 mg/dL	
• Drugs	1 point	▪ Diabetes	
• Alcohol	1 point		
Risk of Major Bleeding		**Risk of Major Bleeding**	
• High risk defined for those with ≥3 points		• Low (0 points = 0.8%/year) • Moderate (1–2 pt = 2.5%) • High (3–4 pt = 10.6%)	

Cr: creatinine; GI: gastrointestinal; Hct: hematocrit; INR: international normalized ratio.

- When choosing an antithrombotic agent, consider the assessment of risks vs. benefits (see Table 9.5).

Table 9.5 Risk/Benefit of Antithrombotic Agents

	Study	Stroke Risk Reduction vs. Placebo	Major Bleeding	Comment
ASA 80–325 mg daily	AFASAK, SPAF, EAFT, ATAFS, PATAF, WASPO ESPS II, LASAF, UK-TIA	22%	1.5%–2.0% yearly	
ASA + Clopidogrel	ACTIVE A, ACTIVE W	43% (28% RRR vs. ASA)	2.0%–2.5% yearly	
Warfarin (INR 2–3)	AFASAK, SPAF, BAATAF, CAFA, PATAF, WASPO, ATAFS, SPINAF, EAFT	64% (43% RRR vs. ASA + Clopidogrel)	2.5%–3.0% yearly	
Dabigatran 110 mg bid	RE-LY	71% (9% RRR vs. W)	20% reduction vs. W	This dose is preferred in those ≥80 years or with eGFR 30–50 mL/min
Rivaroxaban 20 mg die	ROCKET-AF	70% (12% RRR vs. W)	No difference vs. W	Use 15 mg daily if eGFR 30–50 mL/min

(*Continued*)

Table 9.5 (*Continued*)

	Study	Stroke Risk Reduction vs. Placebo	Major Bleeding	Comment
Apixaban 5 mg bid	ARISTOTLE AVERROES	73% (21% RRR vs. W)	31% reduction vs. W	Use 2.5 mg bid if 2 of: • age ≥80 years • weight ≤60 kg • Cr ≥133 mmol/L/ 1.5 mg/dL
Dabigatran 150 mg bid	RE-LY	81% (34% RRR vs. W)	No difference vs. W	

eGFR: estimated glomerular filtration rate; RRR: relative risk reduction; W: warfarin.

- Note: Dabigatran, rivaroxaban, and apixaban are associated with a 10% decrease in all-cause mortality, which is largely due to the 40%–70% reduction in hemorrhagic stroke and ~50% reduction in intracranial hemorrhage (ICH)
- Interrupting anticoagulation
  - Bridge with low-molecular-weight-heparins/unfractionated heparin (LMWH/ UFH) if mechanical heart valve, high risk of stroke, or planned interruption >7 days
  - If short interruption and risk of stroke is not significantly elevated, it is generally acceptable to interrupt oral anticoagulation without bridging LMWH or UFH.

Control of the Ventricular Rate

- Multiple large, randomized trials (AFFIRM, RACE, STAF, PIAF, HOT CAFÉ, AF-CHF) have demonstrated that a strategy of rate control can be at least as effective as rhythm control in properly selected patients.
  - In these studies there was no difference in overall mortality, morbidity, or quality-of-life between rate and rhythm control.
  - The rhythm control groups had an increased rate of hospitalization (usually for cardioversion).
- Clinical factors that may favor a primary strategy of ventricular rate control
  - Patient preference
  - Persistent AF
  - Recurrent AF despite attempts at rhythm control (AAD or ablation)
  - Less symptomatic patients
  - Older patients (age >65 years)
  - Comorbidities that would limit the success of achieving sinus rhythm

- Rate-control targets
  - Resting heart rate <80 bpm (but <100–110 bpm is reasonable if asymptomatic and normal LV function)
  - Alternate targets
    - 24-hour average heart rate <100 bpm
    - Heart rate <110 bpm on 6 minute walk
    - Heart rate <110% age-predicted maximum on exercise stress test
- **Choice of agent**
  - β-blockers and calcium-channel blockers are generally regarded to be equally efficacious, although emerging evidence suggests a relatively greater survival benefit with BB.
    - β-blockers are better rate-control agents (lower heart rate at rest/exercise) with no change or decreased exercise capacity.
    - ND-CCBs are less effective rate-control agents (lesser reduction in heart rate on exertion) but lead to an increase or no change in exercise capacity.
  - Digoxin is considered second line due to its inability to control HR during exertion or stress.
    - As a single agent digoxin is ineffective at controlling ventricular rate in all but the sedentary elderly. The combination of digoxin and β-blockers is more effective than combinations of digoxin and ND-CCB, because of a synergistic effect on the AV node (AVN) (digoxin working well at rest with high vagal but low adrenergic tone, and β-blockers work well with stress with high adrenergic tone and vagal withdrawal).
- **AVN ablation** after permanent pacemaker implanation
  - Indications: Rapid ventricular rate despite medical therapy or significant medication-related side effects
  - Outcome: Improves cardiac symptoms, quality of life, and healthcare utilization
  - Limitations: Loss of AV synchrony (persistent symptoms in hypertrophic cardiomyopathy [HCM], restrictive cardiomyopathy [RCM], or hypertensive heart disease)
  - Note: Consider biventricular pacing in the presence of impaired baseline LV function (e.g., LVEF <40%–50%).

Rhythm Control

- Pharmacotherapy to maintain sinus rhythm may be preferred with:
  - First episode of AF or paroxysmal AF
  - AF due to a reversible cause
  - Highly symptomatic AF
  - Patients of a younger age (<65 years of age)
  - No previous antiarrhythmic drug (AAD) failure
  - Patient preference

Cardioversion

- Cardioversion-related thromboembolism
  - Risk does not differ between modalities (electrical/direct-current cardioversion [DCCV] or pharmacologic).
  - Risk is decreased with adequate anticoagulation prior to cardioversion (<1% vs. 6.1% without anticoagulation).
  - Risk is lowest in the first 12 hours after AF onset (0.3% vs. 0.7% after 12–48 hours).
    - However, 60% of patients will spontaneously convert within 24 hours.
  - Risk of stroke is highest in the first 3–10 days post cardioversion due to atrial stunning.
    - Irrespective of modality, the patient requires 4 weeks of anticoagulation post cardioversion.
- Electrical or synchronized DCCV
  - More effective and preferred for unstable patients
  - Consider starting at higher energy outputs (e.g., > 150 J) in order to limit total energy exposure.
  - Pre-treatment with AAD may enhance the success of DCCV
    - **SAFE-T trial**: Placebo (68% acute success), amiodarone (72%), sotalol (73%)
    - Other options: Flecainide, ibutilide, propafenone
    - β-blockers and verapamil may reduce subacute recurrence only
- Pharmacologic cardioversion
  - More likely to be successful if the AF is recent in onset; however, the success is always inferior to DCCV.

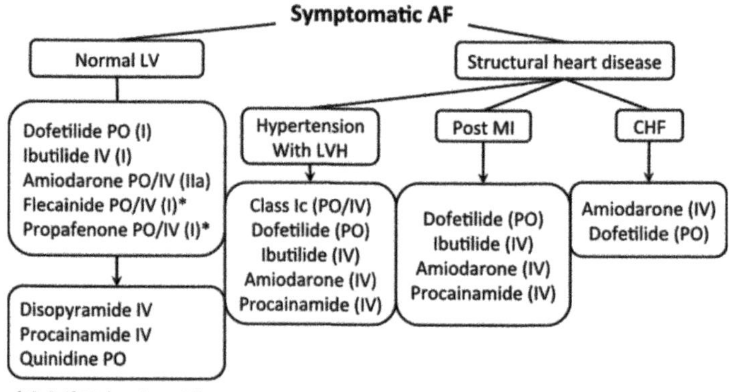

- Choices
  - **Ibutilide**: 1 mg IV infusion over 10 minutes (30%–45% rate of conversion)
  - **Procainamide**: 1 g in 125 cc NS over 30 min IV (30% rate of conversion)
  - **Propafenone**: 450 mg (<70 kg) or 600 mg PO (>70 kg) (50%–80% rate of conversion)
  - **Flecainide**: 200 mg (<70 kg) or 300 mg (>70 kg) (50%–80% rate of conversion)
  - **Amiodarone**: 150 mg IV bolus then infusion (30%–50% rate of conversion)
- A β-blocker or ND-CCB (diltiazem or verapamil) should be given before administering a class I AAD (i.e., procainamide, propafenone, flecainide), because these agents have can potentially slow the atrial rate, resulting in rapid conduction across the AVN (e.g., paradoxical increase in the ventricular rate).

Maintaining Sinus Rhythm Post Cardioversion

- Long-term anti-arrhythmic therapy
  - The goal of AAD therapy is to decrease the frequency, severity, and duration of AF episodes as well as alleviate the associated symptomatology.
    - AF recurrence while taking an AAD is not indicative of treatment failure and does not always necessitate a change in AAD therapy.
    - Anticipated efficacy
      - **CTAF**: 69% sinus at 16 months with amiodarone; 39% with sotalol or propafenone
      - **AFFIRM**: 62% sinus at 1 year with amiodarone; 23% on class I agents
      - **DIAMOND-CHF**: 79% sinus with dofetilide vs. 42% with placebo
  - Choice of AAD should be individualized based on the side-effect profiles, the presence or absence of cardiovascular comorbidities, and underlying renal and hepatic function.

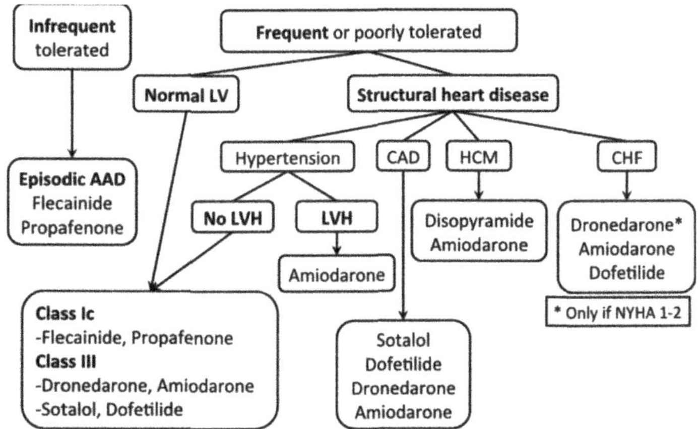

- A β-blocker or ND-CCB (diltiazem or verapamil) should be co-administered with class I AAD (i.e., propafenone, flecainide) because these agents can potentially slow the atrial rate, resulting in rapid conduction across the AVN (e.g., paradoxical increase in the ventricular rate).

- Paroxysmal symptomatic atrial fibrillation: "Pill-in-the-pocket" (PIP)
  - Flecainide or propafenone (doses as above) combined with an AVN agent (β-blocker or ND-CCB)
  - Indications: Patients with <1 episode per month of highly symptomatic but stable paroxysmal AF
  - The first dose must be given in a monitored setting (conversion pauses, bradycardia, pro-arrhythmia).
    - Continuous telemetry for at least 6 hours after medication administration
    - BP monitoring every 30 minutes (for drug-induced hypotension)
    - 12-lead ECG every 2 hours (PIP cannot be utilized if the QRS duration increases by >50% from baseline)
  - Subsequent doses can be taken at home 30 minutes to 1 hour after the onset of the episode.
    - Instruct the patient to rest for 4 hours or until the episode resolves.
    - Instruct the patient to return to hospital if:
      - There is no termination after 6–8 hours.
      - New symptoms develop.
      - There is more than one episode in a 24-hour period.

Ablation

- Surgical ablation (MAZE procedure) ± LAA amputation
  - Generally reserved for patients undergoing surgery for other indications.
- Percutaneous catheter ablation

ATRIAL FIBRILLATION (AF) ABLATION

Indication

- AF that is symptomatic and refractory to ≥1 antiarrhythmic drugs.
- It may be considered as first line therapy in select populations.

Anticipated Success

- Approximately 60% have a 1-year success rate with the first procedure (~60%–70% paroxysmal; ~50–60% persistent).
- Approximately 30% of paroxysmal and 50% of persistent AF patients will need more than one procedure.
- There is approximately 10% added success with the second attempt.

Anticipated Complications

- Death (<0.1%)
- Thromboembolism: Stroke/MI (<1%)
- Perforation/tamponade (1%)
- Pulmonary vein stenosis (0.3%)
- Atrial-esophageal fistula (<1:2000)
- Access site complications (1%–1.5%)
- Phrenic nerve injury/diaphragmatic paralysis (1%–5%; higher with cryoballoon)
- Proarrhythmia (AF or atypical flutter)

Patient Preparation

- Pre-procedure anticoagulation for 1 month prior to ablation, or transesophageal echocardiography to exclude the presence of LAA thrombus.
- Consider stopping all AAD for 5 half-lives before the procedure.
- Anticoagulation: Can be stopped pre-procedure, although emerging evidence suggests it is safe to continue uninterrupted OACs throughout the ablation procedure.
  - Warfarin: Generally continued throughout ablation (uninterrupted warfarin)
  - Dabigatran: Uninterrupted or hold 2 doses if eGFR ≥50, hold 4 doses if eGFR <50
  - Apixaban: Uninterrupted or hold 2 doses if eGFR >30
  - Rivaroxaban: Uninterrupted or hold 1 dose if eGFR >30

Strategies for AF Ablation

- PV isolation (PVI): Most commonly performed ablation procedure for paroxysmal AF
  - Techniques
    - Circumferential antral PVI is preferred to ostial or segmental PVI
    - Cryoballoon ablation
    - Multielectrode circumferential ablation (e.g., pulmonary vein ablation catheter [PVAC], nMARQ)
  - Endpoint: PV isolation with bidirectional (entrance and exit) conduction block
- PVI + defragmentation
  - Techniques
    - PVI + complex fractionated atrial electrogram complex fractionated atrial electrogram (CFAE) ablation
    - Multielectrode ablation (PVAC + Multi-Array Ablation Catheter [MAAC]/ Multi-Array Septal Catheter [MASC])
  - Endpoint: PVI plus elimination of high-grade CFAE
- PVI + linear ablation (compartmentalization of the LA)
  - Techniques:
    - PVI + linear LA ablation: Roof, mitral isthmus, cavotricuspid isthmus (CTI)
    - Multielectrode ablation (PVAC + tip versatile ablation catheter [TVAC])
  - Endpoint: PVI plus bidirectional conduction block across the lines
- PVI + defragmentation + linear ablation (roof ± mitral isthmus): "Stepwise approach"
  - Techniques
    - PVI/LACA + CS and SVC isolation → CFAE → linear ablation
  - Endpoint: PVI plus bidirectional conduction block across the lines

ATRIAL FIBRILLATION (AF) ABLATION — PULMONARY VEIN ISOLATION

Set-Up

- Deflectable decapolar in CS (for differential pacing)

Left Atrial Access

- Single or double transseptal

Circular Mapping Catheter (CMC)

- Types of CMCs
  - Fixed diameter CMCs: 15, 20, and 25 mm diameter
    - CMCs contain 10 (decapolar) or 20 poles (duo-decapolar).
    - When mapping the aim is to keep the shaft at the superior aspect of the PV.
      - For right-sided veins, this will place electrodes 1–5 on the posterior aspect.
      - For left-sided veins, this will place electrodes 1–5 on the anterior aspect.
  - Variable diameter CMCs: 15 to 25 mm diameter
    - CMCs contain 10 (decapolar) or 20 poles (duo-decapolar).
    - The variable diameter allows for better contact and stability in the PV ostium (oversizing) as well as the use in different PV sizes. However, when used in small diameter PVs, there is a possibility of an electrode overlap causing a signal artifact.
    - When mapping, the aim is to keep the shaft at the posterior or superior aspect of the PV.
  - Small caliber CMCs are 15 and 20 mm in diameter.
    - They contain either 6 or 8 electrodes.
- Catheter electrodes
  - Decapolar catheters
    - Widely spaced electrodes are less likely to under-detect PV potentials but are more likely to detect far-field electrical activity necessitating the use of maneuvers to localize the origin of each recorded signal.
  - Duo-decapolar catheters
    - Closely spaced electrodes result in a better ability to differentiate near-field PV potentials from far-field activity.
    - There is a risk of missing near-field potentials as a result of poor tissue contact or partial PVI.

Ablation Catheter

- Irrigated RF: D-curve (medium/blue), F-curve (large/orange), or bi-directional catheter
- Cryoballoon catheter: 23 mm or 28 mm
- Multielectrode catheters: PVAC, nMARQ

Anticoagulation

- IV heparin bolus as soon as LA access is obtained
  - **Empiric bolus dose**: 100 units/kg (warfarin), 120 units/kg (dabigatran), 130 units/kg (rivaroxaban, apixaban)
- Heparin IV infusion to a target activated clotting time (ACT) of 300–350 during the procedure
  - Alternatively bolus heparin q15–30 minutes (depending on ACT)

Sheath Management

- Continuous irrigation with saline (or heparinized saline) at >60 mL/h

Mapping System

- Fluoroscopy (typically only used with cryoballoon and multi-electrode ablation)
- Electroanatomic mapping system

PV Mapping

PV Potentials (PVP)

- PVPs are characterized by:
  - Near-field characteristics: a sharp upstroke, narrow width, and a high dv/dt
  - Extensive or circumferential distribution
  - Proximal-to-distal activation in sinus rhythm
    - A PVP can be traced from the PV ostium distally within the PV.
    - The PVP will exhibit progressive temporal delay without losing its near-field characteristic.
  - PVP cannot be directly captured by low-amplitude extra-PV stimulation.
- Non-PV deflections/potentials
  - Display far-field characteristics: Lower amplitude, wider width, and lower dv/dt
  - Non-circumferential distribution
  - These do not display a proximal-to-distal activation sequence in a sinus rhythm.
    - Reduce in amplitude without an alteration in timing when traced distally within the PV.
  - Can be directly captured by low-amplitude LA, LAA, or SVC stimulation.

PV-specific EGM Interpretation

Table 9.6 PV-specific EGM Interpretation

	Far-Field Source	Distribution of Far-field EGMs	Distinguishing Pacing Maneuver	Recognition in AF, Compare PV to:
LSPV	Posterior LAA	Anterior	Distal CS or LAA pacing	LAA activation
	Adjacent LA	Posterior	Perivenous pacing	Posterior LA
	Ipsilateral PV	Inferior	Ipsilateral PV pacing	Superior LIPV
LIPV	LAA	Anterior	Distal CS or LAA pacing	LAA activation
	Adjacent LA	Posterior	Perivenous pacing	Posterior LA
	Ipsilateral PV	Superior	Ipsilateral PV pacing	Inferior LSPV
RSPV	SVC	Anterior-superior	Sinus rhythm or SVC pacing	Posterior SVC
	Adjacent LA	Posterior	Perivenous pacing	Posterior LA
RIPV	Adjacent LA	Posterior	Perivenous pacing	Posterior LA/RA

- Left superior pulmonary vein (LSPV)
  - **Baseline signal:** Single potential in sinus rhythm in 66%–75%
  - **Signal with pacing**: Double potentials in 100% with LA pacing
  - **PV conduction delay**: Produced by a change of activation at the anterior and inferior LSPV.
    - Maximal when stimulating the LAA directly
- Left inferior pulmonary vein (LIPV)
  - **Baseline signal:** Single potential in sinus rhythm in 66%–75%
  - **Signal with pacing**: Double potentials in 75% with LA pacing
  - **PV conduction delay**: Produced by a change of activation at the anterior and superior LIPV.
    - Maximal when stimulating from the low lateral LA inferior to the LAA base.
- Right superior pulmonary vein (RSPV)
  - **Baseline signal**: Double potentials in sinus rhythm in 25%
    - The first signal (<30 ms from sinus P-wave onset) represents the SVC/RA with the second signal (>30 ms from sinus P-wave onset) representing the local PVP.
    - The **delay** (20–50 ms) between the signals is produced by the time it takes for the impulse to cross the inter-atrial septum via the Bachmann's bundle, and then abruptly change direction to reach the RSPV.
  - **Signal with pacing**: Generally not useful because the SVC's proximity to the sinus node means that no pacing position can further anticipate SVC activation or delay PV activation.
- Right inferior pulmonary vein (RIPV)
  - **Baseline signal**: Single potential in sinus rhythm in 100%
  - Usually there are no non-PV EGM deflections, but may rarely have adjacent LA.

Maneuvers to Differentiate the Source of EGMs Recorded Within the PV

- Decremental pacing
  - Pacing the atrium at an increasingly faster rate, or with a closely coupled extrastimulus, results in a separation of the far-field and PVP signals due to decremental conduction properties present at the LA-PV junction.
  - The usefulness of this maneuver is limited by the observation that:
    - Not all PV ostia demonstrate decremental properties (due myocardial fiber orientation/activation).
    - Decremental conduction may be observed into the LAA with rapid pacing.
    - Rapid pacing may induce AF.

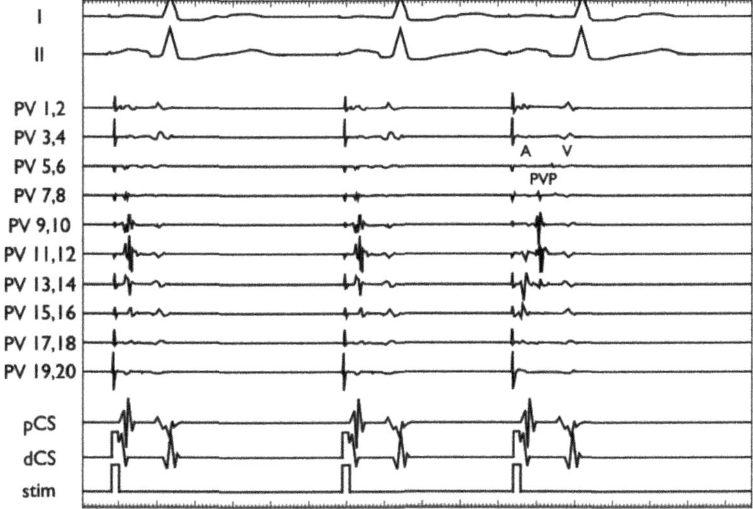

Following a drive train of 600 ms, an atrial extrasystole is delivered from the distal CS catheter resulting in a wider separation between the far-field atrial potential (A) and PVP on the circular mapping catheter positioned in the PV ostium (PV 1–2 to 19–20).

- Differential pacing
  - This results in a separation of the far-field and PVP signals based on the order of activation.
  - The maneuver is most useful for the left-sided PVs.
    - In sinus rhythm, there is near simultaneous activation of the LAA and PV EGM (i.e., signal overlap).
    - Distal CS pacing results in an asynchronous activation or an increase in the relative separation between the LAA and the local PV EGMs by activating the LAA relatively earlier, and delaying PV activation through decremental conduction at the LA-PV junction or a change in activation at the anterior and inferior aspect of the PV.

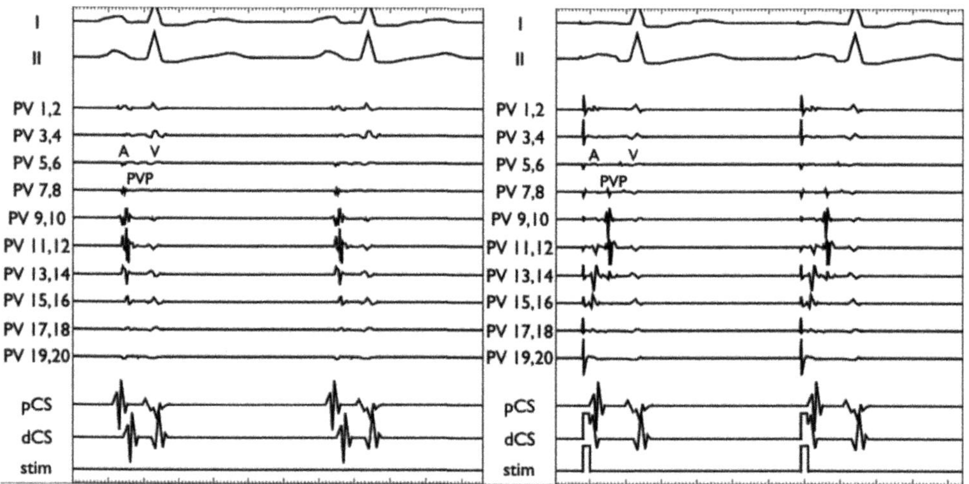

Sinus rhythm: Overlap of far-field LA (A) and pulmonary vein potentials (PVP).

Distal CS pacing: Delay into the PV results in separation of the far-field LA (A) and near field PVPs.

- Site-specific pacing
  - Pacing directly at the proposed far-field source results in:
    - Local EGM is drawn in towards, or merging with, the pacing artifact
    - The PVP is relatively delayed due to decremental conduction at the LA-PV junction.
  - Common far-field sites include:
    - LAA
    - Ipsilateral PV
    - SVC (generally not useful as it is hard for pacing to anticipate SVC activation given its proximity to the sinus node)
    - Peri-venous atrial myocardium
  - Pacing may also be performed from a bipole of the CMC positioned within the PV ostia.
    - The local PV EGM will be drawn into the pacing artifact.
    - The far-field non-PV signal will be delayed due to decremental conduction at the LA-PV junction.
    - Note: Use care to limit pacing outputs in order to avoid direct capture of the non-PV far-field structure.

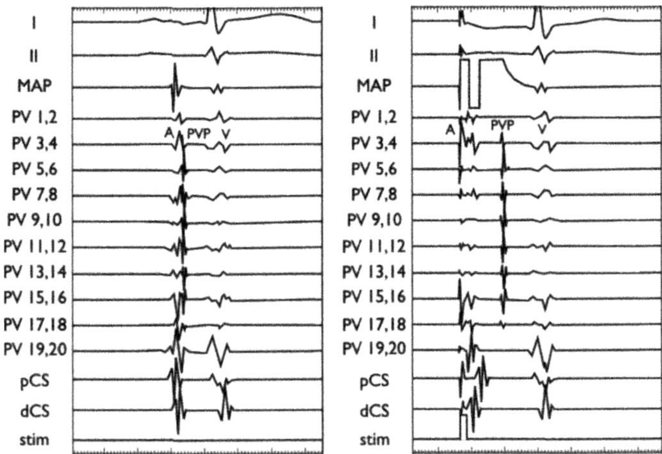

During sinus rhythm (**left panel**) high-frequency EGMs are observed on the CMC (PV). Activation is near simultaneous when compared to the ablation catheter MAP positioned inside the LAA. Pacing performed from the ablation catheter (MAP) in the LAA (**right panel**) advances the far-field LA (A) EGMs and demonstrates clear near field PVPs. In both panels, a ventricular far-field signal (V) simultaneous to the QRS is observed on the circular mapping catheter.

- Pacing the electrical ostium
  - Pacing directly within the vein will draw the PVP towards the pacing spike.
  - Withdrawal of the pacing catheter towards the atrium and across the electrical ostium results in either:
    - Reversal of the PVP-LA activation sequence as the catheter crosses into the LA.
    - Widened separation of the summated LA-PVP EGM as the catheter crosses into the LA.

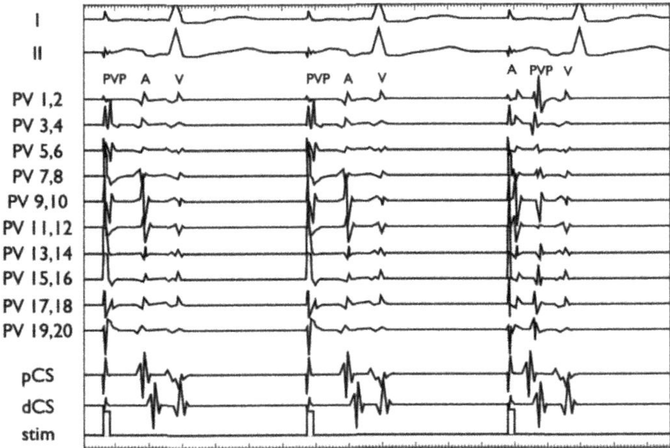

With a circular mapping catheter (PV) positioned inside the PV ositia, pacing is performed from a mapping catheter positioned inside the PV. Initially there is local PV capture followed by conduction to the LA (first two beats). As the catheter is withdrawn into the LA across the electrical ostium, the activation sequence reverses (from PVP – LA to LA – PVP).

AF Ablation — Pulmonary Vein Isolation

- **Irrigated RF**
  - **Power** (maximum): 20–25 Watts (posterior wall), 30–35 Watts (anterior wall)
    - 15–30 Watts (coronary sinus), 35 Watts (LAA-LPV anterior ridge), 35–40 Watts (mitral annulus)
  - **Temperature** (maximum): 43°C
  - **Irrigation**: 8–30 cc/min (during ablation; depending on the catheter), 2 cc/min (during mapping)
  - **Monitoring during RF application**
    - Should see abolition of local EGMs with a decrease in local impedance (~10 Ω).
    - A sudden increase in impedance >20–30 Ω suggests the catheter has slipped into the PV.
- **Cryoballoon ablation**
  - Ablation for 3–4 minutes should be delivered after verification of optimal CB-PV occlusion
  - Occlusion usually assessed through contrast venography; however, alternatives include intracardiac echocardiography (ICE), and analysis of the PV pressure.

Endpoints of Ablation

- Entrance block
  - An entrance block is defined as the stable absence of conduction from the LA into the PV.
  - During ablation, the PVP should delay and disappear.
    - If PVP decreases in amplitude, it suggests the ablation is occurring too deep in the vein and the myocardial sleeve is being directly injured.
    - With "point-by-point" RF ablation the site of early activation progressively shifts until isolation is achieved.
    - With cryoballoon ablation, circumferential isolation occurs simultaneously.
  - Difficulties in assessing entrance block
    - Over-detection of far-field structures may mimic or mask the presence of PV EGMs.
    - Under-detection of PV EGMs ("pseudo-entrance block") may be observed with a relatively distal CMC position, poor CMC-PV tissue contact, and partial PV ablation.

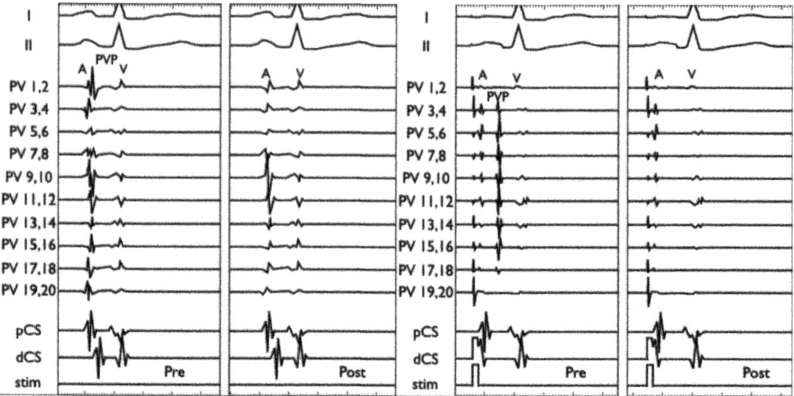

Pre-ablation, a near-field PVP is demonstrated on the CMC positioned at the ostium of the LSPV. Post isolation, only far-field atrial (A) and ventricular (V) EGMs are recorded (**left panel**: sinus rhythm; **right panel**: distal CS pacing).

- Exit block
  - Defined as the stable absence of conduction from the PV into the LA.
  - It is demonstrated via the non-conduction of spontaneous PV discharges or the non-conduction of paced impulses from within the PV to the LA.

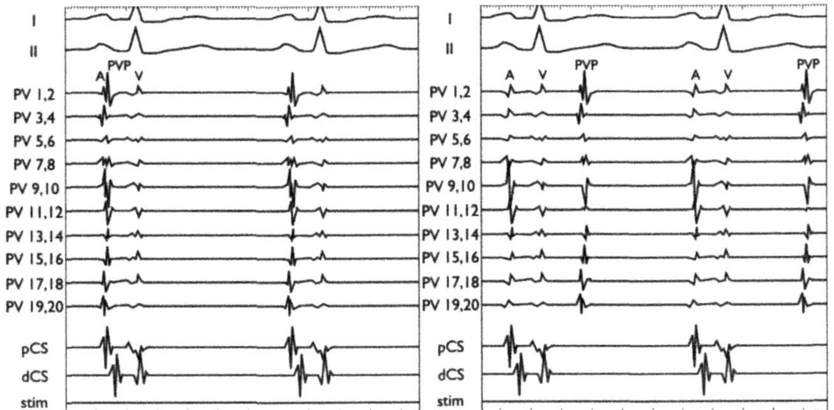

Pre-ablation – Far-field atrial EGMs with associated PVP.

Post-ablation – Spontaneous PVP dissociation.

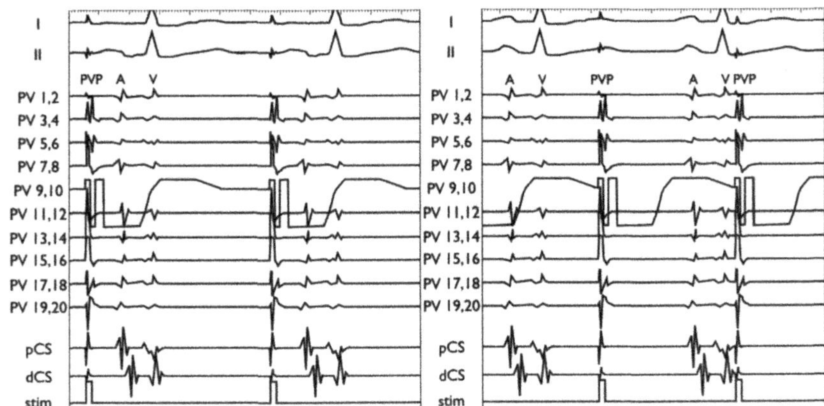

Pre-ablation – Pacing from PV 9–10 captures the PV followed by conduction into the atrium.

Post-ablation – Pacing from PV 9–10 captures the PV without conduction into the atrium.

  - Difficulties in assessing an entrance block with PV pacing
    - The uneven distribution of myocardial sleeves necessitates pacing from all bipoles around the PV circumference to ensure exit block has been achieved.
    - Local PV capture must be verified to differentiate a true exit block from "pseudo-exit block" (apparent exit blok due to PV non-capture).
    - The minimum effective pacing output must be used in order to avoid inadvertent far-field capture, which results in misinterpretation of apparent exit conduction.
      - LAA capture during pacing from the anterior bipoles of the LSPV CMC
      - LA capture during pacing from the posterior bipoles of the LIPV CMC
      - RA/SVC capture during pacing from the anterior bipoles of a RSPV CMC
    - If local PV capture is obscured by the stimulus artifact, programmed stimulation can be performed to unmask the local PV EGM (via decremental conduction at the LA-PV junction).

Determinants of Success

- Post-isolation observation period for spontaneous PV reconnection
  - A minimum 20 minutes is required.
    - There is some evidence suggesting an incremental yield up to 90 minutes.
- Pace capture
  - Procedure
    - High-output pacing (10 mAmp/2ms) from the ablation catheter's distal bipole is performed while slowly moving the catheter along the entire circumference of the index ablation line.
  - Interpretation
    - The presence of a local LA capture indicates incomplete ablation and/or a residual gap in the line.
      - Additional ablation should be delivered until the local capture is no longer elicited.
    - Complete loss of local LA capture correlates with an entrance block in approximately 95%.
      - Note: Local EGM amplitude does not correlate with pace capture sites.
- Adenosine 12–18 mg IV
  - IV adenosine causes PV hyperpolarization resulting in:
    - **No dormant conduction**: The resting membrane potential is hyperpolarized but remains above the threshold; thus, it does not demonstrate a resumption of conduction.
    - **Dormant conduction**: The resting membrane potential is hyperpolarized below the threshold, resulting in a resumption of conduction (i.e., acute PV reconnection).
      - Dormant conduction can be demonstrated in 35%–50% of treated PVs.
      - Its presence is predictive of spontaneous, time-dependent PV reconnection as well 1-year recurrence of AF.
      - Elimination is associated with improved long-term outcomes.
  - Procedure
    - Place the circular mapping catheter in the PV of interest.
    - Administer IV adenosine 12–18 mg with a saline push.
    - Ensure at least one blocked P wave or a sinus pause for ≥3 seconds.
    - Sites of dormant conduction, as defined by the reappearance of PV activity for ≥1 beat, should be targeted for ablation until the dormant conduction can no longer be elicited.
    - These steps should be repeated for each PV.
- Isoproterenol infusion
  - To facilitate the identification of non-PV triggers
    - Potential sites: SVC, LA free wall, LAA, CS os, ligament of Marshall, crista terminalis, RA free wall, interatrial septum, persistent left SVC
  - More frequently found in:
    - Female patients, patients with non-paroxysmal AF, patients with more advanced atrial substrate (i.e., dilated or electrically abnormal atrial tissue), and those with more comorbidities

- Procedure
  - Catheters: CMC in LAA, CMC in SVC, decapolar catheter in CS, decapolar in inferior RA
  - In sinus rhythm, isoproterenol (up to 50 mcg/min) is started until PACs triggering AF are noted (may require BP support).
  - The mapping catheter should be displaced toward the observed trigger origin site.
  - Cardioversion should then be performed.
  - AF re-induction should be repeated until the origin site is located.

Advanced Techniques

- Strategies to improve catheter contact:
  - Conduct an anatomic assessment with pre-procedure imaging.
  - Identify unusual variants, recessed carina, and PV orientation.
    - **LCPV**: If there is a posteriorly directed position, aim for a posterior transseptal puncture.
    - **LSPV**: If there is a high/roof take off, aim for a high transseptal puncture.
    - **RIPV**: If there is a septal position aim for a mid transseptal puncture, and avoid a high or anterior transseptal puncture (results in an inability to reach the PV), or a posterior transseptal puncture (falling into the RA).
  - Use a steerable sheath or a bidirectional catheter.
  - Decrease respiratory movement with either periodic apnea or jet ventilation.
- Mapping sites of PV breakthrough
  - Search for the bipole with the earliest PV activation.
  - At a site of an A-PVP breakthrough, adjacent bipoles will display opposite potentials (positive in one bipole but negative in the adjacent bipole).
  - At the site of an A-PVP breakthrough, the ablation catheter should display a fractionated potential between the local A EGM and the earliest PVP.
- Failure to isolate the PVs
  - LPV–Vein of Marshall Connection
    - High output CS pacing results in simultaneous CS and LA capture followed by a PVP.
    - Low output CS pacing results in a CS-only capture (no LA capture). If PVP occurs with same timing, then a connection other than the LA exists.
  - RA–right PV connection
    - Suspect the RA–right PV connection when PVP is earlier deep in the RSPV with HRA pacing/sinus rhythm.
    - Pace the right PVs and map the exit in the RA; perform ablation at the exit in the RA.

ATRIAL FIBRILLATION (AF) ABLATION — LEFT ATRIAL LINEAR ABLATION

Roof Line

- **Indication**: A roof-dependent peri-venous flutter (MRAT)
- **Goal**: A continuous line between the superior margins of both superior PVs

Set-Up

- 3D mapping system to delineate key landmarks
  - RSPV, LSPV, and LAA
- Circumferential mapping catheter in the appendage
  - Provide a continuous pacing in order to assess conduction across the LA roof on a beat-to-beat basis.
- Irrigated RF with a long sheath
  - This improves stability and facilitates proper catheter orientation (strongly consider using a steerable sheath).

Technique

- Post PVI, a line is extended from the superior margins of the encircling PV lesions.
  - Note: The line is oriented anteriorly to minimize the risk of esophageal injury.
- Possible approaches:
  - **Direct extension** from the LSPV to RSPV using a superiorly oriented catheter (perpendicular to the roof).
    - Extend the line inferiorly and septally via clockwise rotation and catheter flexion.
  - **Large loop** (parallel tip): Catheter is looped around the lateral, inferior, septal, and then cranial walls before entering the LSPV ostia.
    - Withdrawal of the catheter drags a line back from the LSPV to the RSPV.
  - **Small loop** (parallel tip): The catheter is maximally deflected near the left superior PV so that the tip is facing the right PV.
    - Releasing the curve positions the catheter tip adjacent to the right superior PV ostia and allows dragging as the sheath/catheter assembly is pushed toward the LSPV.

Ablation

- **Power**: 30 Watts if catheter tip is perpendicular; 25 Watts if catheter tip is parallel (due to risk of "popping")
- Temperature limit of 43°C with irrigation of 7–30 mL/min
- Catheter stability during ablation is monitored by inspection of EGMs and fluoroscopy.
  - It is important to appreciate an inadvertent displacement of the catheter into the LIPV or LAA to prevent severe complications (PV stenosis or perforation/ tamponade).

Assessment of Complete Linear Block

- Widely separated local double potentials along the length of the ablation line
  - There should be no fractionated activity bridging the double potentials (i.e., gaps).
- Bidirectional block
  - With LAA pacing, the activation sequence of the posterior LA between the PVs should be:
    - Caudocranial (isolated roof line)
    - Caudocranial and right to left (roof + mitral isthmus)
  - With posterior wall pacing, the conduction time to the LAA should shorten as the pacing is moved inferiorly from the ablation line (e.g., down the posterior wall).

Mitral Isthmus Line

- **Indication**: Clockwise or counterclockwise peri-mitral flutter (MRAT)
- **Goal**: Continuous line between the lateral mitral annulus and the left inferior PV
  - This can be difficult to achieve because of the myocardial thickness as well as cooling effect of the CS.

Set-Up

- 3D mapping system to delineate key landmarks
  - LIPV, MV annulus, LAA, and CS
- Multipolar catheter in the CS
  - Anatomic landmark and a method for monitoring the impact of ablation.
  - Try to position it to bridge (or bracket) the proposed site of linear ablation.
  - Continuous pacing is needed to assess the isthmus conduction on a beat-to-beat basis.
- Irrigated RF with a long sheath
  - This improves stability and facilitates proper catheter orientation (strongly consider a steerable sheath).

Technique

- Endocardial
  - The ablation catheter is introduced through a long sheath and positioned on the lateral mitral annulus (4 o'clock in LAO) at an angle between 90° (perpendicular; poor contact) and 180° (parallel; good contact) to the plane of the CS.
  - Lesion is commenced at ventricular aspect of the lateral mitral annulus (AV ratio of 1:1 or 2:1).
  - The sheath and catheter are rotated clockwise to extend the lesion posteriorly to the ostium of the LIPV (approximately 2 o'clock in LAO).
- Epicardial (CS) ablation
  - Required in 50%–60% of cases
  - Should only be performed after complete endocardial ablation in which:
    - Evidence of persistent isthmus conduction exists.
    - Endocardial conduction delay on the ablation catheter is not seen on the adjacent CS bipole.
  - The ablation catheter is advanced into the CS to a site opposite the endocardial ablation lesions.
    - The catheter should be deflected toward the endocardium to maximize contact with the atrial side of the CS and to reduce the risk of left circumflex artery injury.
  - Local EGMs with early and/or fractionated potentials are targeted during peri-mitral flutter or continuous LAA pacing.

Ablation

- **Power**
  - Endocardial: 30–35 Watts near the LIPV; 35–40 Watts near the mitral annulus
  - Epicardial: 15–30 Watts
  - Ablation is performed at each site for 30–60 seconds (or local EGM disappearance).
- **Temperature limit** of 43°C with an irrigation of 7–30 mL/min
- Catheter stability during ablation is monitored by inspection of EGMs and fluoroscopy.
  - During endocardial ablation, it is important to appreciate inadvertent displacement of the catheter into the LIPV or LAA to prevent severe complications (PV stenosis or perforation/tamponade).

Assessment of a Complete Linear Block

- Widely separated local double potentials along the length of the ablation line
  - A short delay (<100 ms) between the adjacent CS pacing artifact and the local atrial potential on the other side of the line suggests the persistence of gaps.
  - There should be no fractionated activity bridging the double potentials.
- Bidirectional block
  - Pacing anterior to the line in the LA (e.g., in the LAA) results in a proximal-to-distal activation sequence along the CS (a distal to proximal CS activation will be present with intact isthmus conduction).
  - Pacing on the posterior aspect of the line via the CS results in late activation on the opposite side.
  - As the CS pacing site is moved further from the ablation line (i.e., toward the septum from distal to proximal CS), the conduction time to the anterior LA (e.g., LAA) should shorten.

Anterior Left Atrial Transsection

- **Indications**
  - Diffusely diseased anterior LA with low-amplitude activity and extensive conduction disturbance
  - Small anterior reentrant circuits that can occur in persistent or permanent AF
- **Goal**: Continuous line between the anterior mitral annulus to either the roof line or the RSPV
  - Note: This may substantially delay activation of the lateral LA and the LAA, resulting in a significant reduction in the contribution of LAA emptying.

Set-Up

- 3D mapping system to delineate key landmarks
  - LIPV, MV annulus, LAA, and CS
- Circumferential mapping catheter in the appendage
  - Continuous pacing is needed in order to assess the isthmus conduction on a beat-to-beat basis
- Irrigated RF with a long sheath
  - This improves stability and facilitates proper catheter orientation (consider a steerable sheath).

Technique

- The lesion is started at the mitral annulus.
- The ablation catheter is progressively withdrawn while the sheath is rotated counterclockwise to increase contact with the anterior and anteroseptal wall of the LA.
- At the level of the transseptal puncture, clockwise rotation is applied to the sheath, and the ablation catheter is progressively extended to the right PVs or to the roof line.

Ablation

- **Power**: 30 Watts
- Temperature limit of 43°C with irrigation of 7–30 mL/min

Assessment of Complete Linear Block

- Widely separated local double potentials along the length of the ablation line
  - There should be no fractionated activity bridging the double potentials (i.e., gaps).
- Bidirectional block
  - Pacing at the anterior LA immediately lateral to the ablation line results in activation propagating laterally and posteriorly around the mitral annulus to reach the septal LA/opposite side of the line.
  - As the anterior pacing site is moved further from the ablation line (toward the lateral LA), the conduction time to the opposite side should correspondingly shorten.

ATRIAL FIBRILLATION (AF) ABLATION — COMPLEX FRACTIONATED ATRIAL ELECTROGRAM (CFAE) ABLATION

- CFAEs are proposed to be critical anatomic regions that perpetuate reentry, and are thought to represent:
  - Regions of delayed conduction or conduction block (representing pivot or anchor points)
  - Sites of autonomic innervation, such as the major **ganglionated plexi** located at:
    - Anterior descending LA: Anterior to the LAA
    - Posterolateral LA: Along the anterior aspect of the left PVs
    - Superior LA: Posterior wall behind the LSPV and the superior LIPV
    - Posteromedial LA: Posterior wall inferior to the right PVs
    - Superior RA: Anterior RA at the RA-SVC junction
    - Posterior RA: Posterior to the RA but anterior to the right PVs

CFAE Localization

- Common CFAE sites include:
  - The interatrial septum (57%)
  - The PV ostia (40%)
  - The LA roof (near appendage; 32%)
  - The proximal CS (32%)
  - The mitral annulus (20%)
  - The posterior LA wall
- Less common sites: Crista terminalis, CTI, LAA

Characterization

- Low-voltage (usually <0.25 mV) multipotential signals with either:
  - Very short CL (<120 ms) with or without multiple potentials
  - Fractionation: Continuous perturbation in the isoelectric line for ≥70 ms
- They should exhibit relative spatial and temporal stability.

Classification

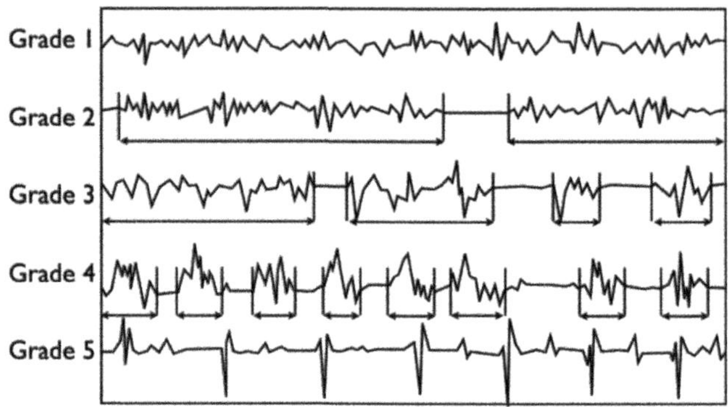

- **Grade 1**: Uninterrupted fractionated activity
  - Fractionation occupying ≥70% of sample ***and*** ≥1 uninterrupted episode lasting ≥1 second
- **Grade 2**: Interrupted fractionated activity
  - Fractionation occupying ≥70% of sample
- **Grade 3**: Intermittent fractionated activity
  - Fractionation occupying 30%–70% of sample
- **Grade 4**: Complex EGMs
  - Discrete (<70 ms) complex (≥5 direction changes) EGMs
  - Fractionation (if present must be <30% of sample)
- **Grade 5**: Normal EGM
  - Discrete (<70 ms) and simple EGMs (≤4 direction changes)
- **Grade 6**: Scar
  - No discernible deflections

Technique

- AF induction
  - Programmed stimulation: Atrial pacing at 20 mA for 5–10 second bursts down to atrial refractoriness
  - This may require pacing from multiple sites or isoproterenol infusion (up to 50 mcg/min).
- Once AF is induced, an electroanatomic map is created
  - CARTO – Interval Confidence Level (ICL)
    - Definition: The number of intervals identified between consecutive complexes identified as CFAE over a specified duration (i.e., 2.5 seconds).
    - Interpretation: The more repetitions observed (higher ICL), the more confident the categorization of CFAE

  - Settings: Threshold (0.05–0.15 mV); interval duration (50–120 ms); internal projection (4–6 mm)
    - ICL Grade: high ≥17; intermediate 10–17; low 3–9
- CARTO – Shortest or average complex interval (SCI or ACI)
  - Definition: The shortest or average interval between consecutive CFAE complexes (in ms) observed over a specified duration (i.e., 2.5 seconds)
  - Interpretation: The shorter the interval, the more confident the categorization of CFAE
  - Settings: Threshold (0.05–0.15 mV); interval duration (50–120 ms); internal projection (4–6 mm)
    - **ACI** Grade: high 50–70; intermediate 70–90; low 90–120
- NavX – Fractionation index
  - Definition: The (time between multiple, discrete deflections (–dV/dT; inter-deflection time intervals) is averaged to calculate a mean CL of the local EGM during AF.
  - Interpretation: The shorter the mean CL, the more rapid and fractionated the local EGM.
  - Settings (see Table 9.7)

Table 9.7 Proposed Settings for Mapping CFAE with NavX

Parameter	Rationale	Setting
Peak-to-peak sensitivity	Minimum detection threshold (used to avoid noise)	0.03–0.05 mV
EGM refractory period	Avoids double-counting of multiphasic EGMs	35–45 ms
EGM width	Avoids detection of broader, far-field EGMs	15–20 ms
EGM segment length	Total recording duration at each point Obtains a mean CL for that point	5 seconds
Interpolation	Maximum distance between points used to assign average values for a vertex	4–6 mm
Internal/external projection	Avoids collection of EGMs from electrodes that are not in good contact with map shell	4–6 mm

Lesion Endpoint

- Ablation should commence at regions with the highest-grade CFAE (shortest CL and greatest degree of fractionation) and continued until the adjacent EGMs have attenuated.
- Note: Ablation at sites of ganglionic plexi may elicit severe bradycardia or even prolonged asystole.
  - The ablation lesion should be completed (if necessary with temporary pacing), because these vagal reactions are generally associated with favorable procedural outcomes.

Procedural Endpoints

- Paroxysmal AF
  - Non-inducibility of sustained AF (>5–10 minutes) or other atrial tachyarrhythmias
- Persistent AF
  - Slowing and termination of AF to sinus rhythm (occurs in <40%) or an organized AT requiring further mapping/ablation to restore sinus rhythm
    - The failure to terminate AF with an ablation does not preclude a successful outcome.
    - Inducibility of AF in persistent cases has limited predictive value.
- If ablation fails to achieve the endpoints, then:
  - Conduct further mapping of less common CFAE sites.
  - Revisit the previously ablated regions to ensure no recovery of conduction.
  - Consider intravenous Ibutilide (1 mg over 10 min) or procainamide (1 g over 10–30 min) to increase the CL of the arrhythmia in bystander regions.

RECURRENT ATRIAL TACHYARRHYTHMIAS AFTER ATRIAL FIBRILLATION (AF) ABLATION

General Information

- Re-do ablation procedures are required in 20%–40% of paroxysmal AF and >50% of persistent AF ablations.
- Causes
  - **PV Reconnection**
  - **Non-PV triggers**
  - **Macroreentrant tachycardia**: CTI, roof, peri-mitral

Classification

- Early recurrence
  - Recurrence appears within the first 1–3 months post ablation.
  - It may represent the sequelae of acute inflammation and tissue healing.
  - It does not implicate treatment failure (50% of those with early recurrence will have no late recurrence).
  - In general, the earlier the early recurrence appears, the better the long-term prognosis.
- Late recurrence
  - Arrhythmia recurrence after 3 months post ablation procedure represents treatment failure.

12-Lead ECG

- Recurrent AF vs. atrial tachycardia

Other Investigations

- As per AT/AF/AFL sections

Management

- As per AT/AF/AFL sections

Ablation of Recurrent Atrial Tachyarrhythmias After AF Ablation

Approach to Arrhythmia Localization

- ECG localization of the arrhythmia focus
  - As per the AT section (See Table 7.1)
- Examine the CS activation sequence (see Table 9.8).

Table 9.8 CS Activation Sequence in FAT and MRAT

	Right Atrium	Left Atrium	
		FAT	MRAT
Proximal to distal	**FAT**: any **MRAT**: any	PV tachycardia (RSPV, RIPV) FAT: Interatrial septum or right-sided LA FAT with previous mitral isthmus line	Counterclockwise peri-mitral flutter Roof-dependent flutter around right PVs
Distal to proximal	–	PV tachycardia (LSPV, LIPV) FAT (left-sided LA)	Clockwise peri-mitral flutter Roof-dependent flutter around left PVs
Flat	–	FAT (roof or posterior wall)	Roof-dependent flutter

FAT: focal atrial tachyarrthmia.

- Assess the CS CL variability
  - **TCL variability** = (longest CL: shortest CL) / mean TCL over 1 minute
  - Interpretation:
    - >15% variability (suggests focal origin)
    - <15% variability (suggests macroreentrant or focal origin)
- Exclude PV reconnection
  - Ensure complete isolation of all four PVs
    - Gaps most often occur in the:
      - Anterior LSPV (adjacent to the LAA)
      - Left PV carina (inferior aspect of the LSPV, superior aspect of the LIPV)
      - RSPV roof and posterior wall
    - Consider adenosine testing pre-ablation to determine if apparently electrically silent PVs are truly isolated
  - If the PV is causal of the AT:
    - The PVP will precede atrial activation (in the other veins it will be A before PVP).
    - PV re-isolation will lead to restoration of sinus rhythm or transition to another AT.
- Activation mapping and entrainment of organized tachycardia
  - As outlined above for the AT section

Approach to Ablation

- Any PV exhibiting reconnection should be re-ablated at antral breakthrough sites.
- Gaps in linear lesions should be mapped and ablated to restore bidirectional conduction block.
- Consider empiric CFAE, linear ablation ("stepwise" approach) and/or targeting of non-PV triggers.

COMPLETE ATRIOVENTRICULAR (AV) NODE ABLATION

Indication

- A complete AVN ablation occurs when the rate control of chronic symptomatic AF is refractory to medical therapy (especially in older individuals).

Anticipated Success

- Palliative procedure (does not eliminate AF)
  - This results in symptom improvement in >85%, but patients are rendered pacemaker dependent.
  - Acute success is seen in 95%–100% with a chronic success in 90%–100%.

Anticipated Complications

- Similar to all invasive ablation procedures
- If left-sided approach required:
  - Arterial bleeding
  - Thromboembolism (myocardial infarction, stroke, systemic)
  - Aortic valve, aorta, or coronary damage
- Polymorphic ventricular tachycardia (VT) and sudden cardiac death (SCD): A rate-related complication may occur in those with a history of rapid, uncontrolled AF.
  - It can be alleviated by pacing at rates >75–80 bpm for ≥2 months post-AVN ablation.

Permanent Pacemaker Management

- Temporary pacing and AV junction ablation followed by permanent pacemaker implantation
  - Prior to AVN ablation, a temporary pacemaker is placed in the RVa.
  - Post AVN ablation, a permanent pacemaker is implanted.
  - Disadvantages
    - Risks are associated with an acute pacemaker malfunction (or acute lead dislodgment) in a patient rendered pacemaker-dependent post AVN ablation.
    - There is a risk of unforeseen problems with pacemaker placement (i.e., inability to implant) in a patient rendered pacemaker-dependent post AVN ablation.
  - A subclavian approach allows a simultaneous pacemaker implant and AV junction ablation without a femoral puncture.
  - After the RV lead placement, the ablation catheter can be advanced through a second sheath in the subclavian vein.

- Permanent pacemaker implantation and subsequent AV junction ablation
  - Implantation of a permanent pacemaker system several weeks prior to AVN ablation
  - Disadvantages
    - There is a risk of displacing the pacemaker lead during the catheter ablation procedure.
    - Delays the achievement of rate control

Set-Up

- Consider a quadripolar catheter in the RV (backup pacing)
- Irrigated or non-irrigated RF catheter: B-curve (small/red), D-curve (medium/blue), or F-curve (large/orange)

Mapping

- Right-sided (venous) approach
  - The D-curve (medium/blue) or F-curve (large/orange) catheter is deflected slightly and advanced into the RV in the RAO projection.
  - In LAO projection, the catheter is relaxed and torqued clockwise to maintain septal contact along the superior-medial TV annulus.
    - **Initial**: In this location, the large atrial, His, and V EGMs should be simultaneously recorded.
  - The catheter is gradually withdrawn towards the atrium to an anatomic position that is proximal and inferior to the standard His bundle recording position.
    - **Final**: In this location, a relatively large A EGM with a small V EGM ($A \geq V$) ± small His (<0.15 mV) should be seen.
  - Note: The catheter tip may again need to be deflected slightly to follow the course of the AV conduction system and to stop the catheter from prolapsing out into the high right atrium.
- Left-sided (arterial) approach
  - A diagnostic catheter is placed on the right side in the His position to guide ablation.
  - The B-curve (small/red) (normal LV) or D-curve (medium/blue) (dilated LV) catheter is positioned across the AV valve via retrograde access.
    - The catheter can be retroverted, rotated towards the septum, and then withdrawn towards the AV to a basal-septal position below the non-coronary cusp.
    - Alternatively, the catheter can be straightened to the inferior apical septum and then withdrawn to a basal-septal position below the non-coronary cusp.
  - Map the area to find a left-sided His (it should occur concurrent to the right-sided His; HV 30–40 ms).
    - Note: The left bundle potential is located 1–1.5 cm below the His; it occurs later (i.e., HV <20 ms), and is associated with an A:V ratio of <1:10 (i.e., absent or very small A EGM).

AVN Ablation During Atrial Fibrillation

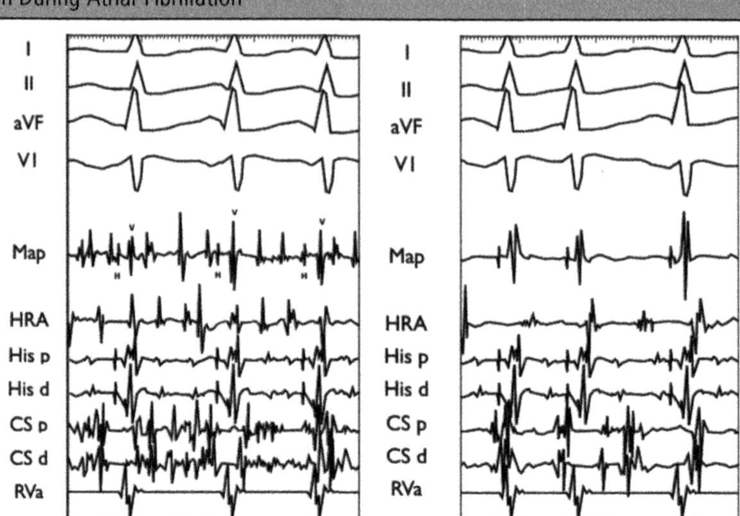

Left panel: Right-sided (venous) approach with a balanced A and V EGM with a small His.
Right panel: Left-sided (arterial) approach with a large V EGM and His with small A.

Ablation

- RF application
  - **Non-irrigated RF**: 50–60 Watts for 30–60 seconds (target temperature 55–65°C)
  - **Irrigated RF**: 25–35 Watts for 30–60 seconds (target temperature 43°C)
- At successful sites, an accelerated junction rhythm appears within a few seconds.
  - Similar to that seen with AVNRT, an initially faster rate is followed by a slowing.
  - A complete heart block usually appears within 5–10 seconds.
  - Ablation can then be consolidated with a further 60 seconds of ablation.

Determinants of Success

- Complete heart block with junctional escape (30–50 bpm)

Advanced Techniques

- Inability to record a clear His signal
  - Causes
    - Anatomic: Intramyocardial course of the His, Scar/fibrosis
    - Electric: Continuous atrial electrical activity in AF may obscure the His.
  - Strategies
    - Cardioversion (if in AF and adequately anticoagulated)
    - Systematically search the superior and inferior septum.
    - Pace from the ablation catheter looking for QRS narrowing (His penetration).

- Anatomic ablation on the right and/or left-side with irrigated/large-tip ablation catheters
  - Aim for a line of ablation along the septum in the vicinity of the AVN tissue.
  - Note: Ineffective ablation lesions may create edema, rendering the His even more difficult to penetrate.

- Failure to achieve complete AV block despite clear His signals
  - Causes and solutions
    - Instability/poor tissue contact: Use a long sheath (right-sided ablation).
    - Distal ablation (i.e., ablation of the right bundle): Perform the ablation more proximally.
    - Ineffective penetration: Do an ablation of both bundle branches or within the non-coronary cusp.

CHAPTER

10

Ventricular Tachycardia

UNDERSTANDING AND MANAGING VENTRICULAR TACHYCARDIA (VT)

General Information

- Tachyarrhythmia of ventricular origin (originates distal to the bifurcation of the bundle of His) at a rate >120 bpm
- **Non-sustained:** ≥3–5 beats in duration but self-terminates within 30 seconds.
- **Sustained:** ≥30 seconds or requires termination due to hemodynamic instability within 30 seconds.
- **Complex ventricular ectopy:** >10 premature ventricular contractions (PVCs)/hour, couplets, triplets, or non-sustained VT
  - Complex ventricular ectopy confers an increased risk of death if found in association with a structurally abnormal heart; there is no increased risk for a normal heart.

Epidemiology and Clinical Features

- Tolerability depends on the rate, cardiac function, and peripheral compensation.
- **Asymptomatic** (with or without electrocardiogram (ECG) changes)
  - Usually due to a slower VT (rate <200 bpm)
- Potential symptoms attributable to ventricular arrhythmias include:
  - **Palpitations**: Usually paroxysmal
  - **Presyncope**: Dizziness, light-headedness, feeling faint, "greying out"
  - **Syncope**: A sudden loss of consciousness with loss of postural tone with spontaneous recovery may be associated with myoclonic jerks mimicking seizure.
  - Chest pain, dyspnea, and/or fatigue are usually related to underlying heart disease.
- Sudden cardiac death

Anatomy and Physiology (Mechanism)

- Pathophysiologic mechanisms of VT (see Table 10.1)

Table 10.1 Mechanisms of Ventricular Tachycardia

	Reentry	Abnormal Automaticity	Triggered Activity
VT morphology	Monomorphic	Monomorphic or polymorphic	Monomorphic or polymorphic
Onset/ termination	Abrupt	"Warm-up/cool-down"	"Warm-up/cool-down"
Inducible at EPS	Inducible • Programmed stimulation	Not inducible	Inducible • Initiated by adrenergic activation and rapid rates • Terminated by verapamil, diltiazem, and/or adenosine
Etiology	Underlying heart disease with myocardial scarring (permanent substrate) or acute ischemia	Metabolic changes • Ischemia, hypoxemia • ↓ Mg, ↓ K • Acid-base disturbances	Pause-dependent • Phase 3 (early afterdepolarization [EAD]) Catecholamine-dependent • Phase 4 (delayed afterdepolarization [DAD])
Risk	Permanent substrate	Reversible substrate	Permanent (genetic or heart disease) or reversible (e.g., due to drug or electrolyte imbalance) substrate

Classification

Monomorphic VT

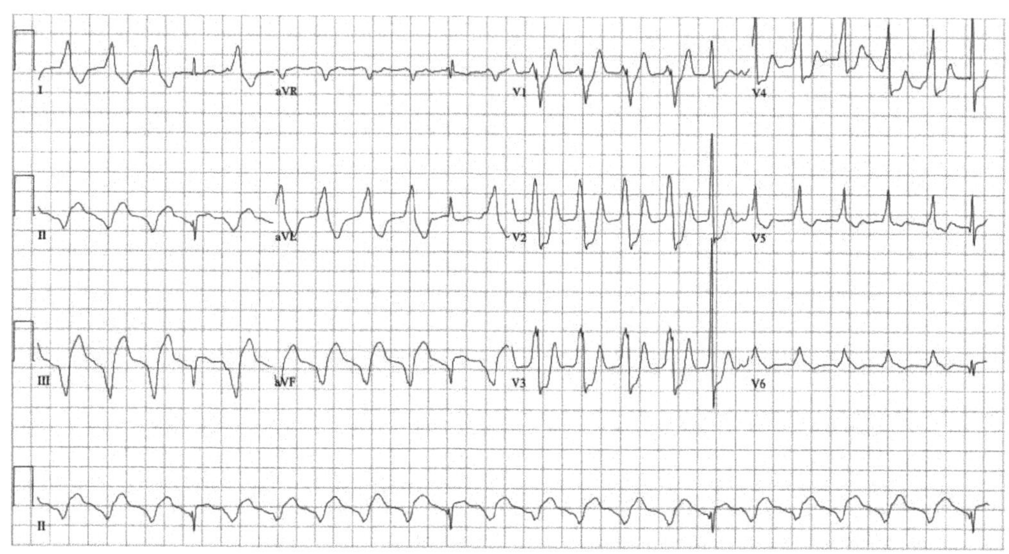

- Single QRS morphology
- Etiology and classification:
  - Reentrant VT
    - Scar-related: Slow conduction from myocardial fibrosis or scar
      - Old myocardial infarction (MI)
      - Dilated cardiomyopathy (DCM)
      - Arrhythmogenic right ventricular cardiomyopathy (ARVC)
      - Congenital heart disease with surgical scar (e.g., Tetralogy of Fallot)
    - Reentry within the conduction system
      - Fascicular VT (left posterior fascicular VT most common)
      - Bundle branch reentry (ischemic cardiomyopathy or non-ischemic DCM with associated His-Purkinje disease)
  - Enhanced automaticity
    - Primary (idiopathic) VT
      - Outflow tract VT (75%): Right ventricular outflow tract (RVOT)-VT, left ventricular outflow tract (LVOT)-VT, aortic cusp VT
      - Non-outflow tract VT: Papillary muscle, mitral annular, tricuspid annular
      - Acute post MI or surgery (myocardial injury)
  - Triggered activity
    - Acute post MI (usually arising near the His-Purkinje system)

Polymorphic VT

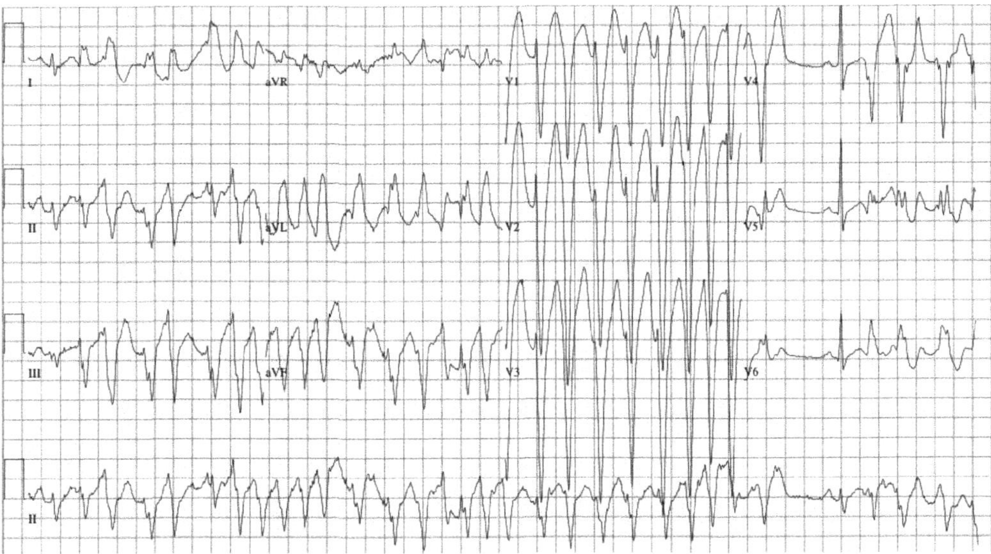

- Unstable VT with beat-to-beat QRS morphology variation (cycle length [CL] between 180 and 600 ms)
- Etiology and classification:
  - Normal baseline QT
    - Pathophysiology
      - Can be due to reentry (e.g., acute MI, often degenerates to ventricular fibrillation [VF]), delayed afterdepolarization (e.g., catecholaminergic polymorphic VT (CPVT))
      - Related to conditions of high sympathetic tone

    - Etiology
        - Acute ischemia (multiple reentrant circuits; abnormal automaticity)
        - Channelopathies: Catecholaminergic polymorphic VT, Brugada syndrome, idiopathic polymorphic VT (PMVT)/VF
- Prolonged baseline QT
    - Torsades de pointes
        - Defined as a PMVT with a QRS amplitude and cardiac axis rotation over a sequence of 5–20 beats.
        - Usually it is not sustained but recurs if the underlying cause is not corrected.
    - Pathophysiology
        - Due to early afterdepolarization
        - **Typical variant:** Initiated by "short-long-short" coupling intervals (pause-dependent, typical for drug-induced)
        - **Short coupled variant:** Initiated by "normal-short" coupling (induced by stress or startle, typical for congenital syndromes, adrenergic dependent)
    - Etiology
        - Acquired prolonged QT: Drugs (class Ia, III antiarrhythmic drug [AAD], phenothiazines, tricyclic antidepressant [TCA]), low Mg, or K
        - Congenital prolonged QT
- Short QT syndrome

Ventricular Fibrillation (VF)

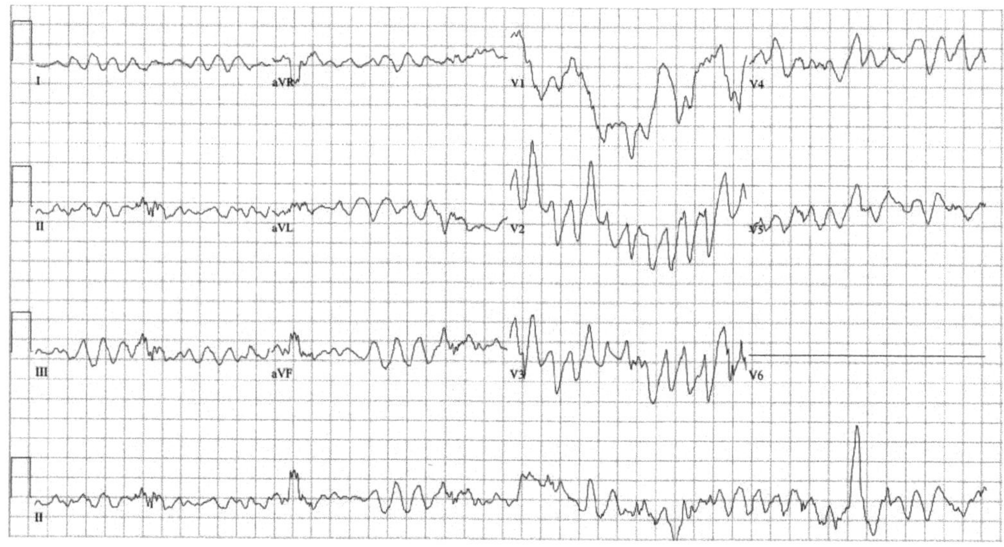

- Chaotic, rapid, disorganized wide-complex tachyarrhythmia (>300 bpm)
- Thought to be due to multiple reentrant wavefronts within the ventricle (wavelet hypothesis).
- All VT may degrade to VF.
- Etiology of primary VF is similar to polymorphic VT.

12-Lead ECG

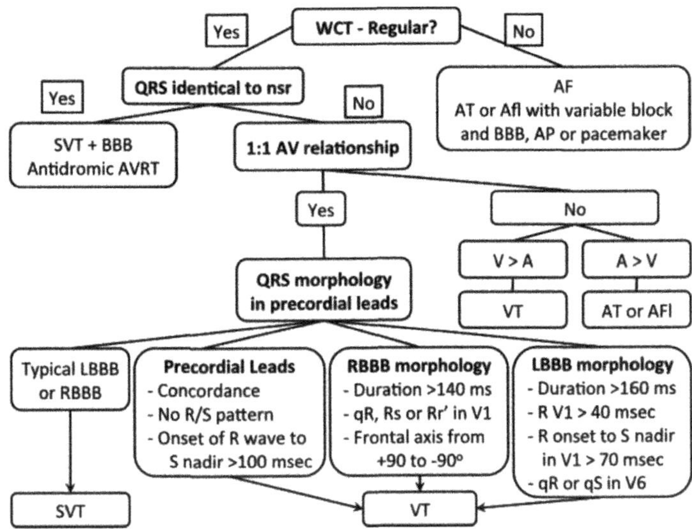

WCT: wide-complex tachycardia; SVT: supraventricular tachycardia; AVRT: atrioventricular reciprocating tachycardia; LBBB: left bundle branch block; RBBB: right bundle branch block.

- Ventricular rate 120–300 bpm (usually around 170)
- P waves
  - AV dissociation (complete AV block) or retrograde P waves (intact VA conduction)
- Axis
  - Change in axis of >40° from baseline or extreme (right superior) axis deviation
- QRS morphology and duration
  - Left bundle branch morphology (Negative QRS complex in V1 – QS, rS) >160 ms
  - Right bundle branch morphology (Positive QRS complex in V1 – qR, R, Rs, RSR′) >140 ms
  - Variable with relatively narrow complexes in fascicular tachycardia (110–140 ms)
    - Right bundle with left axis: Left anterior fascicular tachycardia
    - Right bundle with right axis: Left posterior fascicular tachycardia

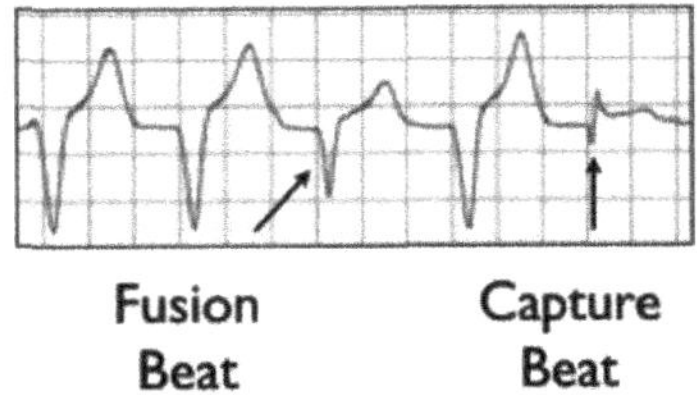

- **Fusion beat** (almost pathognomonic of VT; generally only occurs with rates <160 bpm)
  - A hybrid QRS is a result of the combination of normal atrial conduction down the His-Purkinje system and cell-to-cell conduction of a ventricular impulse.
  - Fusion beats can also occur with PVC, ventricular escape, accelerated idioventricular rhythm, and Wolff-Parkinson-White syndrome (WPW).

- **Capture beat** (pathognomonic of VT; generally only occurs with rates <160 bpm)
  - Atrial impulse induces ventricular activation via the normal conduction system, resulting in a normal narrow QRS that is earlier than expected in the cardiac cycle.
- See page 91 about the differentiation of VT from SVT
- When describing VT, it is important to comment on:
  - **Duration**: Non-sustained or sustained (lasts >30 seconds or associated with hemodynamic instability)
  - **Variability**: Monomorphic or polymorphic
  - **Ventricular rate**
  - **QRS morphology**: Left or right bundle branch block morphology
  - **Axis**: Right/inferior or left/superior

Localizing the Exit Site

- QRS morphology
  - Left bundle morphology (negative QRS complex in V1: QS, rS): RV or LV septum
  - Right bundle morphology (positive QRS complex in V1: qR, R, Rs, RSR′): LV
- Axis
  - Superior (negative in II, III, aVF): Inferior wall or inferior septum
  - Inferior (positive in II, III, aVF): Anterior wall or anterior septum
  - Rightward: Lateral LV wall or apex
- Precordial transition
  - Left bundle morphology VT
    - **≤V3**: Basal LV; RV septum
    - **≥V4**: Apical LV; RV free wall
    - Negative concordance (all negative QRS V1–V6): Apical LV
  - Right bundle morphology VT (reverse transition)
    - ≤V2: Basal LV
    - V3–V4: Mid cavity LV
    - ≥V5: Apical LV
    - Positive concordance (all positive QRS V1–V6): Mitral valve apparatus
- Variants and other features:
  - Outflow tract VT (~LBBB morphology with an inferior axis)
    - V1, V2 R-wave duration
      - >50% of QRS: LVOT (left coronary cusp)
      - <50% of QRS: RVOT or LVOT (right coronary cusp)
    - V2 R:S ratio
      - >1: left ventricular outflow tract (LVOT)
      - <1: right ventricular outflow tract (RVOT)
    - QRS transition in tachycardia compared to normal sinus rhythm (NSR)
      - Earlier transition in NSR: RVOT
      - Earlier transition in PVC/VT: LVOT
    - Localization within the RVOT (see Table 10.2)

Table 10.2 12-Lead ECG Characteristics of VT with a RVOT Focus

	Anterior	Posterior	Middle	Septum	RV Free Wall
Precordial R/S transition	—	—	—	≤V3	≥V4
Lead I and aVL	Neg. (qs or rS)	Pos. (R or Rs)	Pos. (rs or qrs)	Neg.	Pos.
II, III, aVF	—	—	—	Monophasic	Notching

- Localization of LV Basal VT: RBBB morphology (see Table 10.3)

Table 10.3 12-Lead ECG Characteristics of VT with a LV Basal Origin and RBBB Morphology

	Lead I	Lead V1	Precordial Transition
Septal/parahisian	R or Rs	QS or Qr	Early (≤V2)
Aorto-mitral continuity	Rs or rs	qR	Positive concordance
Superior mitral annulus	rs or rS	R or Rs	Positive concordance
Superolateral mitral annulus	rS or QS	R or Rs	Positive concordance
Lateral mitral annulus	rS or rs	R or Rs	Positive concordance
Papillary muscle	No Q	qR or R	

- Epicardial VT
  - QRS duration >198 ms
  - The initial portion of the QRS is delayed.
    - Pseudo-delta wave ≥34 ms (QRS onset to earliest sharp deflection in any lead)
    - Intrinsicoid deflection in V2 ≥85 ms (QRS onset to earliest S wave nadir)
    - RS complex duration >121 ms (QRS onset to earliest R wave peak in any lead)
    - Maximum deflection index >55% (QRS onset to peak R or S wave nadir/ QRS duration)
  - Localizing the epicardial exit site
    - QS in I or aVL: Anterolateral/lateral LV
    - QS in II, III, aVF: Inferior (near the middle cardiac vein)
    - Loss of R from V1 to V2 then prominent R in V3 (near the anterior interventricular vein)

Other Investigations

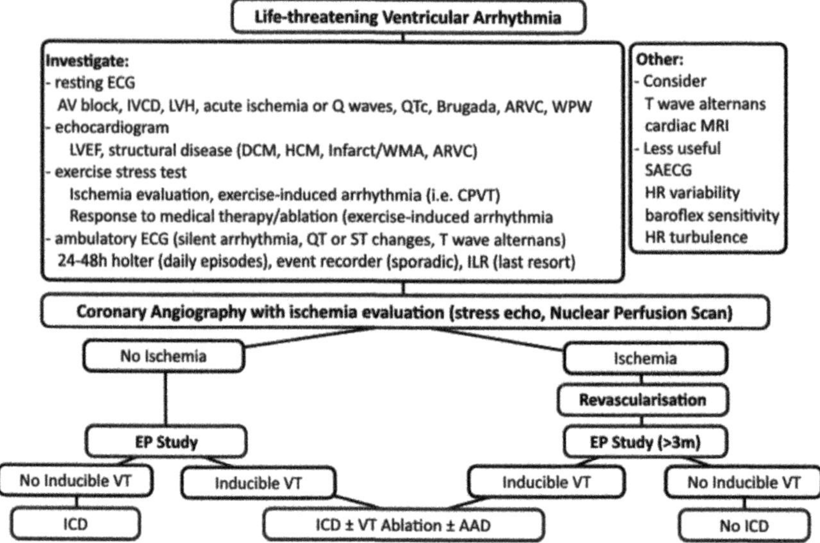

ARVC: arrhythmogenic RV cardiomyopathy; CPVT: catecholaminergic polymorphic ventricular tachycardia; DCM: dilated cardiomyopathy; HCM: hypertrophic cardiomyopathy; HR: heart rate; ILR: insertable looprecorder; IVCD: intraventricular conduction delay; LVEF: LV ejection fraction; LVH: LV hypertrophy; MRI: magnetic resonance imaging; SAECG: signal averaged ECG; WMA: wall motion abnormality; WPW: Wolff-Parkinson-White syndrome.

Management

Acute Management

- Non-sustained VT and PVCs
  - No evidence that suppression of non-sustained VT (NSVT) prolongs life except with very rapid or repetitive (incessant) NSVT that compromises hemodynamic stability.
  - First-line therapy
    - β-blockers
  - Second-line therapy
    - Amiodarone + β-blockers
    - Sotalol
    - Catheter ablation
- Sustained monomorphic VT
  - First-line therapy
    - Direct-current cardioversion (DCCV)
  - Second-line therapy
    - IV procainamide is a reasonable alternative; use with caution if it is congestive heart failure (CHF) or hypotension.
    - IV lidocaine: This is more effective if the cause is ischemic.
    - IV amiodarone
      - Hemodynamically unstable, refractory to cardioversion, or recurrent despite AAD
    - Transvenous pace-termination
      - Refractory to cardioversion, recurrent despite medical therapy
- Polymorphic VT with a normal baseline QTc
  - First-line therapy
    - DCCV

- Adjunctive therapy
  - IV β-blockers
  - IV amiodarone
  - Note: Calcium-channel blockers (CCB) may be effective for DAD (caused by inward calcium current).
  - For Brugada or idiopathic VF consider IV isoproterenol infusion (target HR >100–120 bpm) or PO quinidine.

- Polymorphic VT with a prolonged baseline QTc
  - Treat the underlying cause.
    - Remove offending or unnecessary drugs (including AAD).
    - Treat ischemia.
    - Electrolyte abnormalities (keep K^+ >4.0–4.5 mmol/L)
  - Adjunctive therapy
    - IV magnesium sulfate
      - This is only useful with prolonged baseline QTc.
    - Pacing
      - Overdrive pacing (acute)
      - Chronic pacing: Pause-dependent TdP
    - Isoproterenol
      - IV infusion to a target HR >100–120 bpm
    - IV lidocaine or mexilitine
      - LQT3 with TdP

Chronic Management

Table 10.4 Strategies for Chronic Management of Ventricular Arrhythmias

	Polymorphic VT/VF <48 h After Revascularization or Monomorphic VT in a Structurally Normal Heart	Polymorphic VT/VF >48 h After Revascularization or Monomorphic VT in a Structurally Abnormal Heart (LVEF <40%)
Risk of recurrence	Low	High (20%–30% mortality)
ICD	No benefit (<40d post MI: CABG-PATCH, DINAMIT, IRIS)	Major benefit (CIDS, AVIS, CASH)
Medical therapy	β-blocker (76% RRR) ± amiodarone (CASCADE, EMIAT/CAMIAT: ↓ VF/SCD but did not alter mortality post MI) Sotalol (use with caution in severe CHF or LV dysfunction)	β-blockers (first-line) If arrhythmia/shock • Add amiodarone (load then 200 mg/d: OPTIC) *If resistant:* • Increase amiodarone to 300–400 mg/d *If still resistant:* • Consider catheter ablation (or add mexilitine) *If amiodarone side effects:* • Dofetilide ± class I or β-blockers • Sotalol ± class I
Other	Verapamil > Propafenone	**Catheter ablation** (see below) **Surgical resection** (e.g., LV aneurysm) or transplant

ICD: implantable cardioverter-defibrillator; SCD: sudden cardiac death.

- Non-pharmacologic therapy
  - An ICD may be the only way to reduce the risk of death in the majority of high-risk patients.
  - Primary prevention

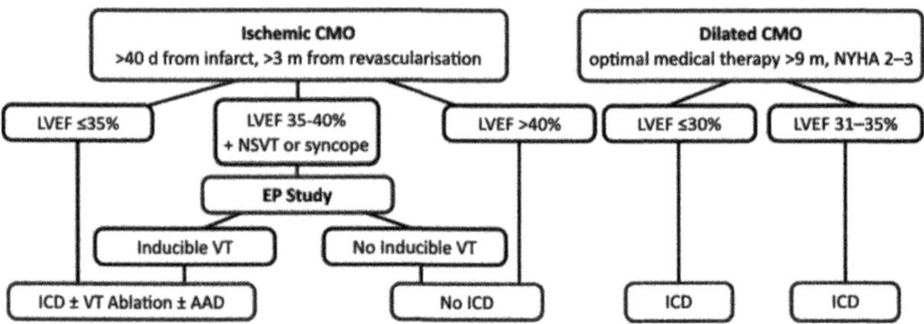

- Pharmacologic therapy
  - Suppression of ventricular ectopy with AADs does not decrease the risk of SCD.
    - **CAST:** Suppression of ambient ventricular ectopy either increased mortality (encainide, flecainide) or had no effect (moricizine).
  - Empiric amiodarone may reduce the arrhythmia burden but it does not generally reduce the risk of SCD.
    - **CHF-STAT**: 674 patients; LVEF <40%; complex ectopy
      - No difference in survival overall vs. placebo (non-ischemic dilated cardiomyopathy [NIDCM] had a trend towards increased survival)
    - **CASCADE**: 228 patients; survivors of VF arrest
      - Amiodarone resulted in less ICD shocks or syncope vs. other AAD
    - **CAMIAT**: 1202 patients; survivors of MI; complex ectopy
      - No survival benefit vs. placebo
    - **EMIAT**: 1500 patients; survivors of MI; LVEF <40%
      - No survival benefit vs. placebo
    - **SCD-HeFT**: 2521 patients; LVEF ≤35%; NYHA 2–3
      - No survival benefit with amiodarone
- Invasive therapy
  - Ablation of reentrant foci is an effective method of treating some types of VT.

CATHETER ABLATION OF VENTRICULAR TACHYCARDIA (VT)

Indications

- Frequent monomorphic PVCs and NSVT
  - This is particularly true if it is associated with LV dysfunction (LV dilatation or decline in LVEF).
- Monomorphic VT: Sustained (class I), non-sustained (class IIa)
  - Patients may be drug resistant or drug intolerant.
  - They do not want a long-term drug therapy.
- Bundle-branch reentrant VT (class I)
- Adjunctive therapy in those with an ICD (class I)
  - Patients receiving multiple shocks as a result of sustained VT that cannot be managed by device programming, changes in AAD therapy, or they do not want long-term drug therapy.

Anticipated Success

- Idiopathic ventricular tachycardia (e.g., RVOT or fascicular VT) 80%–90%, if inducible
- Bundle branch reentry: 80%–90%
- Ischemic VT: 60%–70%
- Dilated cardiomyopathy: 50% (usually requires epicardial ablation)
- ARVC: 70% (usually requires epicardial ablation)

Anticipated Complications

- Similar to all invasive ablation procedures
- 3%–5% major complications
  - Vascular access: hematoma, AV fistula, arterial pseudoaneurysm
  - Catheter manipulation: vascular damage, microemboli/stroke, coronary dissection
  - RF application: cardiac perforation/tamponade, coronary damage, AV block
- Mortality 1%–3%

Patient Preparation

- Use echocardiography (± contrast) to exclude the presence of LV thrombus (if LV ablation is anticipated).
- Stop all AAD for 5 half-lives before the procedure (especially for RVOT VT, fascicular VT).
- Conscious sedation is preferred to general anesthesia due to the risk of rendering the VT non-inducible.

Set-Up

- 3D mapping system
  - **Focal VT:** Set window to 50–80 ms prior to surface QRS onset
  - **Reentrant VT:** Set window to >90% of tachycardia cycle length
- Diagnostic catheters
  - Quadripolar catheters in right ventricular apex (RVa) and at the His
  - Deflectable decapolar in CS (reference and pacing)
- Endocardial RV VT
  - Non-irrigated RF: D-curve (medium/blue), C-curve (green), or bidirectional [D-curve (medium/blue)/F-curve (large/orange)]
  - Irrigated RF: D-curve (medium/blue) or bidirectional [D-curve (medium/blue)/F-curve (large/orange)]
  - Consider long sheath for improved stability in the RVOT (LAMP, SL0, or steerable sheath).
- Endocardial LV VT
  - Irrigated RF ablation: F-curve (large/orange), D-curve (medium/blue), J-curve (extra large/black), or bidirectional (D/F, D/J, F/J)
  - Transseptal with steerable sheath (usually large curve)
  - Arterial access for retrograde approach
- Epicardial VT (see epicardial access below)

Mapping

- Affected area depends on the underlying pathology.
  - Ischemic cardiomyopathy
    - Endocardial (90%): Reentry around the affected area (scar ± functional block)
  - Non-ischemic cardiomyopathy
    - The substrate is more frequently perivalvular or epicardial.
- General approach

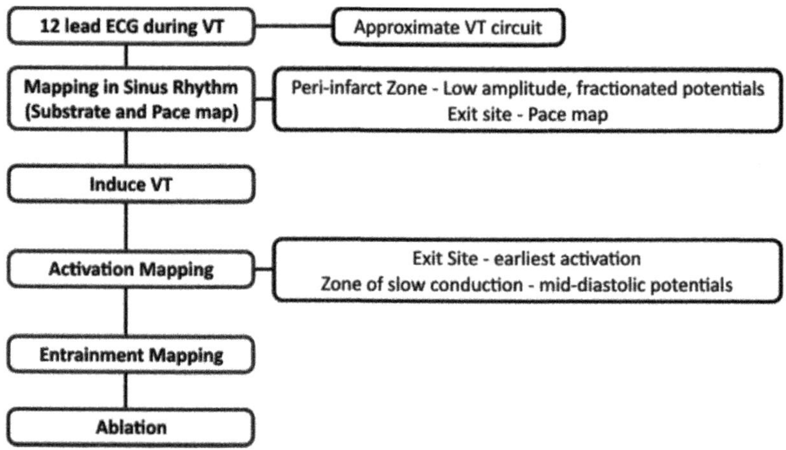

Mapping in Sinus Rhythm

- Substrate (voltage) map to define the scar
  - **Indication**: Non-inducible or hemodynamically unstable VT

Table 10.5 Electrogram-Based Definition of Myocardial Scar

	Dense Scar	Border Zone Scar			Normal
		Endocardial RV	Endocardial LV	Epicardial	
Bipolar EGM	<0.5 mV	0.5 to 1.5 mV	0.5 to 1.6–2.0 mV	0.5 to 1.0 mV	>1.5 mV
Unipolar EGM		0.5 to 5.5 mV	0.7 to 8.3 mV		

  - Adjunctive high-output pacing from ablation catheter over the scar region can help differentiate regions of excitable (viable) tissue within an unexcitable scar.
    - Failure to capture at >10 mA at 2 ms pulse width within a low voltage area may identify electrically unexcitable scars (i.e., circuit border zone).
- Pace map
  - **Indication**: A pace map can be used for any type of VT/PVC but is most useful for focal arrhythmias (idiopathic VT) where the ECG configuration is determined by the sequence of activation.
    - A pace map can be used to approximate the exit site for scar-related VT.

- Process
    - A 12-lead ECG obtained during tachycardia (or of the PVC) is compared to a 12-lead ECG obtained during pacing at the tachycardia CL or PVC coupling interval.
    - Some recording and mapping systems have automated matching algorithms.
- Interpretation
    - Matching QRS in ≥10 leads is considered an adequate pace map for the RF application.

- Late potential and abnormal electrogram (EGM) mapping
    - These include a sharp ventricular potential (high frequency and low amplitude) that is temporally distinct from the far field ventricular (V) EGM.
    - In the sinus, this potential occurs during (or after) the V EGM, but in VT it should occur before the V EGM.
    - This potential represents poorly coupled cells in an area of scar (i.e., slow conduction).

Mapping in Tachycardia

- Time from QRS onset to RVa catheter (RBBB-morphology VT)
    - >120 ms: Suggests LV lateral wall VT
    - <100 ms: Suggests LV septal VT
- Activation mapping
    - **Indication**: Performed during tachycardia (must be hemodynamically stable)
    - The earliest site of ventricular activation (sharp bipolar EGM, or initial negative unipolar deflection) on the distal electrode relative to the surface QRS onset (or stable reference).
        - Ischemic VT: Activation time ≥70 ms before QRS onset are considered early.
        - Idiopathic VT: Rarely have activation times earlier than 40 ms.

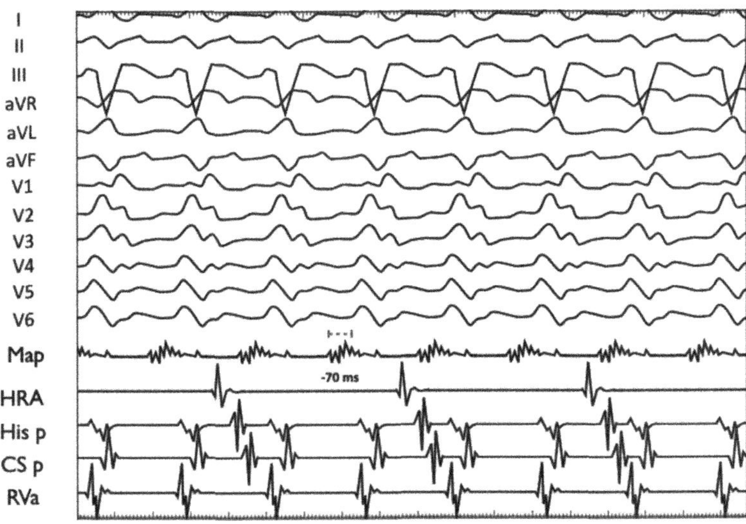

Activation mapping during monomorphic ventricular tachycardia demonstrating a fragmented presystolic electrical activity occurring approximately 70 ms before QRS onset.

- Diastolic potentials
  - Diastolic potentials are discrete (small) electrical signals occurring approximately 10–100 ms before the major ventricular deflection (during the isoelectric segment).
  - They represent the activation of a zone of slow conduction within circuit (the diastolic pathway)
    - The activation should precede all tachycardia complexes during the initiation and reset of tachycardia.
    - There is a loss of potential with termination of the arrhythmia.
    - Note: Continuous activation during the diastolic period represents slow/fractionated conduction in diseased myocardium may not be an essential area of the circuit, thus pacing maneuvers are required for confirmation.

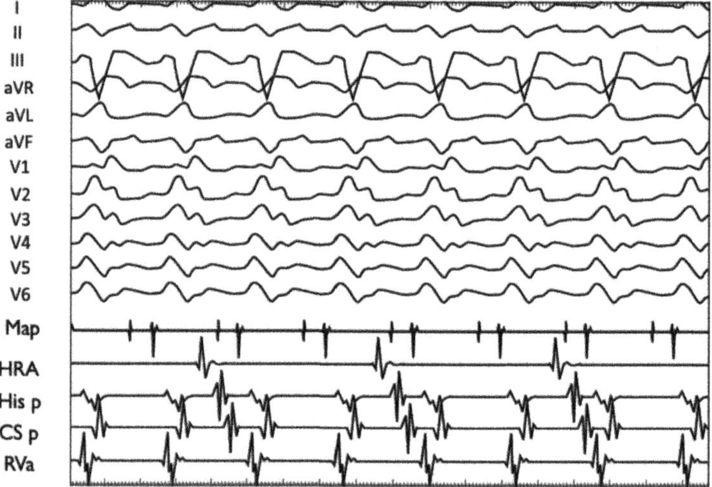

Activation mapping during monomorphic VT demonstrating a mid-diastolic potential separated from the major V EGM by isoelectric intervals.

Maneuvers in Tachycardia

- Entrainment mapping (see Table 10.6)
  - Pacing during tachycardia at rates fast than the TCL (20–30 ms below) captures the ventricle and accelerates the tachycardia to the pacing rate.
    - This confirms the mechanism as reentry.
    - It localizes the reentrant circuit to a particular chamber (or site).
    - It localizes the critical components of the reentrant circuit that sustain tachycardia (i.e., the isthmus of slow conduction or diastolic pathway).
  - Inconsistent post-pacing intervals (PPIs) (PPI variability >30 ms): Automaticity
  - Consistent PPIs (PPI variability <10 ms): Reentry (micro or macro)
    - Concealed entrainment with PPI = TCL: In circuit response
    - Entrainment with fusion and PPI > TCL: Out of circuit response
    - Concealed entrainment with PPI > TCL: Bystander location

Table 10.6 EGM Localization Within the Arrhythmia Circuit

	Local EGM	Concealed Entrainment	Stim-QRS: EGM-QRS	S-QRS: VTCL	PPI – TCL	Pace Map QRS vs. VT	Pace Map S-QRS/ EGM-QRS
Isthmus	Diastolic	yes	=	<0.7	<20	same	=
Inner loop	Diastolic	yes	<	>0.7	<20	same	=
Outer loop	Systolic	no	<	>0.7	<20	different	<
Entrance	Early diastolic	yes	=	<0.7	<20	different	<
Exit	Late diastolic	yes	>	>0.7	<20	same	=
Bystander	Diastolic	yes	>	>0.7	>20	same	>

Ablation Target

- Diastolic pathway
  - Bipolar EGM ≤0.5 mV (fractionated or split)
  - Mid-diastolic potentials (50–70 ms pre QRS)
  - Concealed entrainment during pacing
  - PPI = TCL during VT (or <20–30 ms)
  - Perfect (12/12) pace map
  - Long Stim-QRS (50–70 ms or 30%–50% of TCL)
  - Stim-QRS = EGM-QRS
- The exit site tends to be larger than the diastolic pathway (>1 cm^2).
  - Bipolar EGM 0.5–1.5 mV
  - Pre-systolic potentials (20–50 ms pre QRS)
  - Concealed entrainment during pacing (may occur)
  - PPI = TCL during VT (or <20–30 ms)
  - Perfect (12/12) pace map
  - Short Stim-QRS (<50 ms or <30% of TCL)
  - Stim-QRS = EGM-QRS
- Scar mapping
  - Linear lesions from scar to anatomic barriers
  - Pace mapping at the border zone of the scar
    - Ablation at the closest match (presumed exit)
  - Areas with latency with pacing
  - Areas of normal tissue within the scar (excitable tissue within the scar zone)
  - Areas with abnormal EGMs

RF Application

- **Irrigated RF**: 25–40 Watts for 30–60 seconds

Determinants of Success

- Determination of lesion adequacy
  - Decrease in local impedance by >5–10 Ω
  - Decrease in local EGM amplitude by >75%
  - Doubling in the pacing threshold

- Termination of the tachycardia during RF application (change in CL then break)
- Elimination of inducible tachycardia (at rest and with isoproterenol stimulation)
- Elimination of PVCs (RVOT VT)
- Creation of a RBBB on the surface ECG (bundle branch reentrant VT)

Advanced Techniques

- Non-inducible tachycardia or fast, hemodynamically unstable VT
  - Substrate/scar mapping and ablation in sinus rhythm
  - Use of non-contact mapping (e.g., MEA)
  - Support the blood pressure during VT with positive inotropes, or mechanically.
  - Pharmacologically slow the rate of VT (this may result in non-inducibility)
  - Try high dose isoproterenol (if induction is essential)
- Ablation at a favorable site is unsuccessful:
  - Most often due to inadequate energy delivery (or poor electrode tissue-contact force).
  - Consider mapping in more detail or with different catheter shapes/sizes.
  - Consider changing the access (transseptal or retrograde aortic).
  - Consider an epicardial approach.
- Epicardial VT
  - Pericardial access via a sub-xiphoid approach:
    - Pericardial needle (Tuohy) is introduced between the left subxiphoid border and the lower rib.
    - The needle is oriented towards the left shoulder and flattened to aim for the cardiac margin.
    - Small injections of contrast are used to identify when the needle tip has entered the pericardium.
    - Once in the pericardium, a guide wire is advanced. This wire must cross from left to right in an LAO in order to rule out inadvertent ventricular puncture.
    - Then, a standard sheath or steerable sheath is introduced into the pericardial space.
  - Ablation
    - Irrigated RF is required due to the insulation provided by the epicardial fat and the concomitant lack of cooling (due to absent blood flow); however, the irrigating fluid accumulates and must be drained in order to avoid tamponade (monitor arterial pressure).
  - Anticipated complications:
    - Epicardial coronary artery injury: Perform a coronary angiography pre-epicardial ablation to ensure there are no branches within 1 cm of the potential ablation site.
    - Acute pericarditis: Oral non-steroidal anti-inflammatory medications and/or intrapericardial steroids
    - Vascular perforation or visceral damage
    - Phrenic nerve damage (the left phrenic nerve runs over the anterolateral LV)

IDIOPATHIC RIGHT VENTRICULAR TACHYCARDIA (VT)

Anatomy and Physiology (Mechanism)

- Abnormal automaticity
- Triggered activity: Catecholamine-mediated DAD (phase 4)
  - Intracellular calcium overload: Activation of cyclic AMP by adenylate cyclase results in:
    - Activation of the L-type calcium channel and
    - Release of intracellular calcium from the sarcoplasmic reticulum
  - Facilitated by:
    - Regional denervation
    - Decreased local β-adrenergic receptor concentration
    - Abnormal norepinephrine reuptake
    - Abnormal augmentation of local catecholamine
- Micro-reentry

Epidemiology and Clinical Features

- The most common form of idiopathic VT (60%–75%).
- Typically seen in younger (30–50 years), women (double the rate in men) without a structural heart disease.
- Arrhythmia typically displays a circadian pattern:
  - Peak between 7 to 11 AM and 4 to 8 PM.
- Arrhythmia triggers are typically adrenergic:
  - Triggered by moderate exercise, emotional excitement, and smoking
  - Can be related to menstruation or gestation
- Symptoms
  - Palpitations (80%), light-headedness (50%), atypical chest pain, syncope

Classification

- Repetitive monomorphic VT
  - Short salvoes of NSVT
  - May be suppressed by exercise
- Paroxysmal exercise-induced VT
  - Initiation with or after moderate exercise, emotional excitement
  - Exercise stress test reproduces the clinical VT in 25%–50%.
    - Usually, there is a critical heart rate window for the VT induction.

12-Lead ECG

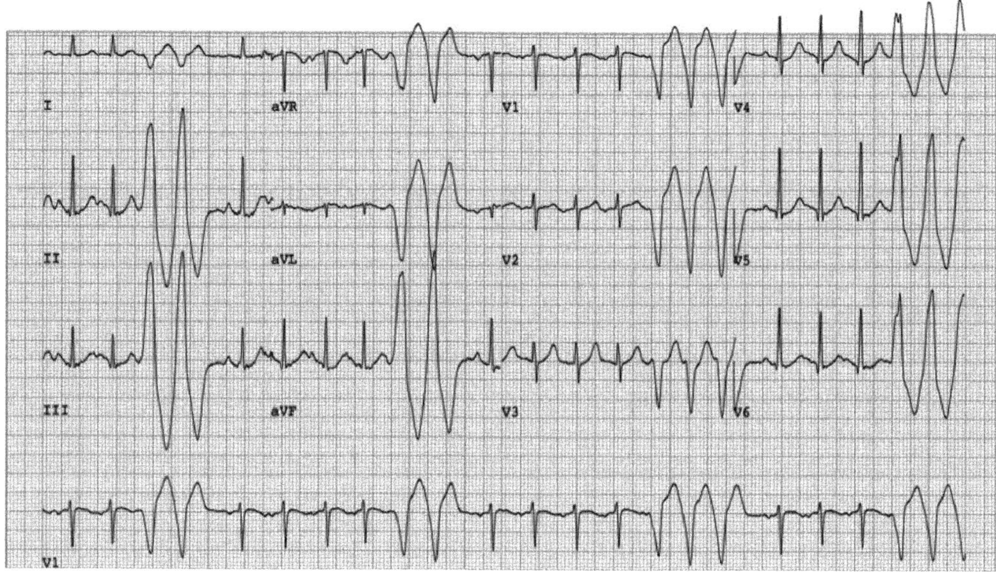

- Baseline ECG
  - Normal QRS axis duration (<110 ms in V1–V3)
  - Upright T wave in V2–V5
- ECG in VT
  - LBBB morphology with an inferior axis
  - VT localization
    - V1, V2 R-wave duration
      - >50% of QRS: LVOT (left coronary cusp)
      - <50% of QRS: RVOT or LVOT (right coronary cusp)
    - V2 R:S ratio
      - >1: LVOT
      - <1: RVOT
    - QRS transition in tachycardia compared to QRS transition in NSR
      - Earlier in NSR: RVOT
      - Earlier in PVC/VT: LVOT
    - Localization within the RVOT (see Table 10.7)

Table 10.7 Localization of VT Within the RVOT

	Anterior	Posterior	Middle	Septum	RV Free Wall
Precordial R/S Transition	—	—	—	≤V3	≥V4
Lead I and aVL	**Neg.** (qs or rS)	**Pos.** (R or Rs)	**Pos.** (rs or qrs)	Neg.	Pos.
II, III, aVF	—	—	—	Monophasic	Notching

Other Investigations

- Holter
  - LBBB morphology PVCs or VT: More frequent when awake (peak between 7–11 am and 4–8 pm) and with exercise
- EGM
  - Usually normal
- Cardiac MRI
  - To rule out ARVC and similar conditions
- Electrophysiology study (EPS): See below.

Management

Acute Management

- Vagal maneuvers, adenosine, β-blockers, verapamil

Chronic Management

- Pharmacologic therapy
  - β-blockers or ND-CCB: Abolishes all symptoms in 25%–50%.
  - ± Class Ic antiarrhythmic (RVOT VT)
- Invasive therapy
  - Catheter ablation: Usually curative; strongly indicated in preference to medical therapy
  - ICD: Sustained VT on medical therapy; usually not indicated due to benign prognosis

Prognosis

- Benign (structurally normal heart)

Catheter Ablation of Outflow Tract VT

Indications

- Drug resistant VT, drug intolerant
- Do not wish long-term drug therapy

Anticipated Success

- A 90% acute and long-term success exists (if inducible at the ablation).

Anticipated Complications

- It is the same as for all invasive procedures.
- RVOT perforation: Especially with high powers and irrigated RF catheters
- Coronary injury: Aortic cusp ablation, septal ablation in the RVOT (left anterior decending [LAD] or left main artery)
- Heart block: This is caused by an inadvertent catheter migration to the His region during ablation.

Anatomy

- The right ventricle lies rightward and anterior to the left ventricle.
- The RVOT is bordered by:
  - The pulmonary valve is superior.
  - The superior margin of the tricuspid valve is inferior.
  - The interventricular septum is posterior.
  - The RV free wall is anterior.
    - Anatomic course
      - Courses anterior and leftward of the LVOT
- The pulmonary valve sits anterior and superior to the aortic valve (5–10 mm).
  - **Right coronary aortic valve cusp**: Adjacent to the posterior septal RVOT
  - **Left coronary aortic valve cusp**: Adjacent to the anterior septal RVOT
- Basal LV/LVOT
  - It consists of the myocardium bordering the mitral valve septally, anteriorly, laterally and inferiorly, and the aortic valve superior and medial.

Pre-Procedure

- Stop all AADs for 5 half-lives before the procedure (especially RVOT VT, fascicular VT).
- Minimal conscious sedation is preferred to general anesthesia because of the risk of rendering the VT non-inducible.

Set-Up

- 3D mapping system: Set the window to 50–80 ms pre-surface QRS.
- Diagnostic catheters
  - Quadripolar catheter in RVa (stimulation)
  - Deflectable decapolar catheter in CS (reference, if required, and pacing)
- Endocardial RVOT
  - Irrigated or non-irrigated RF ablation: D-curve (medium/blue) or C-curve (green/intermediate-small); or bidirectional
  - Consider steerable, LAMP or SL0 sheath (RVOT stability)
- Endocardial LVOT
  - Non-irrigated or irrigated RF ablation: B-curve (small/red) or D-curve (medium/blue) retrograde approach

Mapping

- Use a combination of activation and pace mapping.
- Use non-contact mapping for rare NSVT or ectopy.
  - The MEA is inserted into the RVOT and positioned below the pulmonary valve.

Ideal Ablation Sites

- Local bipolar EGM precedes the surface QRS by at least 30 ms.
- The unipolar EGM displays an initial negative deflection (QS pattern).
- Perfect (12/12) pace map at TCL (if VT) or 400–600 ms (if PVCs).

RF Application

- RVOT
  - **Non-irrigated RF**: 40–60 Watts for 30–60 seconds (target temperature 55–65°C)
  - **Irrigated RF**: 25–35 Watts for 30–60 seconds (target temperature 43°C)
- Coronary cusp
  - Ensure a safe distance from coronary artery ostium (see below).
  - **Irrigated RF**: Start at 10–15 Watts and up-titrate to 25–35 Watts for 30–60 seconds.
- Determinants of success
  - Termination of the tachycardia during RF application
    - Arrhythmia may transiently accelerate before terminating.
    - Transient acceleration without termination suggests proximity to the focus.
  - Absence of spontaneous or isoproterenol induced ectopy after a waiting period (30–60 minutes)

Advanced Techniques

- Coronary cusp ablation
  - Suspect a coronary cusp origin if a broad area of early activation is found in the RVOT adjacent to the aortic cusps.
    - **Right coronary aortic valve cusp**: Adjacent to the posterior septal RVOT
    - **Left coronary aortic valve cusp**: Adjacent to the anterior septal RVOT
  - A coronary angiography must be performed before and after ablation to ensure that the coronary ostia are at least 1 cm from the ablation site, and that no damage has occurred as a result of ablation.
- Multiple RV foci
  - These suggest a more extensive pathologic process (i.e., ARVC) but may be seen with normal hearts.
  - Consider performing a voltage map to define areas of endocardial scar.
- Non-inducible tachycardia or infrequent spontaneous ectopy
  - High dose isoproterenol (up to 30–50 mcg/min)
  - Aminophylline (6 mg/kg IV over 20 minutes followed by 0.5 mcg/min) infusion
  - Epinephrine (25–50 mcg/kg/min)
  - "Cool down" phase: Sudden cessation of infusions
- Large area of early activation
  - Map-related the related tachycardia sites (LVOT, coronary cusps)
  - Use unipolar EGMs to narrow down the optimal site.
- The best site is near the His bundle.
  - Consider the use of cryoablation or alternatively slowly up-titrate the RF energy.
  - Consider ablation from the non-coronary cusp.
- When an ablation at a favorable site is unsuccessful:
  - This is most often due to inadequate energy delivery (use of irrigation/large catheter tips is the solution — it allows greater energy delivery without damaging tissue).
  - Consider mapping in more detail or with different catheter shapes/sizes.
  - Consider related tachycardia sites.
  - Consider an epicardial origin.

BUNDLE BRANCH REENTRANT VENTRICULAR TACHYCARDIA (BBR-VT)

Epidemiology and Clinical Features

- 6% of inducible sustained VT
- Found in association with:
  - Dilated cardiomyopathy (ischemic, valvular, non-ischemic)
  - Myotonic dystrophy
  - Isolated conduction disturbances of the His-Purkinje system

Anatomy and Physiology (Mechanism)

- Conduction system disease creates the substrate for unidirectional block and macroreentry involving the right and left bundles
  - In the most common form (type A), a PVC conducts into the right and left bundle branch
  - Retrograde block occurs in the right bundle branch, which is refractory due to the anterograde beat
  - Retrograde conduction occurs in the left bundle branch due to it having a shorter refractory period than the right
  - If the timing is right, the impulse can conduct anterogradely down the right bundle, activating the ventricle at the termination of the right bundle branch, and then again retrograde.

Classification

Table 10.8 Classification of Bundle Branch Reentrant VT

	Retrograde Conduction	Anterograde Conduction	VT Morphology
Type A	Left bundle	Right bundle	LBBB morphology
Type B	Fascicule of left bundle (ant or post)	Contralateral fascicle	RBBB morphology
Type C	Right bundle	Left bundle	RBBB morphology

12-Lead ECG

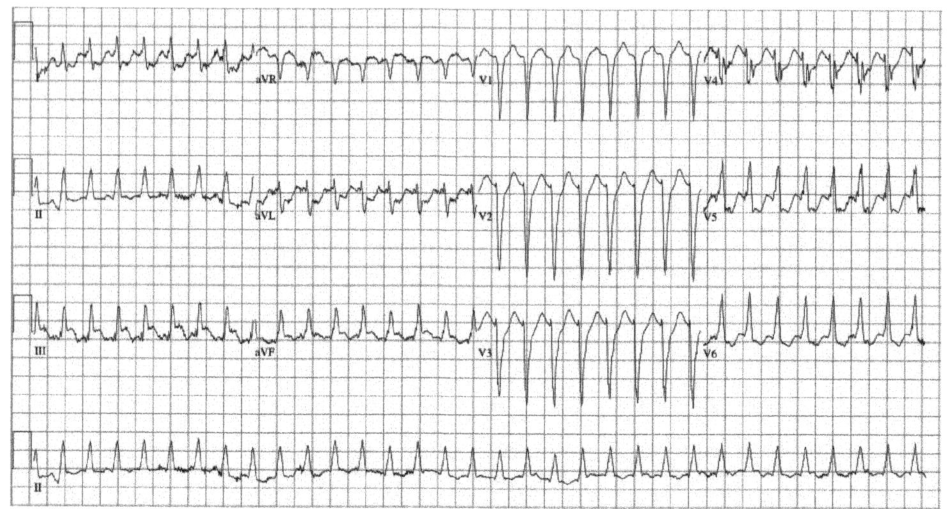

- Baseline: Non-specific IVCD with or without a prolonged PR interval
- VT: Typical LBBB with rapid intrinsicoid deflection (rarely a RBBB pattern)

Other Investigations

- **Echo**: Associated with dilated cardiomyopathy

Management

Acute Management

- May respond to vagal maneuvers, IV verapamil

Chronic Management

- Pharmacologic therapy
  - Usually ineffective
- Invasive therapy
  - Potentially curative: Ablation of the right bundle branch
- Device Therapy
  - There is a high rate of requiring a pacemaker due to the intrinsic conduction system disease prior to ablation.
  - The patient profile may still warrant an ICD placement.

Electrophysiology Study

Substrate

- Anterograde conduction
  - There is a prolonged HV interval or split His (spontaneous or during atrial stimulation/burst pacing).

Tachycardia Induction

- Programmed stimulation from RVa and/or HRA
- It is dependent on achieving a critical conduction delay in the His-Purkinje system.
  - Reproducible initiation of tachycardia with critical V-H interval prolongation

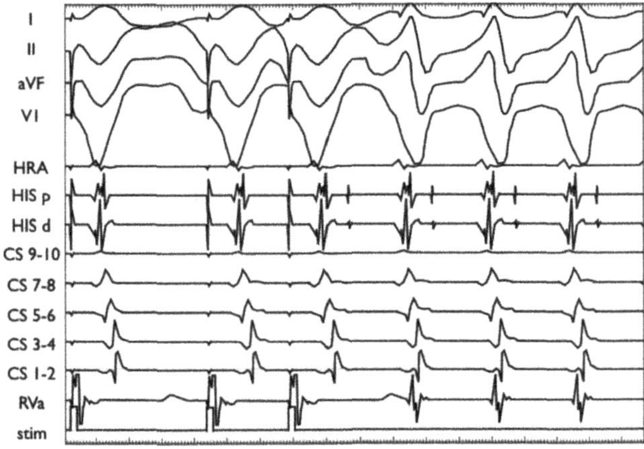

Delay in the VH interval after S2 reveals a His EGM that is subsequently fixed to the following V EGM.

Observations During Tachycardia

- Prolongation of the HV interval
  - **Type A and C**: HV during VT is longer than sinus HV (His is activated in parallel).
  - **Type B**: Tachyarrhythmia HV is shorter (usually <15 ms) than sinus HV.
- The onset of ventricular depolarization is preceded by His, and right- or left-bundle potentials with the appropriate activation sequence (H-RB-V), and stable intervals (HV, RB-V, LB-V).
  - Note: The retrograde His should activate at the same time as the proximal part of the bundle branch serving as the anterograde limb of the reentry circuit.
- Changes in H-H (RB-RB or LB-LB) interval precede changes in the VV interval during VT.

Maneuvers During Tachycardia

- **Entrainment**: Pacing at 10–30 ms shorter than tachyarrhythmia CL
  - Concealed fusion during entrainment by **atrial** stimulation favors BBR-VT
  - Concealed fusion during entrainment by **ventricular** stimulation favors non-BBR reentry, except if the pacing is being performed directly at the breakout site.
- PPI
  - The RVA PPI – TCL should be less than 30 ms (if >30 ms, BBR-VT is unlikely).

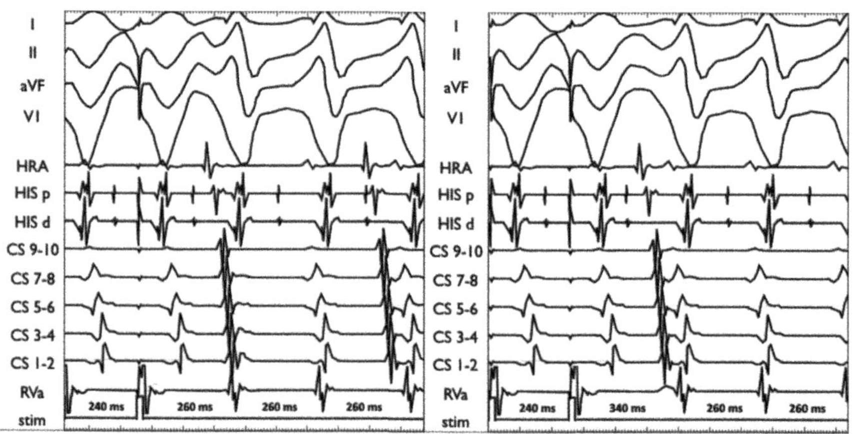

After RVa entrainment at a CL of 240 ms, the PPI is identical to the TCL, suggesting BBR-VT.

After RVa entrainment at a CL of 240 ms, the PPI – TCL is prolonged (120 ms), arguing against BBR-VT.

Termination

- Termination is preceded by spontaneous or pacing-induced block in the His-Purkinje system (HPS).

Differentiation from Other Arrhythmias

- VT due to myocardial reentry will demonstrate:
  - There is a dissociation of the His with atrial pacing.
  - Changes in the V-V CL precede changes in the H-H cycle.

- Pacing maneuvers (RVa entrainment) solidify the diagnosis.
    - RVa PPI – TCL >30 ms after entrainment makes BBR-VT unlikely.
    - Concealed fusion exists during entrainment by ventricular stimulation.
- SVT with aberrancy
  - All SVTs should have proximal followed by distal His activation (BBR-VT is distal then proximal), in addition to the following:
    - AVNRT may have VA dissociation, but entrainment with RVa pacing will have a PPI >30 ms.
    - Junctional ectopic tachycardia (JET) may have a VA dissociation, but is not entrainable with RVa pacing.
    - Intrahisian reentry may have VA dissociation but it is not entrainable with RVa pacing.
    - Orthodromic nodo-ventricular AVRT may have a VA dissociation but is usually not associated with conduction system disease.
    - Orthodromic AVRT has a 1:1 VA conduction; it is entrainable with RVa pacing but PPI must be >30 ms.
    - Anterograde atriofascicular AVRT has 1:1 VA conduction but no/negative HV interval.
    - Focal atrial tachycardia with aberrancy has 1:1 VA conduction, but is not entrainable with RVa pacing.
  - All SVTs should have proximal followed by distal His (BBR-VT is distal then proximal).

Catheter Ablation of BBR-VT

Indication

- Suspected bundle-branch reentrant VT

Anticipated Success

- Acute and long-term success of 95%–100%

Anticipated Complications

- High-grade AV block: **10%–30%**
  - Target the bundle with the worst intrinsic conduction.
  - Consider the need for pacemaker/ICD pre-ablation.

Set-Up

- Quadripolar catheter in RVa (stimulation) ± His (to distinguish His from Purkinje potentials)
- Ablation: Non-irrigated RF is usually sufficient. (If unable to achieve sufficient power use irrigated RF.)
  - **Right bundle**: F-curve (large/orange)
  - **Left bundle**: B-curve (small/red) or D-curve (medium/blue)

Mapping

- Right bundle branch
  - Generally targeted for ablation because:
    - Ablation of the right bundle does not require arterial access.
  - Process
    - The catheter is advanced into the RV at the basal anterior septum near the His bundle.
    - The catheter is advanced apically until a right bundle potential is identified on the distal tip.
    - **Right bundle potential occurs**:
      - Approximately 10–15 ms after the His recording.
      - The A:V ratio is usually <1:10 (or an absent A EGM).

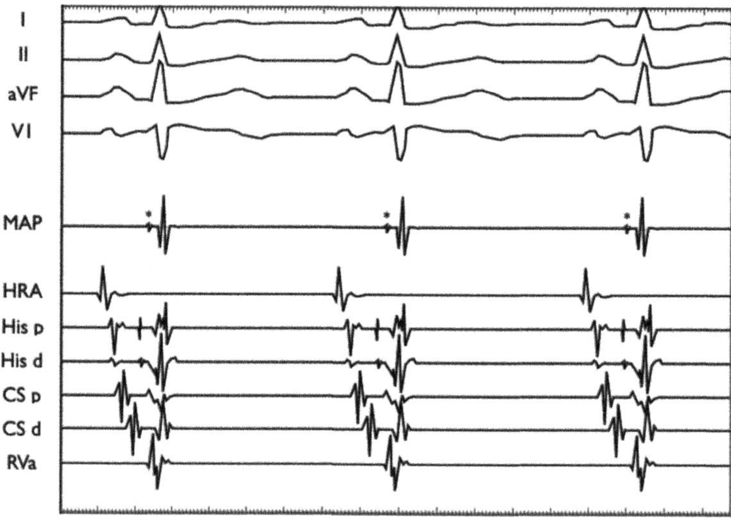

RB potential (*); occurs later than the His potential.

- Left bundle branch
  - Targeted for ablation if:
    - Mechanical trauma to the right bundle induces complete block.
    - Left bundle potentials are recorded intermittently or after the ventricular EGM is in sinus rhythm, suggesting pre-existing complete anterograde block.
  - Process
    - The catheter is advanced towards the LV inferior apical septum via a trans-aortic approach.
    - The catheter is then withdrawn towards the His until a left bundle potential is recorded.
    - **Left bundle potential occurs**:
      - 1–1.5 cm inferior to the His recording site.
      - Approximately 20 ms after the His recording.
      - The A:V ratio is usually <1:10 (i.e., absent or very small A EGM).

Ideal Ablation Sites

- These are located at a complete ablation of the right or left main bundle branch.

RF Application

- **Non-irrigated RF:** 20–60 Watts for 60 seconds (target temperature 55–65°C)
- **Irrigated RF**: 25–35 Watts for 60 seconds (target temperature 43–48°C)
- Determinants of success
  - There is non-inducibility of BBR-VT after a successful RB-ablation.
  - There is an induction of persistent RBBB if targeting the RB, or LBBB if targeting the LB.

Advanced Techniques

- Non-inducible tachycardia
  - Non-inducible tachycardia is usually due to an intermittent complete bidirectional block or insufficient conduction slowing.
  - Try programmed stimulation with short-long-short sequences e.g., S1-S2-S3 of 600-250-400 ms
  - May need:
    - Isoproterenol to sustain tachycardia
    - Class Ia agents (i.e., procainamide) to induce conduction delay
  - Rarely
    - Left ventricular stimulation or atrial pacing protocols are required to induce RBB morphology BBR-VT.
- Unable to record/ablate the right bundle potential
  - Anatomic ablation of the right bundle can be performed by ablating perpendicularly to the axis of the right bundle distal to the His signal.
  - Ablation of the left bundle may require a line of lesions from the anterior superior septum to the inferior basal septum (transecting the anterior and posterior fascicles).
  - Mapping and ablation during VT
- VT remains inducible after successful bundle branch ablation.
  - Consider other mechanisms of the residual VT:
    - Scar-related VT (inducible in 30%–60% after successful ablation of the BBR-VT)
    - Automatic VT
    - Septal VTs in NIDCM can mimic BBR VT; this emphasizes the importance of His and RB/LB EGMs.

FASCICULAR (OR IDIOPATHIC) LEFT VENTRICULAR TACHYCARDIA (VT)

Anatomy and Physiology (Mechanism)

- **Reentry**: Slowly conduct the diastolic segment along the LV aspect of the interventricular septum close to the posterior fascicle (common type).

Classification

- Left posterior fascicle: RBBB pattern and left superior axis (common form; 90%)
- Left anterior fascicle: RBBB pattern and right inferior axis (uncommon form)
- Upper septal fascicle: Narrow QRS and normal axis (rare form)

Epidemiology and Clinical Features

- Presents between 15–40 years; 60%–80% of cases are in men
- Typically sustained monomorphic VT, no PVCs or NSVT

12-Lead ECG

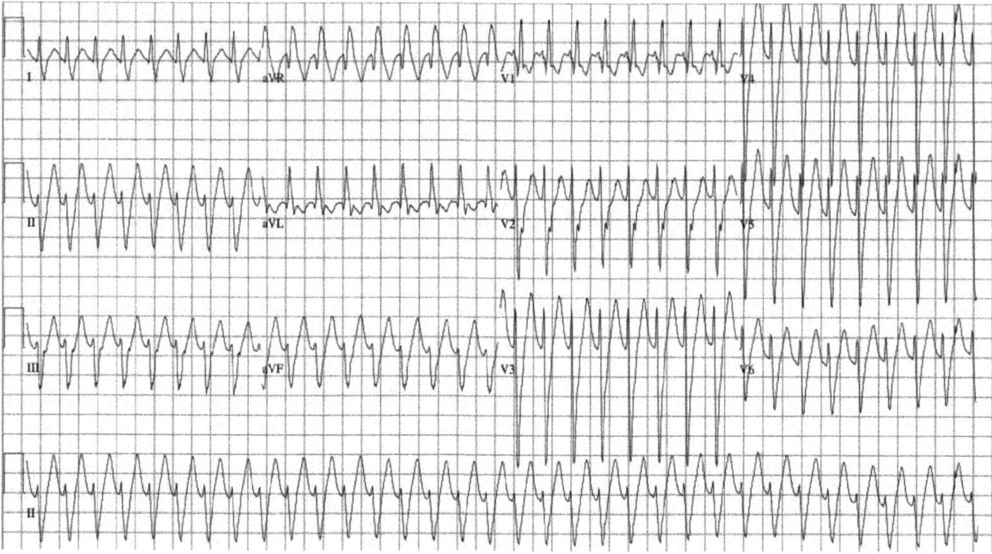

- Baseline ECG is usually normal.
- VT
  - Usually RBBB morphology with relatively narrow QRS (see *Classification*)
  - It may be difficult to differentiate from papillary muscle VT.

Other Investigations

- Echocardiogram is usually normal.

Management

Acute Management

- IV verapamil

Chronic Management

- Pharmacologic therapy
  - PO verapamil
- Invasive therapy
  - Catheter ablation (preferred)

Electrophysiology Study

Substrate

- Discrete (Purkinje) potentials can be observed in the mid-inferoseptal region during sinus rhythm.
  - Late diastolic Purkinje potential (P1) represents a slow conduction in the tissue adjacent to the native fascicle.
    - Usually it is buried within the V EGM but it may occur very late during sinus rhythm as it is activated both anterograde and retrograde.
  - Pre-systolic Purkinje potential (P2) represents an anterograde activation of the posterior fascicle.

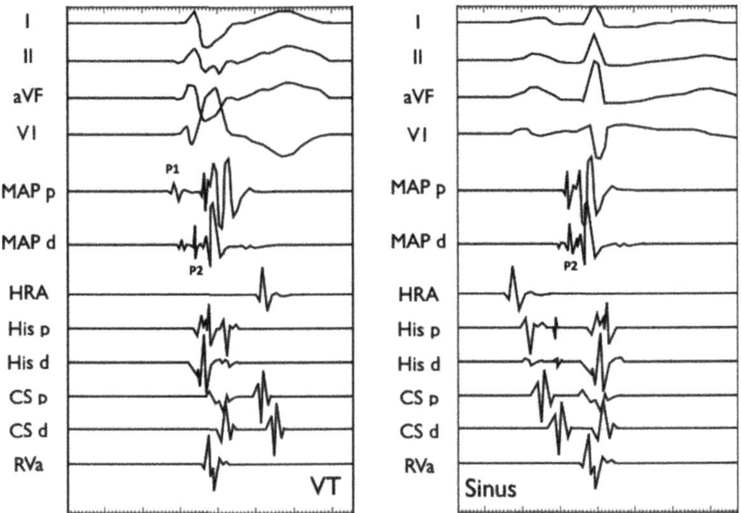

Mapping of the left interventricular septum during VT (**left panel**) and sinus rhythm (**right panel**). During VT, both diastolic (P1) and presystolic (P2) Purkinje potentials are noted, with P2 occurring earlier on the distal electrode but P1 occurring earlier on the proximal electrode. During sinus rhythm, only a presystolic potential (P2) is observed.

Tachycardia Induction

- Induction is programmed stimulation from the RVa (± short-long-short).
- It is dependent on achieving a critical conduction delay in the His-Purkinje system.
  - The ventricular extrasystole blocks in the normal posterior fascicle.
  - It conducts anterograde down the diseased, slowly conducting Purkinje fibers (P1).
  - Then it conducts retrograde via the normal Purkinje fiber (P2).
- Tachycardia also may be induced from atrial pacing.

Observations During Tachycardia

- Discrete (Purkinje) potentials (P1 and P2) can be observed in the mid-septum during tachycardia.
- The HV interval during tachycardia is shorter than the baseline HV interval.

- His activation occurs after left bundle branch (LBB) activation (vs. BBR-VT where His activation precedes activation of the left bundle).
- Earliest ventricular activation:
  - Left posterior VT: The earliest activation is at the mid to apical inferior septum (diastolic potentials in the mid-septum).
  - Left anterior VT: The earliest activation is at the anterolateral LV (diastolic potentials in the mid-septum).
- Onset of ventricular depolarization is preceded by His, right bundle or left bundle potentials with the appropriate activation sequence (H-RB-LB) and stable intervals (HV, RB-V, LB-V).
- Spontaneous variations in V-V are preceded by variations in H-H/RB-RB/LB-LB.

Maneuvers During Tachycardia

- Entrainment can be performed from both the the atria or ventricles.
- The PPI at the site of P1 and P2 will match the TCL.

Catheter Ablation of Fascicular VT

Indication

- VT that is drug resistant, drug-intolerant, or the patient does not wish long-term drug therapy

Anticipated Success

- May be hard to induce in the laboratory (~50%)
- Acute success is 90%–95% (if inducible) with a 5%–10% recurrence.

Anticipated Complications

- LBBB and AV block

Set-Up

- Quadripolar catheter in RVa (stimulation) ± His (to distinguish His from Purkinje potentials)
- Multipolar catheter along the LV septum (if possible; record the left bundle and Purkinje potentials)
- Ablation: Non-irrigated RF is usually sufficient: B-curve (small/red).
  - If unable to achieve sufficient power, use an irrigated RF

Mapping

- The catheter is advanced to the LV via the transaortic approach.
- Once in the LV, the catheter is turned clockwise (while fully deflected) and positioned on apical septum.
- VT is induced and an activation map is performed.

- The aim is to identify the Purkinje potentials (P1 and P2 EGMs).
  - Left posterior VT: The earliest activation is at the mid/apical septum with diastolic potentials in mid-septum.
  - Left anterior VT: The earliest activation is at the anterolateral LV with diastolic potentials in mid-anterior septum.

Ideal Ablation Sites

- Diastolic potential (P1) in the anterograde limb of the VT circuit (mid-septum)
  - This is not necessarily the site of the earliest potential (aim for a P-QRS from 30–130 ms).
  - The more apical the site, the lower the risk of creating a LBBB.
  - Note: If the ablation is ineffective, then move more proximally.
- If P1 cannot be found, a pre-systolic potential (P2) at the VT exit site can be targeted.
- With upper septal fascicular VT:
  - Identify P2 and ablate during sinus rhythm to prevent an inadvertent AV block.
  - Gradually up titrate from low power (10 Watts) while monitoring for junctional rhythm/AV block.

RF Application

- Non-irrigated RF: 40–50 Watts (target temperature 50–60°C) for 60 seconds
- Irrigated RF: 25–35 Watts (target temperature 43°C) for 60 seconds
- Determinants of success
  - Tachycardia slows and terminates within 15 seconds of RF onset.
  - There is non-inducibility of VT with programmed stimulation ± isoproterenol
  - Atrial pacing at different CLs
    - Induction of PVCs with the same morphology as the VT ("ventricular echoes") denotes a unidirectional block.
    - Non-inducibility of PVCs indicates a bidirectional block.
  - The P1 moves from pre-QRS to post-QRS (unidirectional block from P2 to P1).

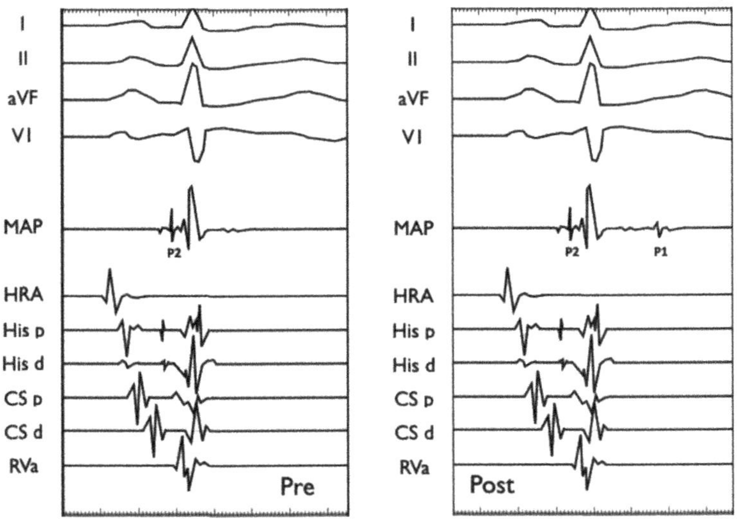

Post ablation, there is a noted delay in the diastolic Purkinje potential (P1) without a change in H-P2 timing (35 ms).

Advanced Techniques

- Non-inducible tachycardia or infrequent spontaneous ectopy
  - High-dose isoproterenol (up to 30 mcg/min) or epinephrine (25–50 ng/kg/min)
  - Wait 30 minutes or more before attempting to reinduce VT (the Purkinje fiber may have been bumped during mapping).
  - Map the ventricular echo beats during atrial pacing.
  - Map and ablate the Purkinje potentials in sinus rhythm.
    - Anatomic ablation where the Purkinje potentials ± pace map
- Unable to find good Purkinje potential EGMs
  - Try a multi-polar catheter.
  - Change the catheter for a different shape/curve.
  - Change the approach from transseptal to transaortic.
  - Perform an anatomic ablation.
    - The linear lesion is at the mid-septum perpendicular to the long axis of the LV.
      - The aim is to transect the middle to distal third of the left fascicular tract.
    - This may be combined with pace mapping.
      - Ablate 10–15 mm proximal to the site of the best QRS by pace mapping.
      - However, the endpoint of this approach is unreliable and difficult to define.
- Poor catheter stability
  - Rapid fascicular VT may result in catheter instability due to excessive cardiac motion.
  - Consider changing the RF catheter, transseptal approach, using cryoablation, or ablating in sinus rhythm.

PREMATURE VENTRICULAR COMPLEXES (PVCs)

Anatomy and Physiology (Mechanism)

Classification

- **Unifocal**: Monomorphic due to a single ventricular focus
- **Multifocal**: Polymorphic with a variable coupling intervals due to multiple ventricular foci
- **Multiformed**: Polymorphic with a fixed coupling interval
  - The impulse originates from a single focus, but the morphology differs because of differing exit sites or ventricular conduction.

Epidemiology and Clinical Features

- In a structurally abnormal heart, complex ventricular ectopy predicts an increased risk of sudden death.
  - 5%–10% 1-year mortality if LVEF is <40%
- In a structurally normal heart, ventricular ectopy holds little prognostic significance.
  - It is seen in 0.5% <20 years of age and 2.2% >50 years of age.
  - In this group there is no evidence to suggest that treatment alters mortality.
- Can be considered benign if:
  - Single
  - Monomorphic
  - Disappears with exercise
  - No associated structural heart disease
- Complex ventricular ectopy:
  - Frequent (>10/h)
  - Consecutive (couplet, triplet, or non-sustained VT)
  - Multifocal (varied sites of origin)
  - Associated with structural heart disease (coronary artery disease, cardiomyopathy), or cardiac obstructive pulmonary disease (COPD)

12-Lead ECG

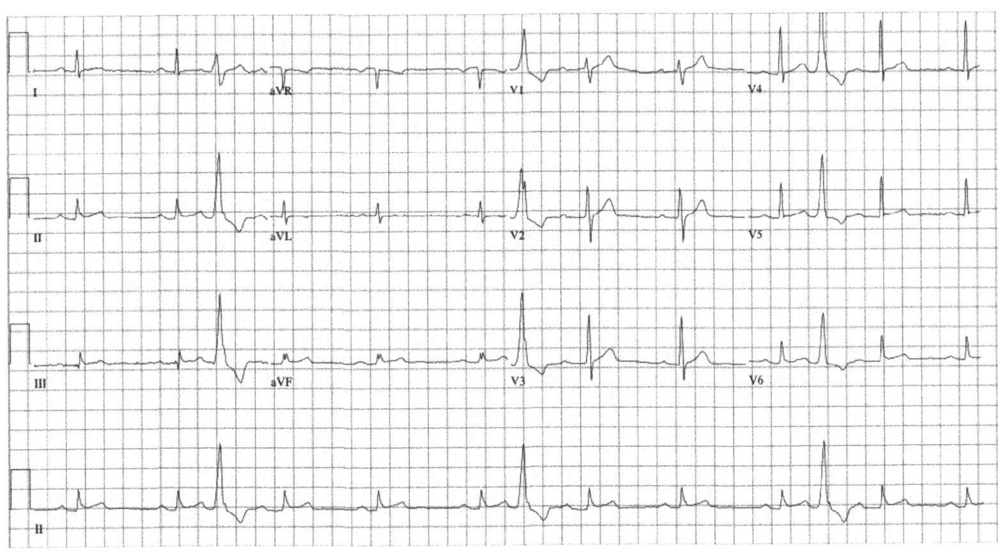

- PVCs have a wide-complex (>120 ms) beat with no preceding P wave (premature in cardiac cycle).
  - Often there is an AV dissociation.
- Fixed coupling: Constant interval between normal complex and wide QRS complex (<0.08 second, favors ventricular origin)
- Usually followed by a complete compensatory pause:
  - The premature beat does not reset the sinus pacemaker due to either VA block or the SA node being refractory at time of premature impulse arrival.
  - The subsequent sinus beat occurs on time based on the underlying sinus rate.
  - PVCs may result in an incomplete compensatory pause if:
    - **Retrograde VA conduction**: Retrograde atrial activation resets the SN (the next beat occurs slightly early).
    - **Interpolated PVC**: PVC occurs so early that it cannot be conducted through a refractory AVN; however, the sinus rate is slow enough to allow the AVN and ventricle to recover prior to the next sinus beat (sinus rhythm continues on time).
    - **Concealed conduction**: Retrograde activation of the AVN by the PVC results in PR prolongation (the AVN is partially refractory). Continued anterograde and retrograde activation may eventually cause an impulse block.
- Localization as per VT section

Other Investigations

- As per VT section

Management

- Non-pharmacologic therapy
  - Reassurance if structurally normal heart and low burden of PVCs (<10%)
  - If >10%–20% PVCs on 24-hour Holter, observe with annual echo and Holter monitor
- Pharmacologic therapy
  - β-blocker, verapamil/diltiazem
  - Alternatives
    - Class Ic (flecainide, propafenone, if no structural heart disease)
    - Class III (sotalol, amiodarone)
- Indications for PVC ablation
  - Symptomatic PVCs: Drug resistant, drug-intolerant, does not wish long-term drug therapy
  - Frequent PVCs (>10%) associated with LV dysfunction (LVEF decline or LV dilatation)
  - Mapping and ablation as per VT section

CHAPTER

11

Sinus Tachycardia

UNDERSTANDING AND MANAGING SINUS TACHYCARDIA (ST)

General Information

Appropriate ST

- Non-paroxysmal ST (heart rate >100 bpm) appropriate to the observed level of physical, emotional, pathological, or pharmacologic stress.
  - Appropriate ST occurs due to increased automaticity in the SA node pacemaker cells as a result of increased sympathetic tone and withdrawn parasympathetic tone.
- Causes
  - Physiologic: Exertion, pain, fever, infection, acute illness, hypovolemia, anemia
  - Psychologic: Stress, anxiety
  - Metabolic: Hypoglycemia
  - Hormonal: Thyrotoxicosis, pheochromocytoma, serotonin-induced
  - Pulmonary: Hypoxemia (pulmonary embolism, chronic obstructive pulmonary disease [COPD], asthma)
  - Drugs
    - Stimulants: Caffeine, alcohol, nicotine
    - Prescription: Salbutamol, catecholamine, theophylline, atropine
    - Illicit: Amphetamine, cocaine, 3,4-methylenedioxy-methamphetamine (MDMA), cannabis
    - Antineoplastic: Doxorubicin (adriamycin), daunorubicin

Inappropriate Sinus Tachycardia (IST)

- Non-paroxysmal "sinus" tachycardia (heart rate >100 bpm) unrelated to, or out of proportion to the level of physical, emotional, pathological, or pharmacologic stress.
  - It is due to an enhanced automaticity within the SA node or crista terminalis.
- Patterns
  - Excessive resting heart rate
  - Excessive heart rates with exercise or stress only
  - Combination

- Causes
  - Intrinsic SA node abnormality (enhanced automaticity)
    - There is an elevated intrinsic heart rate (i.e., in the absence of autonomic influence).
    - IST frequently has an exaggerated heart rate response to epinephrine and exercise.
    - It may have a genetic cause (mutation in gene encoding the ion channels involved in pacemaking).
  - Abnormal autonomic regulation (dysautonomia: ↑ sympathetic nervous system [SNS]/↓ parasympathetic nervous system [PSNS])
    - Onset of illness is often preceded by viral illness or trauma.
    - Non-cardiac symptoms are typical of other dysautonomias.
    - Symptoms of dysautonomia may persist after successful SA node ablation.

Sinus Node Reentrant Tachycardia (SNRT)

- SNRT is a rare paroxysmal (usually non-sustained) tachycardia similar or identical to sinus tachycardia.
- A heterogenous conduction through the SA node complex creates the substrate for a reentrant circuit between the SA node and the RA.

Postural Orthostatic Tachycardia Syndrome (POTS)

- Autonomic disorder is associated with orthostatic intolerance (symptoms on standing).
  - ST only occurs with a postural change.
- Primary forms
  - **Partial dysautonomic form:** The orthostatic heart rate rises >30 bpm above baseline or >120 bpm within 10 minutes of a tilt table test without a decrease in blood pressure (BP; <20/10 mm Hg).
  - **Hyperadrenergic form**: The orthostatic heart rate rise is accompanied by hypertension.
- Secondary dysautonomia due to:
  - Diabetes
  - Amyloidosis
  - Lupus
  - Sarcoidosis

Epidemiology and Clinical Features

IST

- Patients are 90% female; the mean age of presentation is 38 years.
- IST typically begins after a viral illness or trauma.
- Symptoms include palpitations, chest pain, dyspnea, dizziness, lightheadedness, pre-syncope.
  - Associated symptoms include orthostatic presyncope/hypotension, blurred vision, dizziness, tingling, GI disturbances, dyspnea, and sweating.
- The degree of disability varies (asymptomatic to incapacitated).

SNRT

- Symptoms: Palpitations, lightheadedness, pre-syncope (syncope is rare)
- High incidence of underlying organic heart disease

POTS

- Symptoms: Palpitations on standing
- Orthostatic tachycardia (BP and heart rate at 2, 5, and 10 minutes)

12-Lead Electrocardiogram (ECG)

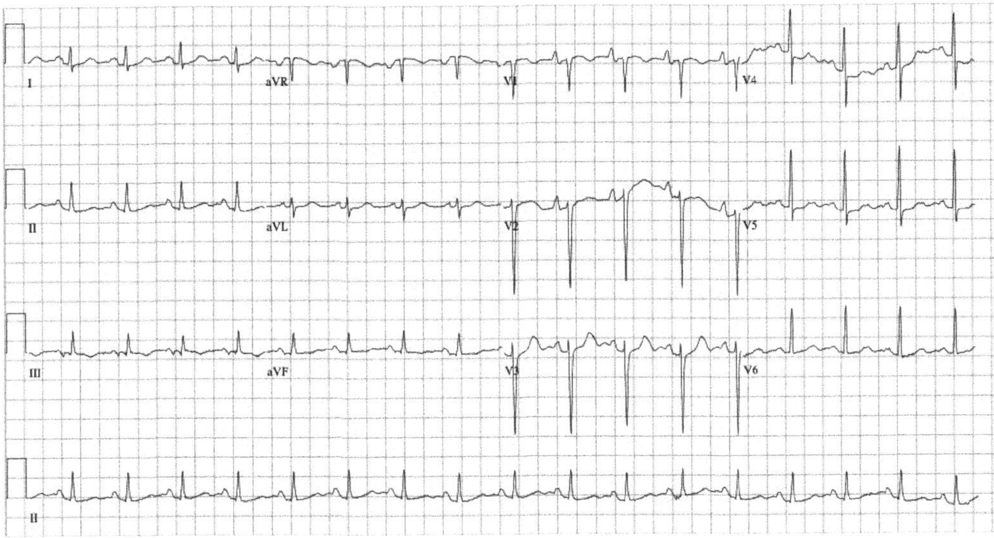

- **Rate**: 100–160 bpm
  - May be faster with thyrotoxicosis or sepsis
  - **IST**: Continuous heart rate >100 bpm or exaggerated response to activity
- **Rhythm**: Regular with some beat-to-beat variability in cycle length (CL)
- **P wave**: P-wave morphology and endocardial activation are identical to sinus.
  - Vector from superior to inferior and from right to left
- **PR**: Usually shortens secondary to the sympathetic tone (accelerated AV conduction)
- **QRS**: Narrow complex unless aberrancy or bundle branch block (BBB).
- **Onset/Termination**:
  - **ST and IST**: Non-paroxysmal (gradual onset and termination)
  - **SNRT**: Paroxysmal (abrupt onset and termination)

Other Investigations

- Investigations into underlying cause (see Etiology)
- **24-hour Holter monitor**
  - **IST**: Persistent ST during the day with nocturnal heart rate normalization
    - Excessive heart rate response to exercise
  - **SNRT**: Paroxysmal bursts of ST (abrupt onset and termination)
- Assessment of intrinsic heart rate (IHR: rarely performed)
  - IV atropine 0.04 mg/kg + IV propranolol 0.2 mg/kg
  - Predicted IHR = 118.1 – [0.57 × age]:
    - High IHR = intrinsic sinus dysfunction
    - Normal IHR = autonomic imbalance
- Echocardiogram
  - Rule out structural heart disease

Management

Acute Management

- POTS may respond to β-blockers, non-dihydropyridine calcium-channel blocker (ND-CCB), and digoxin.
- SNRT may respond to vagal maneuvers, adenosine, and amiodarone.

Chronic Management

- Non-pharmacologic therapy
  - Treat the underlying cause.
- Pharmacologic therapy
  - β-blockers (first line)
  - ND-CCB or ivabradine (second line)
  - Others: Cholinergic (pyridostigmine), antiarrhythmics (sotalol, propafenone)
    - **POTS**: Hydration, fludrocortisone and/or midodrine; clonidine
- Invasive ablation therapy
  - **IST or SNRT:** For frequent or poorly tolerated episodes, refractory to medications
  - Note: Ablation is often unsuccessful and therefore should be used only as last resort.

Electrophysiology Study (EPS)

Substrate

- Anterograde conduction is usually normal decremental AVN conduction.
- Retrograde conduction, if present, will be decremental and concentric.

Tachycardia Induction

- Tachycardia induction may be done via programmed stimulation (atrial extrasystoles or burst atrial pacing—for SNRT) with or without isoproterenol (for IST).
  - IST should not be initiated with atrial or ventricular programmed stimulation.

Observations During Tachycardia

- The AV relationship is usually 1:1 or ≥2:1.
- The VA interval is variable.
- A change in the AA interval precedes change in the HH interval

Maneuvers During Tachycardia

- Ventricular pacing
  - Pacing should not entrain.
  - The atrial activation sequence will differ from tachycardia.
  - AV dissociation will not terminate tachycardia.
  - Post-pacing sequence: VAAV or VAAHV
- Atrial pacing
  - The return VA CL is variable.
  - The AH in pacing at the tachycardia cycle length (TCL) = AH in tachycardia.

Tachycardia Termination

- Arrhythmia ends with a V (stops in the atria).

Catheter Ablation of Sinus Tachycardia (SN Modification/Elimination)

Indication

- IST that is symptomatic, recurrent, or refractory to medical therapy.

Anticipated Success Rate

- 76%–90% acute success rate
- 2%–66% long-term success rate
  - Failure occurs due to re-emergence of pacemaker function along the crista terminalis inferior to the ablation site.

Anticipated Complications

- Sinus bradycardia and sinus pauses can persist for 24–48 hours post ablation.
- Bradycardia requiring pacemaker insertion occurs in 10%–15% of cases.

Set-Up

- Quadripolar catheter in the RV (backup pacing)
- Deflectable decapolar in CS (reference and pacing)
- Irrigated radiofrequency (RF) catheter [F-curve (large/orange)]

Mapping

- Prior to ablation:
  - Determine the baseline response to low-dose isoproterenol (1 mg/min, and 2–3 mg/min).
- Anatomic mapping
  - The catheter is placed in the superior RA along the anterior wall.
  - The SN complex lies in the high RA near the RA-superior vena cava (SVC) junction and extends inferiorly down the lateral RA wall.
    - The most superior-medial aspect of the SA node is responsible for the fastest rate of discharge.
    - This aspect is located near the superior portion of the crista terminalis (anatomic landmark that separates the trabeculated RA from the smooth RA).
- Activation mapping:
  - Target the earliest site of atrial activation.

Ideal Ablation Site

- Ablation is undertaken from the most superior to more inferior locations, which eliminates the fastest rates first leading to downward titration of the SN rate.
  - Note: High-output pacing (20 mA at 2 ms pulse width) should be performed prior to ablation to delineate areas of phrenic nerve capture, given its anatomic proximity to the SN.

RF Application

- **Non-irrigated RF**: 40–60 Watts for 30–60 seconds (target temperature 55–65°C)
- **Irrigated RF**: 25–35 Watts for 30–60 seconds (target temperature 43–48°C)
- Determinants of success
  - During RF: Initial sinus tachycardia followed by a decrease in the sinus rate
  - Post RF
    - Decreased sinus rate (reduction in baseline rate of 20–30 bpm to 60–80 bpm)
    - Blunted response to isoproterenol (rate of less than 100–120 bpm on 2 mg/min)
    - Post-procedure electrocardiogram (ECG) should show a low atrial rhythm (flattened or inverted inferior P waves)

CHAPTER

12

Bradycardia and Blocks

SINUS BRADYCARDIA AND SINOATRIAL (SA) NODE DYSFUNCTION

General Information

- Impairment of the sinoatrial (SA) node ability to generate propagated impulses
  - Consider a 2:1 sinus exit block.

Epidemiology and Clinical Features

- Sinus bradycardia occurs in 1/600 patients over 65 years of age.
- Variable symptoms:
  - Asymptomatic to fatigue, exercise intolerance, dyspnea, presyncope, or syncope.
  - May lead to angina or heart failure.
- Often these patients are highly sensitive to cardiac medications (non-dihydropyridine calcium-channel blocker [ND-CCB], β-blockers, and antiarrhythmic drugs [AAD]).
- Frequently coexists with atrial tachyarrhythmia (atrial fibrillation [AF] and atrial flutter [AFL]).

Etiology

Intrinsic

- Degenerative: Idiopathic age-related fibrosis (most common)
  - SA node fibrosis: Inappropriate sinus bradycardia and exaggerated overdrive suppression
  - Atrial myocardial fibrosis: Propensity to AF or AFL
  - Atrioventricular node (AVN) fibrosis: atrioventricular (AV) block
- Myocardial ischemia
  - SA node: Supplied by right coronary artery (60%) or left circumflex artery (40%)

- Myocardial infiltration
  - Sarcoidosis, amyloidosis, hemochromatosis
- Inflammatory
  - Pericarditis, myocarditis
- Familial diseases
  - Myotonic dystrophy, Friedrich ataxia, Na^+ channel mutations
- Collagen vascular disease
  - Systemic lupus erythematosus, rheumatoid arthritis, scleroderma, ankylosing spondylitis
- Trauma or surgery
  - Valve replacement, ablation, atrial septal defect (ASD) repair, heart transplantation

Extrinsic

- Drugs
  - AADs (class I, class III), β-blockers, diltiazem/verapamil, digoxin, ivabradine
  - Sympatholytic (reserpine, methyldopa, clonidine), alcohol, lithium
- Electrolyte imbalances
  - Potassium, calcium, or magnesium
- Metabolic
  - Hypothyroidism, hypothermia
- Myocardial ischemia
  - Inferior myocardial infarction (MI): Neural reflex
- Autonomic-mediated syndromes
  - Neurocardiogenic syncope, carotid-sinus hypersensitivity
  - Situational: Coughing, micturition, defecation, vomiting
- Infection
  - Chagas, endocarditis, *Salmonella,* diphtheria, rheumatic fever, viral myocarditis

Classification

- **Inappropriate sinus bradycardia**
  - Sinus bradycardia in the absence of an appropriate cause or that results in symptoms
- **Tachycardia-bradycardia syndrome**
  - Atrial tachycardia (AT; usually AF) alternating with sinus bradycardia, sinus pauses, and/or an AV block
- **Intermittent sinus pauses include**:
  - **Sinus arrest**: Transient cessation of SA node firing (>2 seconds)
  - **Sinoatrial (SA) exit block**: Depolarization fails to exit the SA node (the RR interval is unchanged).
    - Type 1 (Mobitz): The time between sinus firing and when the atrial capture progressively prolongs leading to gradual shortening in the PP intervals before the pause (pause PP < two preceding PP).
    - Type 2 (Mobitz): The PP interval is constant before and after the pause and is a multiple (2×, 3×…) of the basic PP interval.

- **Chronotropic incompetence**: Inappropriately low heart rate response during exercise.
  - **Absolute**: Inability to increase heart rate to 60% age-predicted target (220 – age) or to >100–120 bpm.
  - **Relative**: Able to reach target heart rate but at a significant delay with reduced exercise tolerance.

12-Lead ECG

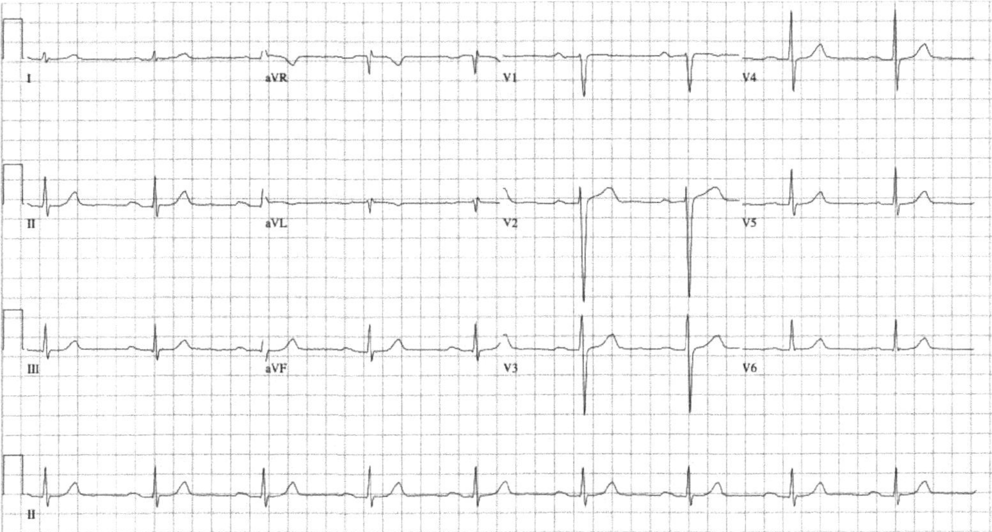

- Heart rate <60 bpm with characteristics of sinus rhythm
  - 1:1 P:QRS relationship
    - Every P wave is followed by a QRS complex and every QRS complex is preceded by a P wave.
  - Sinus P-wave morphology and axis
    - Upright in I, II, aVF, and V2–V6 (best seen in II)
    - Inverted in aVR
    - Upright or biphasic in V1 and V2; upright in V3–V6

Other Investigations

- Carotid sinus massage or tilt table testing to identify neurocardiogenic causes
- Treadmill stress test
  - Assesses the chronotropic response to exercise
- Ambulatory electrocardiogram (ECG) monitoring (Holter, event monitor, ILR)
  - Correlates symptoms with the electrical disorder
- Assessment of intrinsic heart rate (IHR: Rarely performed)
  - IV atropine 0.04 mg/kg + IV propranolol 0.2 mg/kg
  - Predicted IHR = 118.1 – [0.57 × age]:
    - Low IHR = intrinsic sinus node dysfunction (SND)
    - Normal IHR = autonomic imbalance
- Electrophysiology study (see *Assessment of SA Node Function* section)

Management

Acute Management

- Atropine or isoproterenol

Chronic Management

- Stop medications that suppress the SA node (e.g., β-blockers, verapamil/diltiazem, digoxin).
- Pacemaker indications:
  - Chronic bradycardia (if secondary to essential drug therapy)
    - Clear association of bradycardia with symptoms exists (class I).
    - Clear association with symptoms has *not* been documented (class IIa)
    - Minimally symptomatic with heart rate <40 bpm while awake (class IIb)
  - Tachycardia-bradycardia syndrome
    - Tachycardia-bradycardia syndrome is defined as symptomatic AF with a slow ventricular response (heart rate <40 bpm), pauses (≥1 pause of ≥5 seconds), or as a result of essential drug therapy for which there is no alternative (class I).
  - Sinus arrest, SA nodal exit block
    - Frequent symptomatic sinus pauses (>3 seconds: class I)
  - Chronotropic incompetence
    - Symptomatic (class I)

Prognosis

- Sinus bradycardia is generally benign if it is asymptomatic.
  - It has a 2%/year risk of developing AVN dysfunction.

FIRST-DEGREE ATRIOVENTRICULAR (AV) NODE CONDUCTION BLOCK

General Information

- All impulses are conducted to the ventricles but with a prolonged conduction time.
  - The site of conduction delay may be intra-atrial in the AVN and/or His-bundle conduction.

Etiology

- High vagal tone (usually accompanied by sinus bradycardia and/or sinus pauses)
- Age-related conduction system degeneration

- Myocardial ischemia
  - Inferior ischemia: AVN ischemia
  - Anterior ischemia: His-Purkinje ischemia
- Drugs (digoxin, β-blockers, verapamil/diltiazem)
- Inflammatory disorders (acute rheumatic fever, myocarditis)
- Trauma (catheter-induced, AVN ablation)
- Infection (i.e., *Salmonella,* Chagas)
- Endocarditis (aortic root abscess)

12-Lead ECG

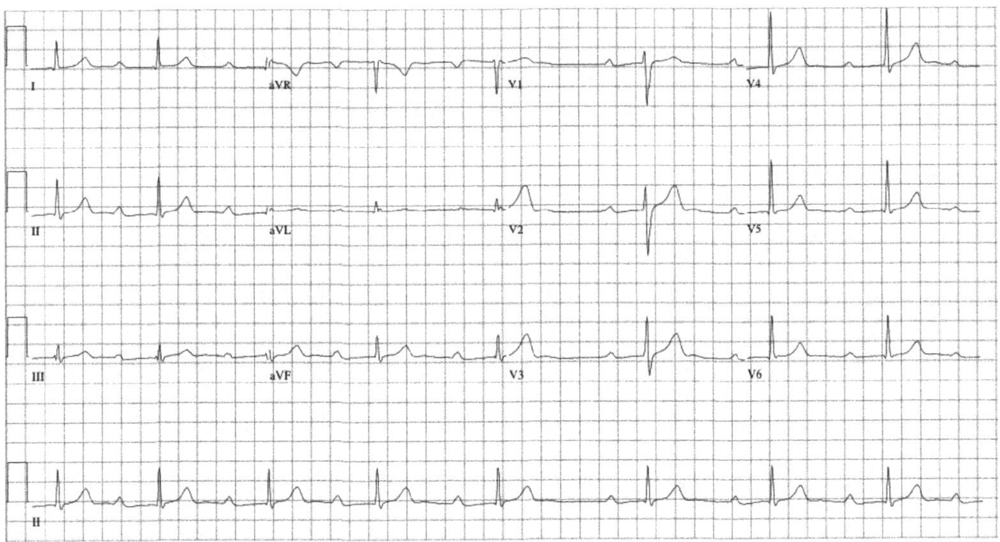

- PR interval >200 ms with heart rates >60 bpm (or >220 ms if the HR is <60 bpm)
- "Marked first-degree AV block" if the PR interval is >300 ms

Other Investigations

- Directed at the underlying cause
- An electrophysiology study (EPS) is usually not indicated.
  - See "Assessment of AVN Function" section.

Management

- In the absence of other cardiac pathology or symptoms, it does not affect prognosis, is of no clinical significance, and does not require specific treatment.
- However, evidence from the Framingham study suggests that a prolonged PR interval (>200 ms) is associated with an elevated risk of:
  - Mortality (HR 1.44).
  - Pacemaker implantation (HR 2.89).
  - AF (HR 2.06).

Pacemaker Indications

- Symptomatic (pacemaker syndrome or hemodynamic compromise: class IIa)
- Marked first-degree AV block (PR >0.3 second) in patients with LV dysfunction and heart failure symptoms in whom a shorter AV interval results in hemodynamic improvement (class IIb)

Prognosis

- A first degree block within the AVN (85%) tends to be benign and non-progressive.
- A first degree block below the AVN (wide QRS) tends to progress to higher-degree AV block.

SECOND-DEGREE ATRIOVENTRICULAR (AV) NODE CONDUCTION BLOCK

General Information

- Intermittent failure of AV conduction
  - Not every P is followed by QRS, but some form of AV relationship exists.
- Nomenclature
  - Based on the ratio of conducted to blocked beats (1:1 block, 2:1 block, variable block)
  - **High-grade block**: Block persists for ≥2 sequential beats

Mobitz Type 1 (Wenckebach)

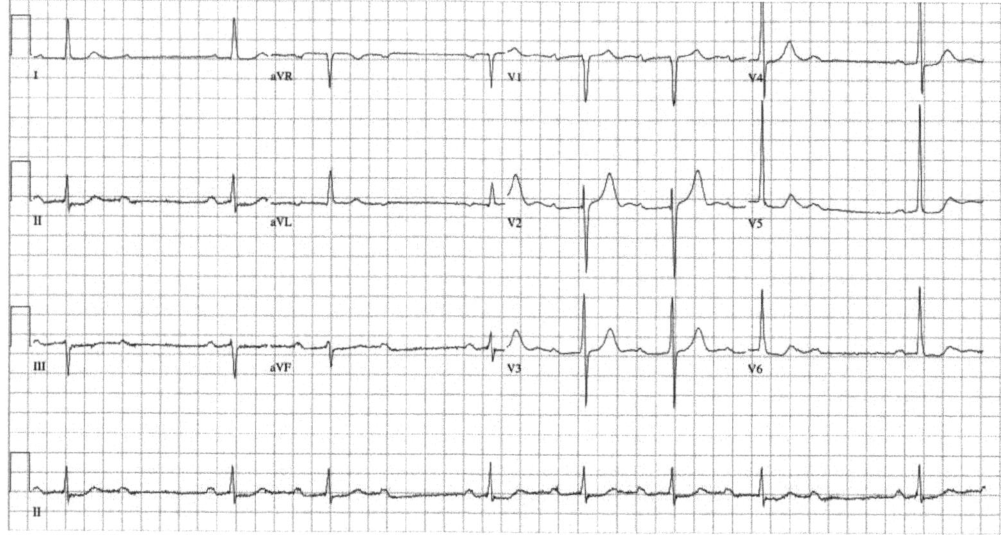

General Information

- Gradual prolongation in the PR interval (Wenckebach sequence) following a non-conducted beat (Luciani phenomenon).
  - The PR interval following the dropped beat is shorter than the last conducted beat.
  - As the PR interval prolongs, there is reciprocal RP interval shortening.

- Clinical features and epidemiology
    - Mobitz type 1 usually occurs due to a block at the level of the AVN.
    - Mobitz type 1 is observed in 6%–11% of healthy people.

Etiology

- High vagal tone (usually accompanied by sinus bradycardia and/or sinus pauses)
- Age-related conduction system degeneration
- Myocardial ischemia
    - Inferior ischemia: AVN
    - Anterior ischemia: His-Purkinje
- Drugs (i.e., digoxin, β-blockers, diltiazem, verapamil)
- Post-AVN modification (edema or direct injury)
- Myocarditis
- Infection (i.e., *Salmonella*, Chagas)
- Endocarditis (aortic root abscess)

Management

- None unless symptomatic
- Acute symptomatic bradycardia:
    - Atropine IV
    - Isoproterenol infusion
- Pacemaker indications:
    - Symptomatic bradycardia (class I) or pacemaker syndrome (class IIa)
    - Asymptomatic: Intra-/infrahisian delay demonstrated at EPS

Prognosis

- Only rarely will it progress to a Mobitz II or third-degree AV block.

Mobitz Type 2 (Hay)

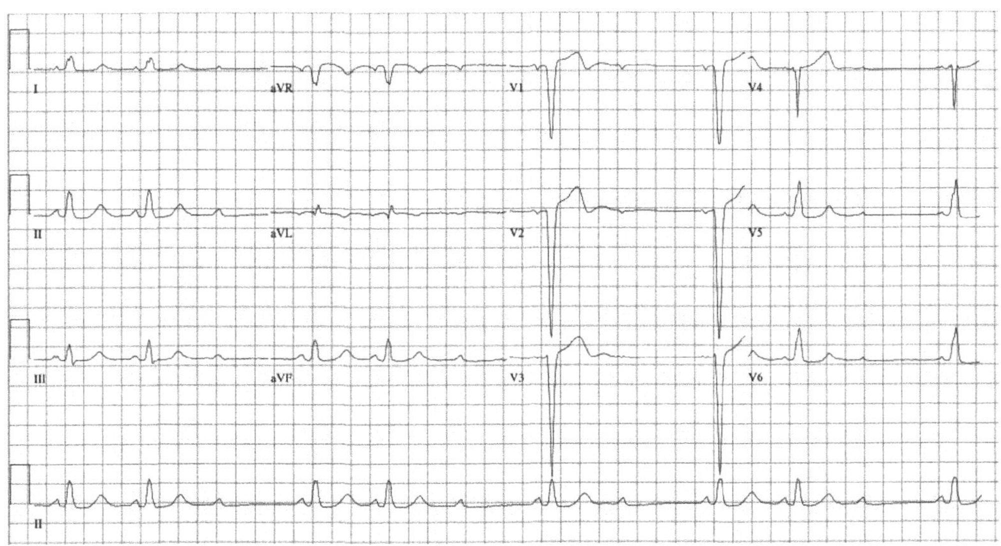

General Information

- All-or-none conduction:
  - There is a stable PR and RP interval with the occasional dropped QRS.
  - It can be regular (e.g., 2:1) or irregular.
- It occurs due to a block at the level of the His-Purkinje system (almost always indicates distal block).

Etiology

- Age-related conduction-system degeneration
- Myocardial ischemia
  - Inferior ischemia: AVN
  - Anterior ischemia: His-Purkinje
- Drugs (i.e., amiodarone, procainamide)
- Interventional
  - Surgical (i.e., aortic valve replacement, atrial septal defect/ventricular septal defect [ASD/VSD] closure)
  - Post AVN modification (i.e., edema or direct injury)
  - Post alcohol ablation (hypertrophic cardiomyopathy [HCM])
- Myocardial infiltration (i.e., sarcoid, myxedema, hemochromatosis)
- Systemic inflammatory disorders (i.e., ankylosing spondylitis, Reiter syndrome)
- Myocarditis
- Infection (i.e., *Salmonella,* Chagas, lyme)
- Endocarditis (aortic root abscess)

Management

- Acute symptomatic bradycardia:
  - Atropine IV
  - Transcutaneous or transvenous pacing
- Pacemaker indications:
  - Symptomatic bradycardia (class I) or pacemaker syndrome (class IIa)
  - Asymptomatic: Intra-/infrahisian delay demonstrated at EPS
  - Exercise induced (but non-ischemic) second- or third-degree AV block (class I)

Prognosis

- Significant risk of abruptly developing syncope or third-degree AV block

2:1 AV Block

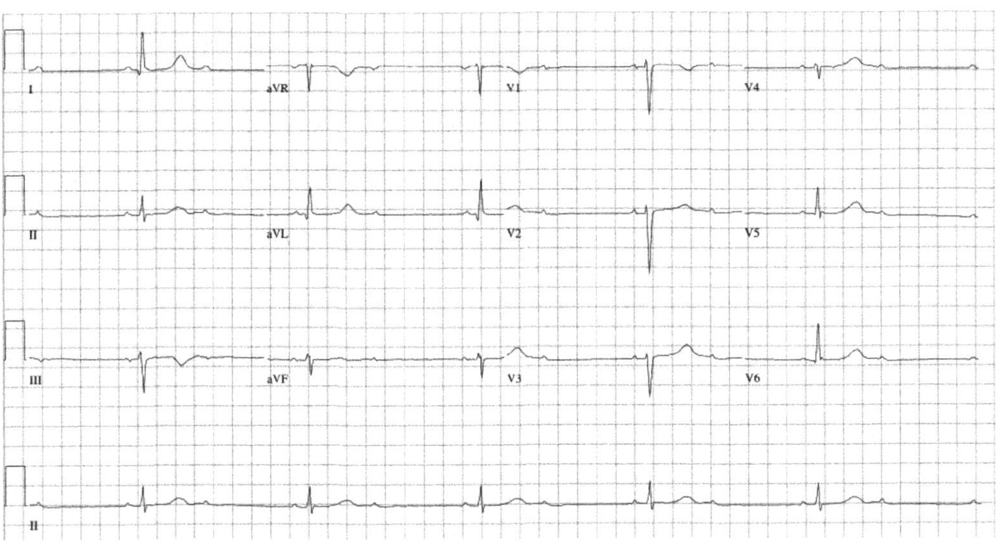

General Information

- It is difficult to know if a 2:1 AV block represents an underlying Mobitz type 1 or 2 block.
  - Type 1 is suggested by a narrow QRS complex and variable PR interval.
    - The AV block improves (moving from 2:1 to 3:2 block) with atropine, isoproterenol, and exercise.
    - The AV block worsens with vagal maneuver; that is, an increased number of P waves results in *more* conduction down to the ventricles.
  - Type 2 is suggested by a wide QRS complex.
    - The AV block is worsened (moving from 2:1 to 3:1 block) with atropine, isoproterenol, and exercise.
    - The AV block does not change with a vagal maneuver; that is, the increased number of P waves results in *less* conduction down to the ventricles.
- A 2:1 AV block may be associated with a ventriculophasic rhythm.
  - The interval between two consecutive P waves in which the first was blocked (PP) is wider than the interval between two consecutive P waves that resulted in AV conduction (P-QRS-P) due to variations in neurohormonal control.

High-Grade Block

- An AV block that persists for ≥2 sequential beats

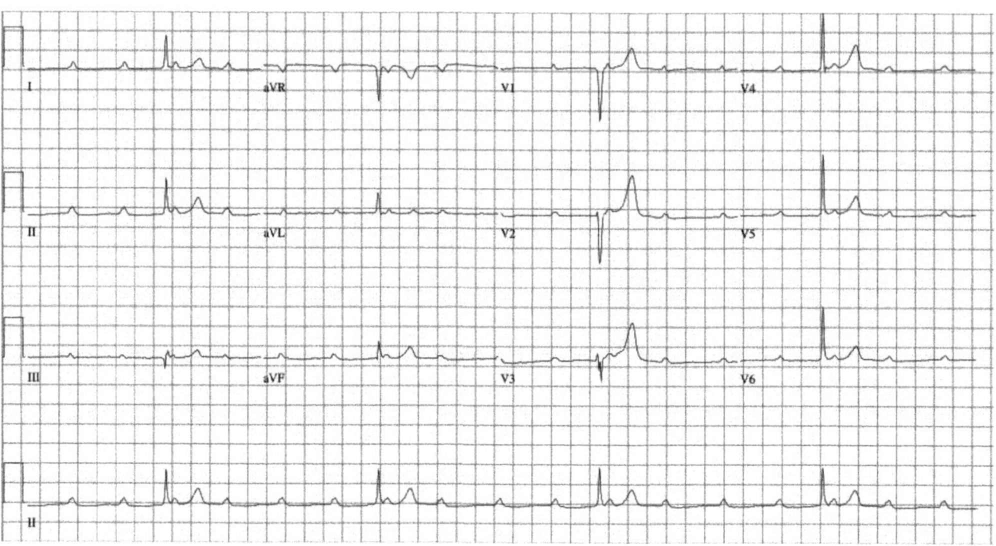

THIRD-DEGREE (COMPLETE) ATRIOVENTRICULAR (AV) NODE CONDUCTION BLOCK

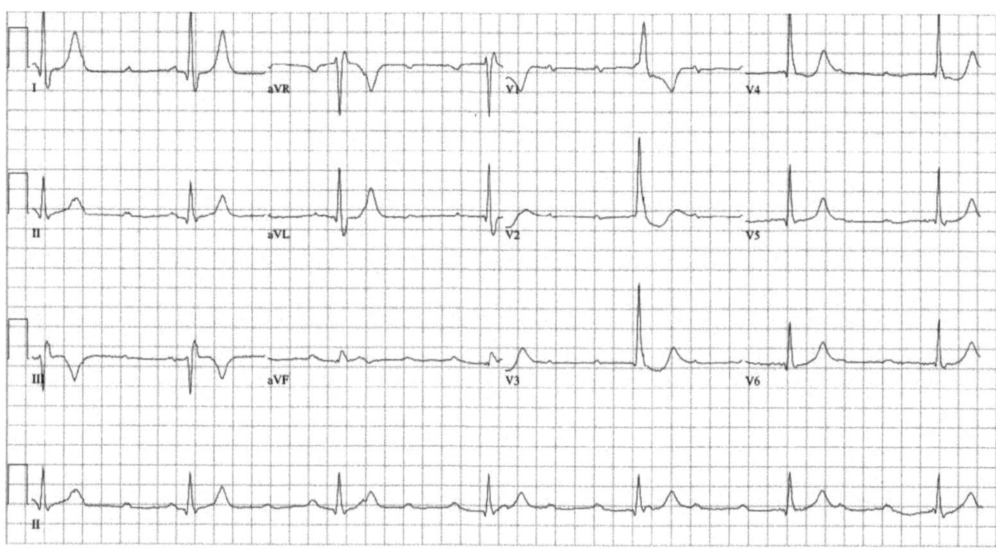

General Information

- This is a complete failure of AV conduction with independent atria and ventricles (**AV dissociation**)
  - P waves are not conducted and never produce a QRS.
    - A compensatory increase may be seen in the sinus rate secondary to the slow ventricular rate.

- Escape rhythm is dependent on the function of subsidiary pacemakers distal to the block.
  - A narrow junctional rhythm (40–55 bpm) suggests the block is within the AVN.
  - A wide ventricular rhythm (20–40 bpm) suggests the block is inferior to the AVN.
- Subtle variation in P-P and R-R intervals are common due to ventriculophasic modulation.

Etiology

- High vagal tone (usually accompanied by sinus pauses)
- Age-related conduction system degeneration
- Myocardial ischemia
  - The AVN is supplied by the AV nodal artery, which arises from the right coronary artery (RCA; 90%) and the left circumflex artery (LCX) (10%).
  - The His bundle is supplied by AVN artery with a small contribution from left anterior descending (LAD) septal perforator.
  - The right bundle is supplied by septal perforators of the LAD with collaterals from RCA and LCX.
  - The left anterior fascicle is supplied by septal perforators of the LAD.
  - The proximal left posterior fascicle is supplied by the AVN artery and LAD septal perforators.
  - The distal left posterior fascicle is supplied by anterior and posterior septal perforators.
- Drugs (i.e., digoxin, β-blockers, diltiazem, verapamil)
- Post AVN modification (edema or direct injury)
- Myocarditis
- Infection (i.e., *Salmonella,* Chagas)
- Endocarditis (aortic root abscess)
- Congenital (<0.04%): Neonatal lupus is associated with 60%–90% of cases (maternal anti-Ro antibody)

Management

- Acute symptomatic bradycardia
  - Atropine IV and isoproterenol infusion are likely ineffective.
  - Transcutaneous followed by transvenous pacing if unstable escape.

Pacemaker Indications

- Symptomatic (Class I)
- Post cardiovascular surgery or AVN ablation (class I)
- Asymptomatic
  - Asystole >3 seconds, escape rhythm <40 bpm or escape/block below the AVN (class I)
  - Narrow escape >40 bpm (class I if cardiomegaly/LV dysfunction; otherwise, class IIa)
  - Exercise-induced (but non-ischemic) second- or third-degree AV block (class I)

Prognosis

- Annual mortality ~50%

CHAPTER

13

Cardiac Implantable Electronic Devices

PERMANENT PACEMAKERS

Cardiac implantable electronic devices (CIEDs) sense intrinsic cardiac electric potentials and, if too infrequent, transmit electrical impulses to the heart to stimulate cardiac contraction.

- **Sensing**: Sensing is the ability of the pacemaker to appreciate an intrinsic electrical signal. The response to sensing can be:
  - **Inhibition**: The pacemaker stimulus is suppressed due to a spontaneous intrinsic event sensed before the end of the sensing (alert) period.
  - **Triggering**: The pacemaker stimulus is generated due to a spontaneous intrinsic event sensed before the end of the sensing (alert) period.
- **Capture**: The ability of a pacemaker to trigger a cardiac depolarization and resultant mechanical myocardial contraction (atrial or ventricular).
  - Pacemaker output pulses can be understood by considering Ohms law: Current = voltage / resistance.
    - Voltage (V): The force moving current (measured in volts)
    - Current (I): The volume of flow of electricity (measured in amperes)
    - Impedance (R): Resistance to flow (in the circuit and patient; measured in ohms)

CIED NOMENCLATURE (NBG Code)

Table 13.1 Standard CIED Nomenclature

First Position	Second Position	Third Position	Fourth Position	Fifth Position
Chamber Paced	**Chamber Sensed**	**Response to Sensing**	**Rate Modulation**	**Multisite Pacing**
A	A	T	O	O
V	V	I	R	A
D	D	D		V
	O	O		D

NBG: NASPE/BPEG Generic.

The Clinical Cardiac Electrophysiology Handbook © 2016 Jason Andrade.
Cardiotext Publishing, ISBN: 978-1-942909-00-2.

- The first letter indicates the chamber(s) paced.
  - A: Atrial
  - V: Ventricular
  - D: Dual-chamber (atrial and ventricular)
- The second letter indicates the chamber in which electrical activity is sensed.
  - A, V, or D
  - O is used when the pacemaker discharge is not dependent on sensing.
- The third letter refers to the response to a sensed electric signal.
  - T: Triggering of pacing function
  - I: Inhibition of pacing function
  - D: Dual response (i.e., any spontaneous atrial or ventricular activity will inhibit that chamber's pacing function but lone atrial activity will trigger a paced ventricular response)
  - O: No response to an underlying electric signal
- The fourth letter represents rate modulation.
  - R: Rate-response ("physiologic") pacing
  - O: No programmability or rate modulation
- The fifth letter represents multisite pacing
  - A, V, or D

Programming Modes

- AOO or VOO: Paces regardless of intrinsic activity (i.e. no sensing or inhibition)
- AAI: Pacing and sensing in the atrium only (reserved for pure SA node disease)
- VVI: Pacing and sensing in the ventricle only, usually used with permanent atrial fibrillation (AF)
- VDD: Usually single lead device that senses atria and paces ventricle
- DDD: Dual chamber (atrial and ventricular) sensing and pacing
- AAT or VVT: Diagnostic (tests sensing thresholds or etiology of inhibitory signal–lead/muscle)

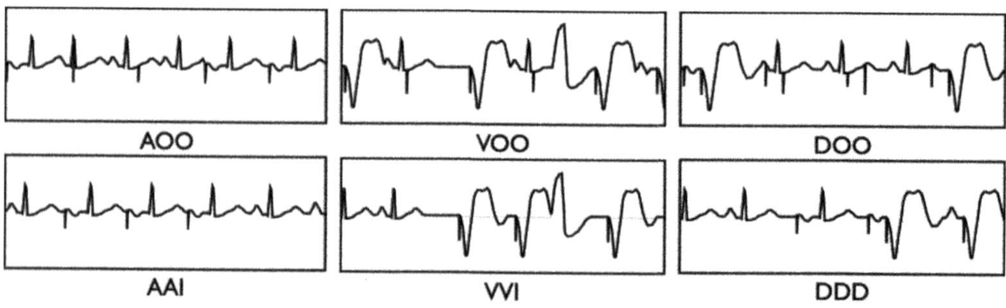

A Basic CIED System

Pulse Generator

- The pulse generator is placed subcutaneous (pre-pectoral) or submuscular in the chest wall.
- Consists of:
  - **Casing** (a.k.a., "can"): Titanium (biocompatible, strong, and lightweight)
  - **Connector**: An epoxy "header" containing the lead connector ports.
  - **Components** (sensing, timing, and output circuits)
    - Diodes: Keep current going the right direction
    - Resistors: Impede flow in an effort to channel the current
    - Crystal oscillator: The "time clock" of the pulse generator
    - Microchips: Memory and "intelligence" functions
  - **Battery** (usually lithium iodide): The largest component inside the pulse generator

Pacing Leads

- Endocardial leads are inserted transvenously to the atrium, RV, and/or the coronary sinus (CS).
- Epicardial leads can be inserted via thoracotomy and are fixed to the exterior of the heart.
- Endocardial leads are implanted into the myocardium via:
  - **Active fixation** (distal screw)
    - Advantages
      - Easy fixation, with the ability to reposition
      - Lower rate of dislodgement
      - Chronic removability
    - Disadvantages
      - More expensive
      - More complicated implantation procedure
  - **Passive fixation** (distal fins or tines designed to snag/entangle the trabeculae)
    - Advantages
      - Less expensive
      - Minimal trauma to patient
      - Potentially lower thresholds
    - Disadvantages
      - Higher rate of acute dislodgement
      - It is more difficult to remove a chronic lead.
- Pacing leads can be:
  - **Bipolar**: Two conductor coils (electrodes) on the distal portion of the lead, and separated by 2–3 cm of insulation on the distal portion of the lead.
    - The **stimulating cathode** (negative pole) is the distal electrode (distal tip).
    - The **receiving anode** (positive pole) is the proximal electrode (proximal ring).
    - Advantages
      - Less oversensing (far field, myopotentials, electromagnetic interference)
      - No pocket (pectoral muscle) stimulation
      - May be programmed to a unipolar configuration
    - Disadvantages
      - Larger diameter with a stiffer lead body

- **Unipolar**: Single conductor coil and electrode tip
  - The **stimulating cathode** (negative pole) is intracardiac (distal tip).
  - The **receiving anode** (positive pole) is extracardiac (the pulse generator).
  - Advantages
    - It has a smaller diameter lead.
    - Theoretically it is more reliable (single coil within the lead).
    - There is a larger paced electrogram (EGM) amplitude due to larger field.
  - Disadvantages
    - It is limited to a unipolar configuration.
    - It has a tendency to oversense (far field, myopotentials, electromagnetic interference).
    - Pacing may result in pocket stimulation.
    - It cannot be used with implantable cardioverter-defibrillators (ICDs).

CARDIAC IMPLANTABLE ELECTRONIC DEVICES (CIEDs) TIMING CYCLES

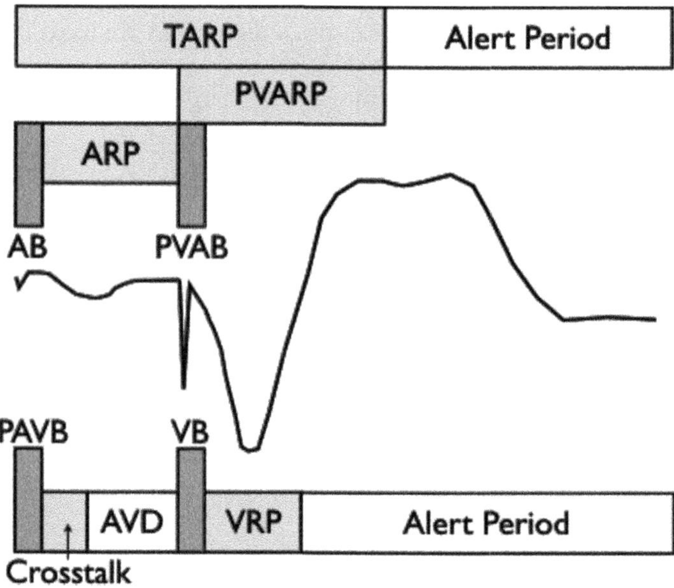

See text for terminology.

- General terminology
  - **Refractory period** (300 ms): Interval during which the CIED does not respond to intrinsic signals
    - This keeps the pacemaker from resetting the timing cycle with inappropriate signals.
    - **Absolute refractory period** "Blanking" (30–50 ms)
      - The CIED does not "see" intrinsic signals.
    - **Relative refractory period**
      - The CIED "sees" and counts intrinsic events but does not respond to them.

- Alert period
  - This is the time after the refractory period that sensor is open and looking for signals.
- **Lower rate limit** (LRL): The slowest rate of pacemaker stimulation.
  - This is analogous to the pacing interval, which is the time period in milliseconds between two consecutive paced events in the same chamber without an intervening sensed event.
- **Upper rate limit** (URL)
  - This is the fastest rate the pacemaker will stimulate the heart (i.e. the maximum tracking rate if a dual chamber device; or the maximum sensor rate if rate response is turned on).

- Atrial channel
  - AV delay (AVD)
    - Time from native/paced atrial event to the subsequent ventricular impulse (native or paced)
  - Atrial blanking period (ABP) and post-ventricular atrial blanking period (PVABP; a.k.a. far-field blanking)
    - Period of blanking post intrinsic or paced atrial impulse (ABP) or ventricular pacing (PVABP)
    - Prevents the atrial channel from oversensing the paced impulses in atria/ventricle, respectively
  - Atrial refractory period (ARP) and and post-ventricular atrial refractory period (PVARP)
    - Time that the atrial channel is refractory
    - Initiated by intrinsic or paced atrial impulse (ARP) or ventricular pacing (PVARP)
    - Prevents the pacemaker from restarting the timing cycle to inappropriate signals
      - ARP: Device is able to count intrinsic atrial impulses and extrinsic noise
      - PVARP: prevents the device from tracking ventricular depolarization and retrograde P waves.
  - Total atrial refractory period (TARP)
    - Sum of ABP + ARP (AV Delay [AVD]) and post-ventricular atrial refractory period (PVARP)
      - Atrial sensed events during TARP do not affect the timing cycle but will trigger the mode-switch.
    - The length of TARP will limit the URL (maximum tracking rate or maximum sensor rate).
      - If TARP is ≥ URL, there will be 2:1 behavior (abruptly "hitting the wall").
      - If TARP is < URL, then Wenckebach phenomena will be observed ("Wenckebach window").
  - Atrial alert period
    - This is the time after the refractory period when the atrial sensor is looking for stimuli.
- Ventricular channel
  - Ventricular blanking period (VBP) and post-atrial ventricular blanking period (PAVBP)
    - This is the period of blanking post-intrinsic or -paced ventricular impulse (VBP) or atrial pacing (PAVBP).
    - It prevents the ventricular channel from sensing the paced impulses.

- **Ventricular triggering period** ("cross-talk sensing window")
  - When a ventricular sensed event occurs during this period (typically 100–120 ms), it would trigger "safety pacing" (ventricular pacing at an interval that is shorter than the AVD).
- Ventricular refractory period (VRP)
  - This is the time period that ventricular channel is refractory.
  - It is initiated by an intrinsic or paced ventricular impulse.
  - It prevents the pacemaker from restarting the timing cycle to inappropriate signals.
- Ventricular alert period
  - It is the period after the VRP where the ventricular sensor is looking for stimuli.

- Timing cycles
  - VV timing (pacer keeps constant VV interval) is the most common.
  - AA timing (pacer keeps constant AA interval) is also used.

Other Pacemaker Functions

- Rate-response/rate-adaptive pacing
  - A sensor within the pacemaker increases and decreases the pacing rate based on "physiologic need."
    - Essentially, this sensor acts as a surrogate for normal SN variability.
    - The minimum and maximum heart rate, and "aggressiveness" can be programmed.
    - This function is useful for patients with chronotropic incompetence.
  - Types of sensors:
    - **Vibration sensors** react to vibration using a piezoelectric crystal.
      - Pro: They have a quick response, need no special lead, provide easy programming, and are self-powered.
      - Con: The sensor is not specific to exercise and is easily influenced by external vibration (i.e., tremor, bumpy car rides); the response is not proportional to the work load, and they are hard to optimize.
    - The **accelerometer** reacts to forward/backward activity at specific frequencies.
      - Pro: As per vibration, it is less susceptible to external influences; it is proportional to the workload.
      - Con: It can be fooled by certain motions (rocking chair), and it is not sensitive to external demand.
    - **Minute ventilation sensors** react to transthoracic impedance (resistance across the chest).
      - Pro: They are slow to respond, sensitive to workload, and immune to the environment.
      - Con: They are unable to use a unipolar lead; arm motion/speech influences the sensor.
    - **Evoked response sensors** react to a decrease in the measured QRS depolarization area.
      - Note: These sensors only work when the device is pacing.
    - **QT interval sensors** react to a decrease in QT interval (measured from pacing spike to evoked T wave).
      - Note: They only work when the device is pacing.
    - **Closed-loop sensors** assess cardiac inotropy via the variations of intracardiac impedance on a beat-to-beat basis during the systolic phase of the cardiac cycle at the apex of the right ventricle.

- Hysteresis
  - The pacemaker allows the rate to fall below the programmed LRL following the sensing of an intrinsic beat in the alert period (kicks in at a programmable rate lower than LRL).
    - It is used to encourage native cardiac activity and prolong battery life.
  - **Search/scan hysteresis** temporarily decreases the rate to allow intrinsic cardiac activity. This can occur with:
    - **AV conduction** (↑ AVD to allow native conduction) or ventricular activity (rate < base rate)
    - **Reverse hysteresis** (↓ the AVD in order to speed conduction in response to a short pulse rate)
      - Essentially, this works to force ventricular pacing; it is only useful with cardiac resynchronization therapy (CRT) devices

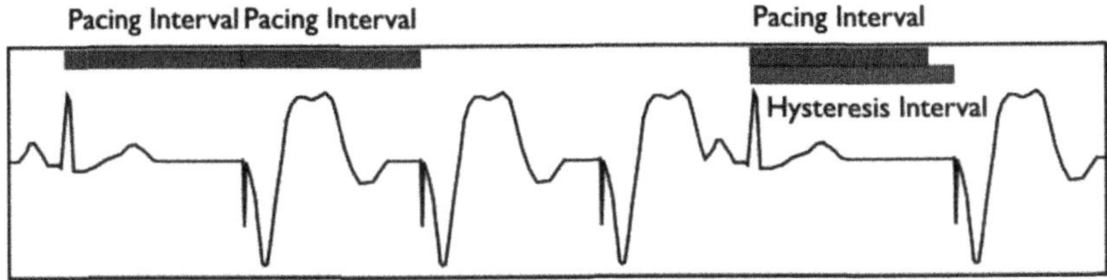

- Rate-adaptive AV delay
  - The AVD can shorten from a programmed baseline to a programmed minimum AVD as the atrial rate increases (mimics normal physiology).
    - Allows atrial tracking at faster rates because of a shorter TARP (AVD + PVARP).
  - It is performed through either linear or stepwise shortening of the AVD.
- Mode switching
  - Rapid atrial rates sensed by the pacemaker induce a switch from dual- to single-chamber pacing to avoid tracking of atrial arrhythmia and pacing the ventricle at unnecessarily high rates.
- Active capture control/autocapture
  - The pacemaker periodically starts at maximum amplitude and works down to the minimum effective capture threshold in order to minimize device output.
- Rate fading
  - This smooths the heart rate to prevent abrupt change (exercise-induced ↓ heart rate, mode-switching).

IMPLANTABLE CARDIOVERTER-DEFIBRILLATOR (ICD)

- An ICD is a specialized device designed to directly treat a cardiac tachyarrhythmia.
- The basic system does not fundamentally differ from a pacing system, except that:
  - The generator has a larger volume (to house the high-voltage power supply and a shock capacitor).
  - The RV pacing lead has a larger diameter owing to the defibrillation function.

- In general, the ICD has all of the sensing and pacing capabilities of a conventional pacemaker but in addition is designed to detect potentially harmful ventricular arrhythmias and to deliver therapies as follows:
  - **Anti-tachycardia pacing (ATP)** results in the device delivering a preset number of rapid pulses in succession in an attempt to terminate the arrhythmia.
    - Types of ATP
      - **Burst**: RV pacing is at a fixed rate. Usually, it is set as a percent of the ventricular tachycardia cycle length (CL).
      - **Ramp**: The RV pacing rate progressively increases within the drive train.
      - **Scan**: This provides burst RV pacing at progressively faster rates. The rate is altered between drive trains, resulting in the next burst being faster than the last.
      - **Ramp-scan**: This is a combination of the above.
    - Programmable
      - Coupling interval: Timing of the first pulse is after the VT beat.
      - Cycle length: Generally, it is set at 81%–88% of the tachyarrhythmia cycle length.
      - Burst length: It is the number of beats in the drive train (usually 8).
    - Outcomes
      - Generally, there is a >90% success for arrhythmia termination (70% for fast VT).
      - This improves the quality of life and potentially survival (when compared to ICD shocks).
  - If unsuccessful, the device will perform a **cardioversion or defibrillation**, a low- or high-voltage, biphasic shock between the defibrillation coil and generator
    - Programmable
      - Energy: In Joules (voltage × current × time)
      - Waveform: Monophasic (shock is delivered to the heart from one vector) or biphasic (shock is delivered via two vectors; more effective).
      - Vector: RV Coil (B) to can (A) and SVC coil (X); RV coil to can; RV coil to SVC coil
      - Direction: Normal = Coil to can (B to AX); reversed = Can to coil (AX to B)
- It is important to note that the "ventricular tachycardia/ventricular fibrillation" (VT/VF) detection is based on the heart rate sensed from the RV electrode.
  - If a set duration of tachycardia is exceeded, then the arrhythmia is "detected."
    - Thereafter, discriminators can be used to differentiate ventricular from supraventricular origin (note: descriminators are only applied in the VT zone and cannot be programmed in the VF zone).
    - However, in the absence of discriminators, the rate and duration of tachycardia define the arrhythmia "zone" and elicit programmed therapies. As such, fast SVT may result in therapies being delivered due to the ventricular rate exceeding the predefined trigger.
- Up to three ventricular rate-detection zones can be programmed to allow delivery of different ICD therapies depending on the tachyarrhythmia rate.
  - The slow VT zone is usually set between 170 and 188–200 bpm.
    - In primary prevention, this may be set to monitor only (no therapies delivered) or to include a variable number of anti-tachycardia pacing (ATP) therapies prior to cardioversion or DC shock.
      - In general, ATP therapy is more effective for slower VTs.

    - The fast VT zone is usually set between 188–200 and 222–250 bpm and usually includes 1 or 2 sets of ATP therapies prior to cardioversion or direct current (DC) shock.
    - The VF zone is usually set for rates faster than 222–250 bpm and may include ATP during charging.
- Redetection: After the ICD delivers therapy, it needs to check the rhythm again to determine if the arrhythmia has terminated.
    - The ICD searches for sinus rhythm (which is defined by the ICD only by heart rate).
    - If the ICD cannot determine a return to sinus rhythm, it concludes the arrhythmia is ongoing and delivers more therapy.

ICD Therapies

- Detection, assessment, and treatment of tachyarrhythmia is progressive and depends on several steps.

Step 1. Sensing

- The most important step in the detection of tachyarrhythmia is the ability of the device to sense it.
    - Tachyarrhythmia is fundamentally different to bradyarrhythmia detection, needing to differentiate signals over a wide range of amplitudes (e.g., a sinus rhythm R wave 10 mV, but a VF R wave of VF 0.2 mV) while avoiding oversensing other signals (e.g., T wave).
    - While the EGM amplitude may be adequate in sinus rhythm, there may be variable sensitivity during tachycardia due to rapid changes in the EGM amplitude.
    - This may result in some signals being underdetected ("drop-out").
    - If enough are underdetected, then the rate trigger or counters may not meet criteria to diagnose a tachyarrhythmia, and thus therapy would not be delivered.
- In general, ICDs automatically adjust sensitivity relative to the signal amplitude, or automatically adjust the signal amplitude (gain) relative to the sensitivity.
    - Automatic/adaptive sensing threshold adjustment starts with a low baseline sensitivity (typically 0.3 mV), which increases to a percentage of the R-wave amplitude (typically 50% to 80%).
        - The sensitivity then decays linearly, exponentially, or with an initial constant then linear.
    - **Band pass frequency**: Narrow the frequency to remove the sensing of noise.
    - **Dynamic noise algorithm** can raise the sensing to stay above noise.

Step 2. Detection Criteria

- **Rate**: The first step in determining if an arrhythmia is present is merely determining the frequency of the tachycardia. Based on the rate, a zone (e.g., VT or VF) is determined for subsequent therapies.
- **Duration**: The second criterion for detection is the duration of tachycardia. This is used as a surrogate to determine whether the arrhythmia is sustained or non-sustained.
    - It is programmed as a series of counters, e.g., 18/24 beats of tachycardia > the rate detection threshold.

Step 3. Algorithms for Discrimination of SVT from VT

- Note: Descriminators do not apply in the VF zone.
- SVT detection ("Rate Branch")
  - The atrial and ventricular rates are compared.
    - If the rates are equal (**V = A**) or the atrial rate is greater than the ventricular rate (**A > V**), then further discriminators are applied.
    - If the ventricular rate is greater than the atrial rate (**V > A**), then therapy is delivered.
- Therapy inhibitors
  - **Morphology**: The device composes templates of EGM morphology in baseline (e.g., normal sinus) rhythm.
    - Using vector timing and correlation, the device compares these baseline templates to tachycardia with the expectation that they will differ significantly from those registered during a ventricular arrhythmia: e.g., SVT looks like sinus (>94% correlation) or VT doesn't look like sinus (<94% correlation).
    - These templates are especially useful in single-chamber devices due to the lack of atrial lead.
    - These templates should not be used in patients with bundle branch block (BBB) or rate-dependent EGM changes.
  - **Sudden onset**: This compares the RR interval at tachycardia onset to the average RR interval in the preceding beats – nominal deemed sudden if the difference is greater than 100 ms.
  - This helps differentiate sinus tachcyardia (gradual onset) from VT (sudden onset)
    - Discriminator function
      - If the measured delta is greater than the programmed delta, therapy is not inhibited (i.e., VT).
      - If the measured delta is less than the programmed delta, therapy is inhibited (i.e., SVT).
    - **Programming**:
      - It is possible to inhibit therapy by adjusting the delta to a smaller value, which makes the device more sensitive to detect VT; e.g., a smaller change or jump in arrhythmia onset is required to qualify as VT.
    - **Limitations of this discriminator**:
      - It may fail if VT occurs during sinus or supraventricular tachycardia. That leads to a smaller decrease in the RR interval compared to the preceding beats.
      - It may fail if VT accelerates gradually into (from below) detection zone. This is particularly challenging when VT crosses in and out of detection zones.
  - **Rate/interval stability**: The device examines the RR intervals between tachycardia beats and determines whether the tachycardia is regular or irregular based on programmed criteria.
    - This helps differentiate AF (irregular/unstable cycle length) from VT (regular/stable cycle).
    - Discriminator function
      - During tachyarrhythmia, the delta between the second-longest and the second-shortest intervals in the interval stability window (nominal 12) is measured.
      - If the measured delta is less than the programmed stability delta (nominal 80 ms), therapy is not inhibited (e.g., deemed stable and therefore VT).

- If the measured delta is greater than the programmed stability delta (nominal 80 ms), therapy is inhibited (e.g., deemed stable and therefore AF).
- **Programming**: Adjusting the delta to a smaller value makes the device less sensitive to detecting VT (smaller variations in rate required to qualify as AF).
- **Limitations of this discriminator**: It may fail if irregular VT or pseudo-regular AF exists.

- **A-V association**: Assesses the AV ratio by evaluating the number and timing of P waves between R waves.
  - The AV association and pattern/timing is used to define AV versus VA conduction, e.g., VT with retrograde conduction.
  - Used in conjunction with stability, onset, and morphology in dual-chamber devices.
  - Discriminator function
    - During tachycardia, the delta between the second-longest and second-shortest AV intervals in the stability window is measured (nominal 12).
    - If the measured delta is less than the programmed AVA delta (nominal 60 ms), an association between A and V events is determined and SVT is diagnosed.
    - If the measured delta is greater than the programmed AVA delta (nominal 60 ms), dissociation between A and V events is determined and VT is confirmed.

- Inhibitor override
  - **Sustained rate duration** delivers therapy after a programmable time interval even if the episode has been classified as SVT.
    - This aims to prevent VT therapies from being are erroneously inhibited by discriminators.
    - **Limitations**: It may result in inappropriate shocks for sustained SVT.
- Therapy accelerator
  - **Shock if unstable**: Therapy is delivered if the device determines the VT is polymorphic in nature.

COMPLICATIONS OF DEVICES

Early

- Venous access (<1%)
  - Pneumothorax, hemothorax, air embolism
- Lead
  - Myocardial or cardiac perforation (<1%)
  - Malposition or inability to place (inability to obtain satisfactory thresholds, phrenic stimulation)
  - Dislodgment (1%–5%; RV < RA < LV/CS); usually <3 days but may occur up to 3 months post procedure
- Pocket
  - Hematoma (<5%; ↑ with anticoagulation or dual antiplatelet therapy)
  - Infection (1%–3%): These include superficial, wound dehiscence, deep (pocket), or systemic (endocarditis).
  - Pain: Suspect an infection if it occurs remote from the implant or improves and then recurs.
- Generator
  - Loose set screw

Delayed

- Venous Access
  - Venous thrombosis, or SVC syndrome (0.5%)
- Lead
  - Exit block
  - Insulation or conductor (pacing/high voltage coil) failure (0.5%/year)
  - Pacemaker lead endocarditis
- Generator
  - Erosion, migration, or pocket infection
  - Twiddler's syndrome
  - Externally damaged: Trauma, radiation, lithotripsy, defibrillation/cardioversion
  - Failure: Battery depletion, component malfunction
- Device malfunction
  - Pacing/sensing: Over- or undersensing, cross-talk, pacemaker-mediated tachyarrhythmia
  - Electromagnetic interference
  - CIED system component (device or lead) advisory (2%)
- Device proarrhythmia
  - Lead arrhythmogenicity
    - **Early**: Local myocardial mechanical stimulation or irritation
    - **Late**: Lead fibrosis creating arrhythmogenic substrate
  - Ventricular undersensing
    - Inappropriate pacing during a vulnerable period of repolarization.
  - "Normal" right ventricular pacing
    - Normal "short-long-short" (bradycardia) pacing leading to ventricular tachyarrhythmia
    - "Dyssynchrony" leading to ↑ heart failure leading to ↑ ventricular arrhythmias
    - Reentry at the site of a prior infarction
  - "Normal" biventricular pacing
    - Abnormal depolarization/repolarization leading to ↑ heterogeneity and/or dispersion of refractoriness

ICD-Specific Complications

- Failure to deliver therapy
  - Programming: The threshold for tachycardia is set too high, or SVT discriminators may need adjustment.
  - Drop-out: Undersensing may result in misclassification of a rate below the detection cut-off.
  - Electromagnetic interference: ICD therapies may be inhibited by the magnet response.
- Appropriate therapy creates complications such as:
  - Psychological reactions may occur in patient or family members.
  - An increase in episodes of appropriate therapy is associated with decreased LV function/worsening of heart failure and increased mortality.
- Inappropriate or unnecessary therapy
- Ineffective therapy

ASSESSMENT OF THE CARDIAC IMPLANTABLE ELECTRONIC DEVICE (CIED) PATIENT

Clinical Evaluation

Symptoms

- Shortness of breath/effort intolerance
- Palpitations
- Presyncope/syncope
- Infectious symptoms

Change in Medical Status

- Stroke
- Heart failure (NYHA functional class)
- Angina/myocardial infarction (CCS Class)

Medication Assessment

- Current medications
- Recent medication changes
- Particularly note diuretics, antiarrhythmic medications

Device History

- Report the index indication for CIED therapy.
- Specify type of device: Single, dual, resynchronization, and defibrillator.
- Specify model and leads: Manufacturer; active/passive fixation leads; bipolar/unipolar leads.
- History of therapies: Appropriate and inappropriate

12-Lead ECG

- Identify the underlying rate/rhythm.
- Specify the **type of device**: Single- or dual-chamber pacing.
- **Programming**: Determine if it is a small spike (bipolar) or large spike (unipolar).
- **Capture:** Assure there is a cardiac depolarization for every pacemaker output (i.e., P wave or QRS after every spike)
- **Sensing**: Native complexes appropriately inhibit pacemaker activity.
- Location of the ventricular wire:
  - "Left bundle branch block (LBBB) morphology": RV apex (negative inferior leads), RVOT (positive inferior leads)
  - "Right bundle branch block (RBBB) morphology": LV apex (negative inferior leads), LVOT (positive inferior leads)
    - Note: If RBBB morphology exists, rule out perforation, patent foramen ovale/atrial septal defects (PFO/ASD), and epicardial/coronary sinus lead.

Other Investigations to Consider

- Chest radiograph
  - Check lead placement (compare to old chest x-ray [CXR] to ensure no migration has occurred).
  - Exclude lead fractures (typically these occur at the junction of the clavicle and first rib).

APPROACH TO PACEMAKER AND IMPLANTABLE CARDIOVERTER-DEFIBRILLATOR (ICD) INTERROGATION

Identify the Device

- Identify the generator: make and model.
- Identify the lead(s): number, position, make, and model.
- Are there any advisories/recalls for the leads or generators?

Assess the Intrinisic or Underlying Rate and Rhythm

- Observe the intracardiac EGM for the presenting/underlying rhythm.
- Baseline device parameters:
  - LRL and URL
  - Intervals: AV/PV delay, TARP, PVARP, blanking periods
  - Programmed pacing mode (e.g., DDD, VVI)
  - Mode switching: On or off, and parameters for mode switching
  - Tachyarrhythmia zones and programmed therapies (if ICD)
- Assess battery status
  - Check the current battery voltage and impedance.
  - Check the elective replacement indicator (ERI).
  - Check the charge time and date of last charge (if ICD).

Assess Lead Function

- Pacemaker leads are expected to fail at 0.5%/year; ICD leads at 0.6%–5%/year (see Table 13.2).

Table 13.2 Signs of Lead Failure in Pacemakers and ICDs

Pacemaker	ICD
• Failure to capture (33%) • High pacing threshold (14%–30%) • Abnormal impedance: High (5%), low (12%) • Abnormal sensing: Under (13%), over (12%) • Failure in sensing and capture (13%–15%)	• Inappropriate shocks (33% to 76%) • Abnormal high-voltage lead impedance (56%) • Increased capture threshold (22%)

Sensing

- The ability of the CIED to detect intrinsic myocardial depolarization (i.e., the potential difference between the lead's cathodal and anodal electrodes)
  - Defined by the smallest intrinsic myocardial signal that can be consistently detected by the CIED
  - Influenced by the rate of change of the local EGM voltage (**slew rate**)
- How to interrogate and determine sensing:
  - Sensing is automatically measured by the interrogator/device.
  - Decrease the paced rate to allow underlying rhythm to manifest.
- Assessment of device sensing:
  - The key to sensing is stability, as after the acute phase (3 months) the height of P and R waves should not change dramatically over follow-up.
    - At implant, R waves should be > 5 mV and P waves >1.5–2 mV.
    - Chronic R waves should be >5–10 mV and chronic P waves >2–5 mV.

- Programming changes to adjust sensing:
  - Programmed as the "bar" above which the device detects a signal.
    - **Lowering** the mV setting makes the device **more** sensitive (to pick up missing signals).
    - **Increasing** the mV setting makes the device **less** sensitive (to avoid detecting signals).
  - Usual settings:
    - P-wave amplitude is normally set at 1/3 of sensed P waves (~0.5 mV).
    - R-wave amplitude is normally set at 1/2 of sensed R waves (~3 mV).

Capture Threshold

- Minimum amount of current required to reliably stimulate contraction.
- How to interrogate and determine the threshold:
  - Increase the pacing rate above the underlying rate.
    - For the A lead, consider AAI if there is intrinsic conduction or DDD with long AV delay if there is underlying heart block; during testing look for a lack of atrial response (e.g., an absence surface P wave, or intracardiac AR/AS after AP).
    - For the V lead, consider VVI unless that is intolerable, in which case use DDD with a short AV delay; look for a lack of ventricular response (surface QRS complex or VR/VS after VP).
  - Reduce the impulse energy (voltage) until loss of capture.
    - Note: Threshold is usually lower in the ventricle secondary to better electrode-myocardial contact.
- Assessment of capture threshold:
  - The key to threshold is stability.
  - The threshold generally increases and peaks over the first 2–6 weeks after implant due to the inflammatory response at the distal electrode.
    - This may be overcome by the elution of steroid from the distal electrode.
  - After the acute phase (3 months), the threshold should not change dramatically.
    - At implant, the threshold should be <1.0–1.5 V in the atrium and ventricle.
    - The chronic threshold should be <1.5–2.0 V in the atrium and ventricle.
- Programming to adjust capture threshold:
  - The initial threshold is typically set at 5–6× above the implant threshold.
  - Chronic threshold:
    - Typically it is set at 2–3× the tested threshold.
    - The exception is in the patient with complete heart block who is pacemaker dependent. In these patients, the threshold may be set much higher to offer a larger safety margin.

Lead Impedance

- Lead impedance is a measure of the resistance to current flow with pacing.
  - It reflects the combined effect of capacitance, resistance, and inductance.

- Related to the inherent characteristics of the lead as well as factors related to implantation:
  - The inherent resistance of the conductor coils
  - The size and shape of the electrode tip (higher with smaller-diameter and bipolar leads)
  - The electrode/myocardial interface
- How to interrogate and determine the lead impedance
  - Lead impedance is automatically measured by the interrogator/device.
    - Normal high-voltage coil impedance is roughly 20–100 Ω.
    - Normal pacing lead impedance is roughly 200–1500 Ω.
- Assessment of lead impedance
  - The key to lead impedances is stability.
  - While there is a normal trend in pace/sense lead impedance to decrease over time, a >30% change from baseline or an acute change >200 Ω (pacing) or >12 Ω (HV) is worrisome.
  - Significant increase suggests:
    - **Early**: Lead dislodgment, perforation, or header-connector problem
    - **Late:** Lead conductor fracture; change in the local myocardial substrate (e.g., ischemia, or infarct at lead tip); changes in myocardial conductance (e.g., pharmacologic agents, electrolytes)
  - A significant decrease suggests lead or adaptor insulation failure (i.e., the energy is dissipating into the tissue).

Special Tests

- Retrograde conduction test
  - Overstimulate the ventricle and check for VA conduction.
- Measure Wenckebach point
  - Overstimulate atria and check for AV conduction.
- Provocative maneuvers
  - Arm abduction/adduction/rotation, Valsalva, or pocket manipulation during real-time telemetry (intracardiac EGM/marker channels) if an abnormal lead impedance or oversensing due to lead failure or myopotentials is suspected.

Note: Provocative maneuvers should only be performed in ICD patients after inactivation of tachyarrhythmia therapies (risk of inappropriate shock).

Observations/Events/Diagnostics

- Rate histograms
  - Flat rate histograms suggest relative inactivity or the need for a rate-response function assessment.
- Episode data
  - The general approach to interpreting arrhythmia episodes relies on it being a systematic approach and interpretation of all the available information starting with the "A and V dot plots," followed by direct interpretation of the intracardiac EGMs.
    - Atrial high-rate episodes
    - Ventricular high-rate episodes
    - Noise reversion
    - Pacemaker-mediated tachycardia

Programming and Print

- After the device has been interrogated, programming changes should be made.
- A printed copy of the device settings should be placed in the medical record and provided to the patient.

PROBLEM SOLVING CARDIAC IMPLANTABLE ELECTRONIC DEVICES (CIEDs)

Failure to Sense ("Undersensing")

- **Definition**: Failure to recognize and appropriately respond to intrinsic signals.
  - This results in pacing despite the presence of intrinsic activity.
- Causes
  - Programming
    - Programmed in a non-sensing mode (i.e., AOO, VOO, or DOO)
    - The sensitivity set too low (the device does not see the intrinsic signals)
    - Prolonged refractory or blanking period
  - Change in sensed signal
    - Deterioration in signal over time
      - Lead maturation (inflammation or fibrosis at the electrode tip)
      - Disease progression (ischemia/infarct, cardiomyopathy)
      - New bundle branch block (results in electrical vector changes)
      - Respiratory or motion variation
    - Transient decrease in signal amplitude
      - Post cardioversion/defibrillation
      - Metabolic/electrolyte abnormality (hypothyroidism, medications)
  - Generator failure
    - Impending battery depletion
    - Component malfunction (sensing circuit abnormality, stuck reed switch)
    - Magnet application
  - Lead failure
    - Lead dislodgement or perforation (early)
    - Air in the pocket (unipolar only)
    - Insulation failure (associated with decreased impedance)
    - Lead conductor coil fracture
  - Pseudo malfunction
    - Recording artifact (i.e., false pacemaker spikes on the recording system)
    - Triggered mode or safety pacing
    - Fusion and pseudofusion beats
    - Functional undersensing (undersensing due to event falling on the refractory period)
- Initial management
  - Consider placement of a magnet to enable asynchronous pacing.
- Treatment of the underlying cause
  - Correct electrolyte abnormalities, treat ischemia, and remove non-essential medications.

- Programming changes
  - Increase the sensitivity.
- Device changes
  - Lead revision and/or insertion (if a lead problem)

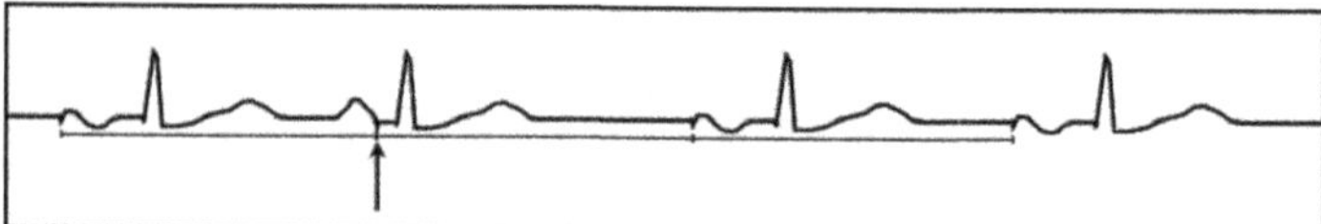

Failure to Pace

- **Definition**: Failure to deliver stimulation when it would be otherwise anticipated
- Causes
  - Programming ("oversensing")
    - An inappropriate event results in the inhibition of pacing and/or inappropriate therapies.
      - The pacemaker inappropriately "thinks" that it sees intrinsic activity that is not there.
    - Internal interference
      - T-wave oversensing (T wave misclassified as an R wave on the ventricular channel)
      - R-wave oversensing (R wave misclassified as a P wave on the atrial channel)
    - External interference
      - Electromagnetic interference
      - Myopotential (unipolar devices)
      - Lead noise (sensed "make-break" signals)
        - Crosstalk (interaction between the active lead and abandoned leads)
        - Insulation failure between anodal and cathodal conductor coils (bipolar system)
        - Conductor coil fracture
        - Loose set screw
        - Loose distal fixation helix or screw
  - Generator failure
    - Total battery depletion (more common than circuitry failure)
    - Generator component failure
  - Lead failure
    - Lead disconnection (incompatibility between lead and pulse generator)
    - Conductor failure (associated with increased impedance)
    - Insulation failure (associated with decreased impedance)
  - Pseudomalfunction
    - Programming (hysteresis, sleep or rest mode, PVARP extension after a PVC, mode switch)
- Initial management
  - If the patient is not pacemaker dependent, then monitoring may be appropriate pending elucidation of the underlying cause and provision of a definitive treatment.
  - If the patient is pacemaker dependent, then IV isoproterenol may be attempted prior to placement of a transvenous temporary pacemaker lead.

- Programming changes
  - Lower the sensitivity (if ICD and T wave are oversensing, then ensure sensing of low-amplitude VF)
  - Lengthening of the blanking or refractory period (if ICD, then may limit the detection of VT)
  - Changing sensing decay algorithm (not available in all devices)
- Device changes
  - Generator change (if a generator/battery problem)
  - Lead revision and/or insertion (if a lead problem)

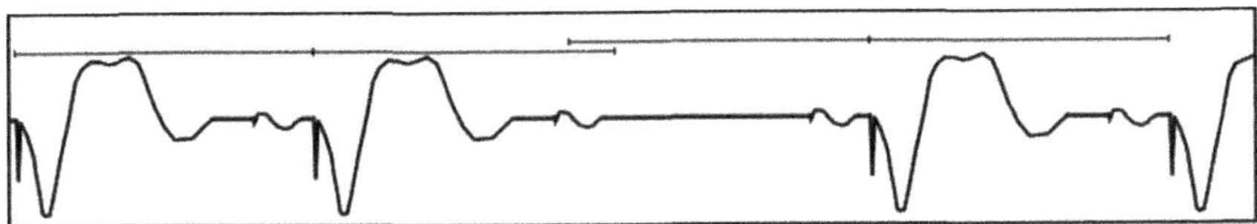

Failure to Capture

- Definition: The pacing artifact is not followed by an atrial or a ventricular complex.
- Causes
  - Programming
    - The output is set too low.
  - Capture threshold elevation
    - Deterioration in the capture threshold occurs over time.
      - Lead maturation (exit block due to early inflammation or late fibrosis at electrode tip)
      - Progression of the underlying cardiomyopathy (infarction, infiltrative cardiomyopathy)
    - A transient change in the capture threshold occurs.
      - Metabolic/electrolyte abnormality (hyperkalemia, acidosis, hypoxemia)
    - Drugs
      - Increased pacing threshold with class I and class III antiarrhythmic drugs
      - Decreased pacing threshold with steroids, isoproterenol
  - A lead failure occurs.
    - Lead dislodgement or perforation (early)
    - Air in the pocket (unipolar only)
    - Insulation failure (↓ impedance if current loss to other sources)
    - Conductor failure (↑ impedance if crush between clavicle and first rib, or wire fracture)
  - Pseudomalfunction occurs.
    - Recording artifact mimicking malfunction
    - Functional non-capture (output delivered in refractory period)
    - Isoelectric evoked potential
    - Latency

- Initial management
  - If the patient is not pacemaker dependent, then monitoring may be appropriate pending elucidation of the underlying cause and provision of definitive treatment.
  - If the patient is pacemaker dependent, then IV isoproterenol 0.5–5.0 mcg/min infusion (to increase heart rate) may be attempted prior to placement of a transvenous temporary pacemaker lead.
- Treatment of the underlying cause:
  - Correct the electrolyte abnormalities.
  - Treat ischemia.
  - Remove non-essential medications.
- Programming changes include:
  - Increase the pacing output/pulse width to facilitate a reliable capture, pending definitive treatment.
- Device changes include:
  - Lead revision and/or insertion (if a lead problem).

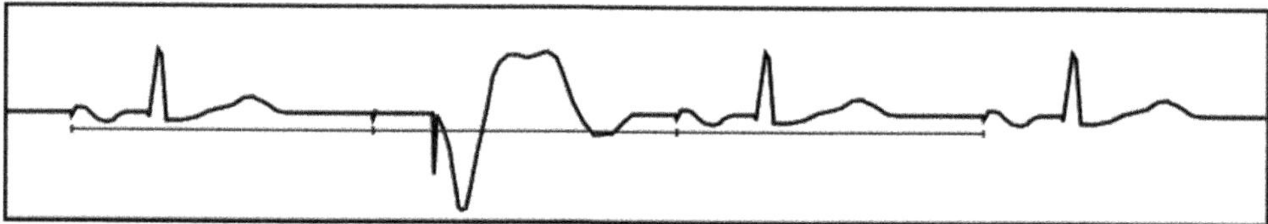

MANAGING THE PATIENT WITH AN IMPLANTABLE CARDIOVERTER-DEFIBRILLATOR (ICD) THERAPY

Background

- Approximately 30%–60% of patients will have a shock within 2 years of implantation; 60% are appropriate.

Clinical Assessment

- See *Assessment of the CIED Patient*

Investigations

- Laboratory
  - Electrolytes (potassium, magnesium) should always be checked.
  - Check for myocardial ischemia (cardiac troponins, creatine kinase-MB [CK-MB]) and heart failure (brain natriuretic peptide [BNP]).
  - Test the thyroid function (TSH ± free T3/T4).
  - Test the renal function (creatinine, estimated glomerular filtration rate [eGFR]).
  - Test for drug intoxication (i.e., digoxin, theophylline, barbiturates, cocaine, amphetamines).
- **Echocardiography**: For patients with appropriate shocks, this rules out deterioration in LV function.
- **Consider an ischemia evaluation** (stress test/myocardial perfusion [MIBI] scan, angiography).
- Perform a 12-lead electrocardiogram (ECG) and a chest x-ray.

Device Interrogation

- See *Approach to Pacemaker and ICD Interrogation*

Determine Type of Shock

- Appropriate shock (VT or VF) due to:
  - Modification of, or non-compliance to drug therapy
  - New or worsened heart failure
  - New or worsened myocardial ischemia
  - Underlying cardiac pathology
    - Severe LV dysfunction
    - Remote infarction
    - Channelopathy (Brugada, LQT)
    - Idiopathic VF
  - Metabolic derangements:
    - Electrolyte abnormalities (K^+, Mg^{2+})
    - Hyperthyroidism
  - Alcohol excess or drug abuse
  - Device proarrhythmia
- Unnecessary shocks
  - Hemodynamically tolerated/slow VT, non-sustained VT or ATP-sensitive VT
- Inappropriate shock due to:
  - **Failure to discriminate SVT** (with or without aberrancy): AF, AFL, AT, AVNRT/AVRT
  - Programming problem:
    - Thresholds set too low
    - T-wave oversensing
    - Atrial far-field sensing
  - Artifact
    - Myopotential
    - Lead failure
    - Insulation break
    - Electromagnetic interference
  - **Implant problem**: Loose set screw
    - Phantom shock

Management (Depends on Cause)

- Repetitive ICD shocks in the absence of tachyarrhythmia or due to tachyarrhythmia (atrial or ventricular) that is hemodynamically tolerated:
  - Place a magnet over the device to inhibit further shock delivery.
  - Note: Continuous telemetry must be maintained during magnet application.
- Evaluate and treat reversible causes.
  - Replete electrolytes (K^+ to 4.0–4.5 mmol/L and IV $MgSO_4$ if QTc is prolonged).
  - Treat myocardial ischemia.
  - Remove unnecessary drugs (including antiarrhythmics and vasopressors).
- Treat the underlying cause.
  - Add/modify therapies directed at the primary pathology.
- Optimize β-blocker therapy.
  - First-line therapy for patients receiving appropriate ICD therapies:
    - If it is an appropriate shock, β-blockers can decrease the probability of recurrent shocks and treat the underlying cardiac condition
    - If it is an inappropriate shock, β-blockers may decrease the ventricular rate during SVT, thus decreasing the probability device therapy.
- Add/modify AAD therapy.
  - Further AAD choices should be based on the underlying arrhythmia.
    - If it is an appropriate shock, then AADs may slow the VT, increasing the likelihood of an ATP success.
    - If it is an inappropriate shock, then AADs may help maintain sinus rhythm.
- Consider reprogramming the device.
  - ATP settings (more or less aggressive depending on the underlying cause of the shock)
  - Detection rates (based on the clinical arrhythmia history)
  - Discriminators (if SVT is causing inappropriate shocks)
- Consider catheter ablation.
  - SVT ablation for SVT-induced inappropriate shocks
  - VT ablation for VT-induced appropriate shocks
- Post discharge care:
  - In general, patients are restricted from private driving for a period of:
    - 6 months after an appropriate ICD therapy that results in hemodynamic compromise
    - 3 months after an appropriate ICD therapy not associated with hemodynamic compromise, but LVEF <30%
    - 1 month after an appropriate ICD therapy not associated with hemodynamic compromise, but LVEF >30%
  - Note: Restrictions are region-specific and consultation with the local agency is recommended.
- Prognosis
  - ICD shocks are associated with increased all-cause mortality:
    - 6× increase for appropriate shocks
    - 2× increase for inappropriate shocks
    - 20% increased relative risk (RR) of death for each shocked episode
  - High levels of depression/anxiety
    - Generally related to the number and recency of shocks received
    - Management: Cognitive behavior therapy

ARRHYTHMIC OR ELECTRICAL STORM

Definition: Three or more distinct episodes of sustained or device-terminated VT and/or VF within a 24-hour period

Background

- Electrical storm occurs in 10%–40% of patients with secondary prevention devices (rare in primary prevention).
- An electrical storm results from a complex interplay between arrhythmogenic substrates and acute perturbations in autonomic tone and cellular milieu.
  - No independent predictors have been reproducibly identified.

Assessment and Investigations

- As above

Management

- Evaluate and treat reversible causes.
  - As above
- β-blockers
  - β-blockers are first-line therapy for patients with an electrical storm.
  - Non-selective β-blockers (such as propranolol) are preferred due to the role of β_2-receptors in the perpetuation of electrical storm.
  - Note: If there are concerns regarding hemodynamic instability, consider the use of IV esmolol.
- Antiarrhythmic drug therapy
  - IV Amiodarone is the preferred first line AAD (especially in combination with β-blocker).
  - Second-line or alternatives:
    - IV procainamide
    - Lidocaine, especially if associated with acute ischemia
  - For storm related to Brugada syndrome, the use of isoproterenol or quinidine may terminate incessant arrhythmias.
- Optimize device programming
  - Modify ATP settings to minimize the need for DC shock.
  - Consider overdrive pacing if related to bradycardia-induced torsade de pointes.
- Sedation
  - Deep sedation and, if necessary, intubation/ventilation can be essential to reduce adrenergic stress.
- Provide circulatory mechanical support if refractory ventricular arrhythmias result in hemodynamic compromise.

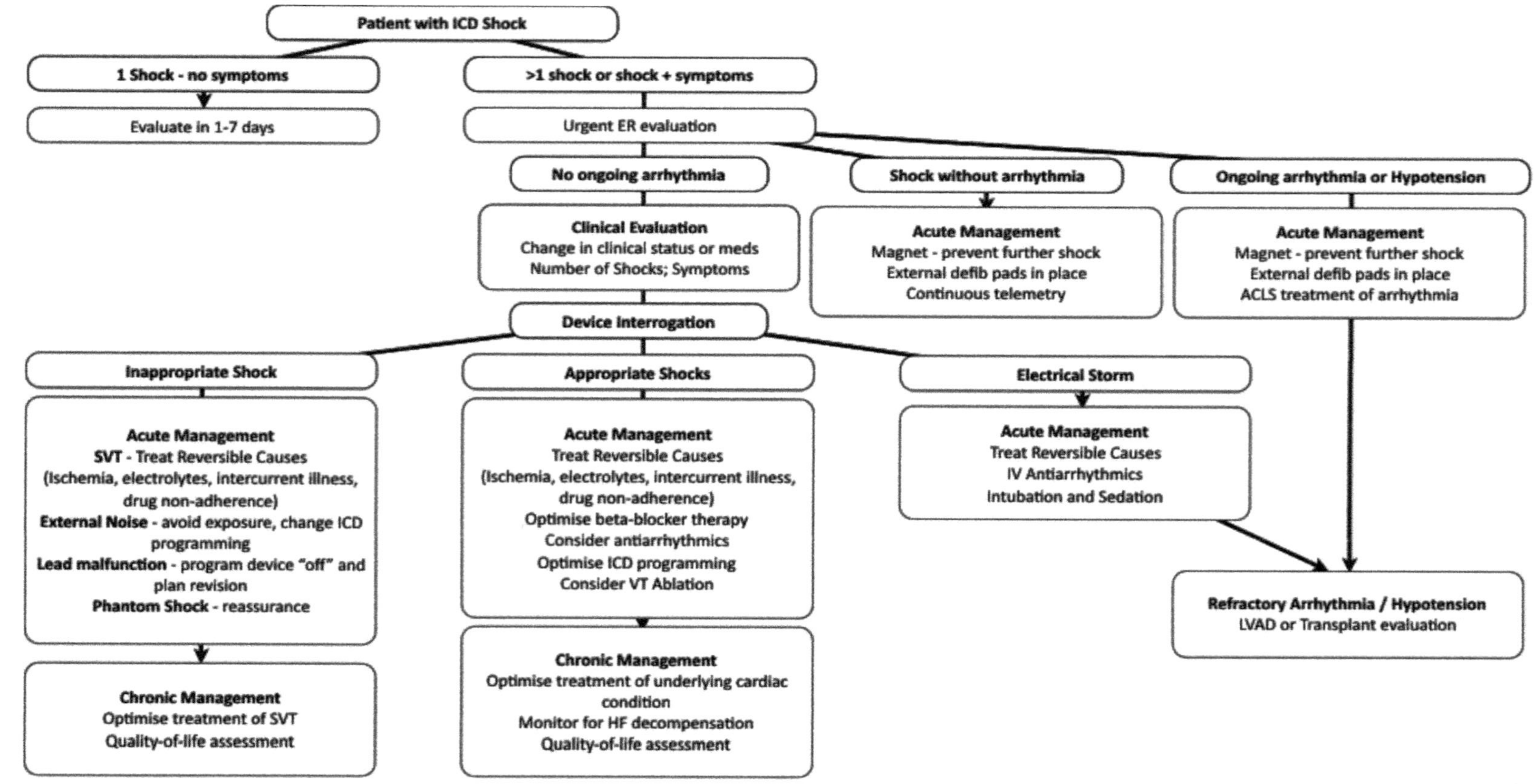
Patient with ICD Shock
1 Shock - no symptoms
Evaluate in 1-7 days
>1 shock or shock + symptoms
Urgent ER evaluation
No ongoing arrhythmia
Clinical Evaluation
Change in clinical status or meds
Number of Shocks; Symptoms
Shock without arrhythmia
Acute Management
Magnet - prevent further shock
External defib pads in place
Continuous telemetry
Ongoing arrhythmia or Hypotension
Acute Management
Magnet - prevent further shock
External defib pads in place
ACLS treatment of arrhythmia
Device Interrogation
Inappropriate Shock
Acute Management
SVT - Treat Reversible Causes
(Ischemia, electrolytes, intercurrent illness, drug non-adherence)
External Noise - avoid exposure, change ICD programming
Lead malfunction - program device "off" and plan revision
Phantom Shock - reassurance
Chronic Management
Optimise treatment of SVT
Quality-of-life assessment
Appropriate Shocks
Acute Management
Treat Reversible Causes
(Ischemia, electrolytes, intercurrent illness, drug non-adherence)
Optimise beta-blocker therapy
Consider antiarrhythmics
Optimise ICD programming
Consider VT Ablation
Chronic Management
Optimise treatment of underlying cardiac condition
Monitor for HF decompensation
Quality-of-life assessment
Electrical Storm
Acute Management
Treat Reversible Causes
IV Antiarrhythmics
Intubation and Sedation
Refractory Arrhythmia / Hypotension
LVAD or Transplant evaluation

CARDIAC IMPLANTABLE ELECTRONIC DEVICES (CIEDs): SPECIAL CONSIDERATIONS

Magnet Response

- Pacemakers
  - In most devices, placing a magnet over a pacemaker temporarily turns off the sensing, causing the device to pace in an asynchronous mode at a fixed heart rate.
    - The majority switch to high-rate, asynchronous pacing (80–100 bpm); some pace at the programmed rate, and a minority pace at a slow rate (~60 bpm).
- ICDs
  - In most devices, placing a magnet over an ICD results in a transient inhibition of arrhythmia detection and therapy delivery, which lasts as long as the magnet is positioned over the device.
    - Note: For some Boston Scientific devices, a magnet application for >30 seconds results in deactivation of the device if the "change tachy mode with magnet" function is enabled (i.e., the ICD remains inactive even after the magnet is removed).
  - In contrast to pacemakers, when a magnet is applied to an ICD, the pacing function is unaltered.
  - During magnet mode, it is essential to maintain continuous ECG monitoring in order to detect potentially life-threatening ventricular tachyarrhythmia.
- Caveats
  - Some devices can be programmed to not respond to magnet application.
    - Because of this variability, it is critical to verify the device programming.
  - Also, there are some differences between manufacturers with respect to proper magnet position.
    - Medtronic devices: Magnet should be placed directly over the ICD.
    - St. Jude Medical devices: The magnet should be placed off-center such that the curve of the magnet is over the top or bottom end of the device.

Radiotherapy

- Delivery of radiotherapy for cancer can lead to a number of issues:
- **Inability to deliver radiotherapy**: The CIED may result in mechanical obstruction of the radiotherapy field.
  - Consider repositioning the CIED system if necessary.
- **Oversensing**: If the radiotherapy average dose rate at the device exceeds 1 cGy/min, the CIED may inappropriately sense direct or scattered radiation as cardiac activity during the procedure.
  - Consider programing the device to an asynchronous pacing mode.
  - Consider temporarily suspending tachyarrhythmia therapies and detection.
- **Device damage**: Exposing the device to high doses of direct or scattered radiation with an accumulated dose greater than 100–500 cGy may damage the device.
  - Consider using appropriate shielding during the procedure.
  - Consider the accumulated dose to the device for patients undergoing multiple treatments.

- Device operational errors:
  - Exposing the device to scattered neutrons may cause an electrical reset of the device, errors in device functionality, errors in diagnostic data, or loss of diagnostic data.
  - Consider delivering radiotherapy treatment by using photon beam energies ≤10 mV (conventional x-ray shielding does not protect the device from the effects of the neutrons).

Surgery

- General
  - Cautery use should be minimized, and the grounding pad should be kept distant from CIED site.
- Pacemakers
  - If a patient is pacemaker dependent the device can be programmed in an asynchronous mode (e.g., DOO or VOO) with the base rate increased to greater than the intrinsic rate
  - Monitor the heart rate with telemetry or pulse oximetry.
- ICDs
  - The main concern is the risk for inappropriate shock due to the sensing of external noise.
  - Pre-operatively, the ICD function should be verified, and therapies and detection programmed off.
  - Postoperatively, the device should be re-verified to ensure no damage to the device or leads has occurred, and the previous therapies re-enabled.

Resuscitation

- Advanced cardiac life support (ACLS) protocols should be initiated if a patient enters a life-threatening cardiac arrhythmia.
- Chest compressions should be continued regardless of the presence of a CIED.
- If the ICD delivers a therapy, some of the defibrillation current may enter the rescuer.
  - Minor discomfort (i.e., slight tingle in the skin) can be prevented by wearing latex gloves.
  - If rescuers are uncomfortable during resuscitations, the ICD can be deactivated with a magnet.
- Note: VT or VF refractory to ICD therapy requires external defibrillation and/or AADs as dictated by ACLS.

External Cardioversion and Defibrillation

- Clinically appropriate energy output should be used regardless of the presence of a CIED.
- The external pads or paddles should be positioned distant from the CIED pulse generator (10-15 cm away from the generator with an anterior–posterior vector).

- Patients who receive external shock must have their CIED interrogated afterwards to ensure that device function and/or programming have not been altered.
  - Pacing thresholds may rise after the external energy delivery, leading to loss of capture.
  - External energy delivery that affects the generator rarely may cause a total device failure.

Central Line Placement

- Insertion of central venous lines and pulmonary artery catheters requires special care in CIED patients.
- Central lines
  - Subclavian venipuncture should be avoided ipsilateral to an implanted device due to:
    - The risk of the needle injuring the insulation of indwelling leads.
    - The possibility of ipsilateral venous occlusion (occurs in up to 20% at 2 years).
  - The metal guidewire may contact the lead system during placement.
    - Such contact may generate artifact that may inhibit pacing or trigger an inappropriate shock.
    - Consider avoiding a metal guidewire or deactivating the ICD during placement.
- Pulmonary artery (PA) catheters
  - There is a risk of lead dislodgment in passing PA catheters through the RA and RV.
    - This is a significant concern in patients with CRT devices because of the risk to the LV lead.
  - If the decision is made to proceed, then the PA catheter should be placed under fluoroscopic guidance.

Overpacing in the RV

- Chronic RV pacing may result in the deterioration of ventricular function due to mechanical dyssynchrony.
  - It occurs in up to 10% of patients within one year of implantation (up to 15% long-term).
  - It is more common in those with reduced baseline left ventricle ejection fraction (LVEF <40%), and frequent pacing (>40%).
- Management
  - Extend the AV delay (AVD).
    - Doing so may only be 20%–50% effective.
    - It requires reliable AVN conduction.
    - It limits the 2:1 block point due to increased TARP.
    - AF recognition delays or requires the abandonment of mode-switching.
    - Susceptibility to pacemaker-mediated tachycardia (PMT) increases; this is reduced with rate-adaptive AVD.
  - AAI pacing
    - This strategy requires reliable AV conduction (1%–3% annual incidence of third-degree AVB in isolated SND).
    - It is ineffectual for bradyarrhythmia related to AF.

- DDIR mode: This mode permits a long AVD without tracking during AF.
  - Limitations:
    - The DDIR mode is operationally VVIR during AV block if the sinus rate is less than the lower rate limit.
    - Competitive atrial pacing may precipitate AF.
  - Novel "minimize ventricular pacing" algorithms (e.g., Managed Ventricular Pacing or SafeR mode)
    - These may be more effective than the above methods at reducing V-pacing with SND.
    - They may reduce the ventricular pacing percentage from >90% to <10% in selected populations.

Pacemaker-Mediated Tachycardia (PMT)

- PMT is an endless loop tachycardia in dual-chamber devices (DDD and VDD as required in atrial tracking modes).

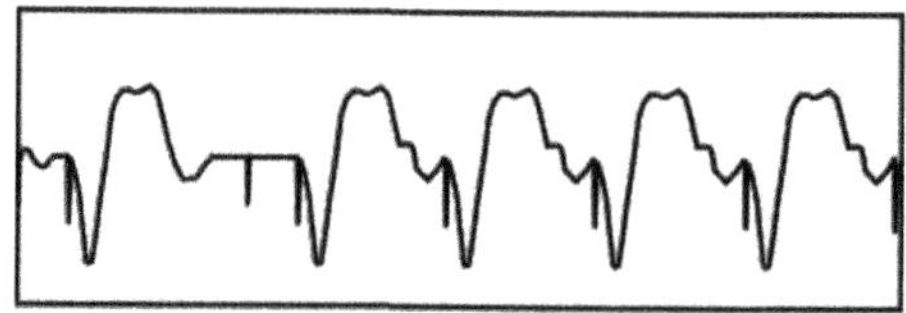

- Retrograde atrial activation is detected by the atrial sensor, which then stimulates the ventricle.
  - Ventricular depolarization without an immediately preceding atrial event, such as:
    - Isolated ventricular depolarization (PVC)
      - PVC with intact retrograde conduction (most common mechanism).
    - Ventricular pace without preceding atrial depolarization
      - Atrial loss of capture
      - Atrial oversensing (far-field signal, myopotentials)
    - Atrial undersensing of anterograde P waves (preserved sensing of retrograde P waves)
    - Atrial threshold testing (sub-threshold atrial stimulation)
  - Ventricular pace preceded by atrial event with sufficient time for atrial repolarization, leading to:
    - Non-conducted PAC
    - PAC with AVI prolongation to conform to lower rate interval (LRI)
    - Excessively long AVI
- The rate of this tachycardia is limited by the pacemaker's programmed upper limit.
  - Tachycardia cycle time = VA conduction time (V pace to retro P) + functional PV delay
- Testing for PMT substrate:
  - Retrograde conduction test at implantation (VDI mode)
    - 60% SSS and 25% AVB have the retained ability for retrograde conduction

- Management
  - Immediate
    - The application of a magnet will result in asynchronous pacing and terminate the PMT.
  - Device programming
    - Treat the cause
      - Loss of atrial capture, atrial undersensing, atrial oversensing
    - Most pacemakers have algorithms to terminate PMT.
      - After a number of VA intervals, the device extends the VA interval.
      - If there is lengthening, the pacer confirms PMT and increases TARP to break the circuit.
      - However, in some cases they may be programmed off or ineffective.
    - Increase the PVARP or TARP (blind the atria to all post-PVC events).
      - This limits the maximum tracking rate, causing a 2:1 block with activity.
      - "Post-PVC management" will increase PVARP/TARP for only one cycle post PVC.
    - Decrease the sensitivity of the atrial lead.
      - Retrograde P waves are often small amplitude compared to normal P waves.
      - Note: Programming the dynamic P-wave amplitude limits this strategy.

Atrial Fibrillation

- Mechanism
  - Postulated to be related to tricuspid regurgitation or AV dyssynchrony leading to increased RA pressure and dilatation
- Prevention
  - Atrial or dual chamber pacing
  - Atrial preventative pacing algorithms:
    - Atrial pacing above intrinsic rate
    - Accelerated atrial pacing rate following PAC
    - Post mode switch overdrive pacing
  - Anti-tachycardia pacing in response to atrial tachyarrhythmias
    - More effective for slow cycle length AT or AFL

Pacemaker Syndrome

- Intrinsic atrial impulses occur during or just after ventricular pacing in single chamber devices.
  - Impulses cause the atria to contract against closed AV valves.
  - This results in the reflux of blood back into the vena cavae and lungs.
- Symptoms include:
  - Dyspnea, palpitations, nausea, chest pain/fullness, headache, lethargy, neck throbbing
- Management
  - Upgrade to a dual-chamber (DDD) pacemaker and reprogram the AV delays.

Runaway Pacemaker

- A runaway pacemaker is a rare medical emergency.
- It is due to the total failure of a pacemaker generator, resulting in rapid tachycardia.
- A magnet application is usually ineffective.
  - Often the device must be manually disabled manual (disconnection of the lead from the generator).

DEFIBRILLATOR THRESHOLD TESTING

- Indications
  - Concern regarding arrhythmia underdetection (small R waves)
  - Concern regarding inability to defibrillate (e.g., right-sided implant)
  - Concern regarding ineffective therapies
    - Medications that increase defibrillator threshold (DFT):
      - Flecainide, lidocaine, mexilitine, phenytoin, quinidine, amiodarone
      - Diltiazem/verapamil (IV), propranolol
    - Medications that decrease DFT:
      - Azimilide, dofetilide, ibutilide, procainamide, sotalol
- Contraindications
  - AF/flutter AFL with uncertain or subtherapeutic anticoagulation
- Risks include:
  - Death (<1%)
  - Stroke/systemic thromboembolism (<1%)
  - Heart failure or hypotension necessitating inotropic support
  - Cardiac arrest, non-elective intubation, chest compressions
- Procedure
  - Ensure external "hands-free" defibrillation pads are correctly applied.
  - Verify adequate device function:
    - Verify impedance (pacing and high-voltage), sensing (P and R waves), and thresholds are normal and stable.
    - Ensure there is no T-wave or far-field R-wave oversensing.
  - Reprogram the device
    - A low sensitivity (typically ~1.2 mV) can assess VF detection with a "worst-case scenario" sensing.
    - Use a tachyarrhythmia detection zone (i.e., VF only) at a reasonable number of intervals.
    - Ensure that the ATP is programmed off.
  - Protocols for programming the DFT:
    - **Step down**: Reduce the shock amplitude until a shock fails to defibrillate the heart; i.e., start at 35 J, then decreases to 25 J, then 15 J. Lowest successful shock level is then called the DFT.
    - **Step up**: Increase the shock amplitude until a shock successfully defibrillates the heart; i.e., program 3 shocks at 15 J, 25 J, and 35 J. The lowest successful shock level is then called the DFT.
    - **Step down/step-up**: "Step down" until failure, and then "step up" until successful again.
  - Sedate the patient and perform a synchronized 1-2 J test shock via the external defibrillation.

- Induce VF
  - T-shock: Start with a 6–8 beat drive train at 400 ms with a T-shock (1–2J) at 300 ms.
    - If there is a BBB, delay the S2 by 10–30 ms.
    - If unsuccessful: Progressively increase or decrease the T-shock by 10 ms and change the drive train to a different rate (e.g., 350 ms).
  - 50-Hz burst: Rapid pulse delivery (20 ms) for 10 seconds.
- After DFT testing, the device will need to be reprogrammed.
  - Tachyarrhythmia detection zones, intervals, and therapies, discriminators, sensitivity, pacing

NON-RESPONDERS TO CARDIAC RESYNCHRONIZATION THERAPY (CRT)

Epidemiology

- Non-response to CRT is estimated at 30%–40% of patients, depending on the definition used.

Causes

- Suboptimal percentage of biventricular pacing (i.e., <95% pacing)
  - Suboptimal AV timing
  - Arrhythmia (PACs/PVCs, AF: ~30%)
- Suboptimal LV lead position (~10%–20%)
- Anemia (~30%)
- Suboptimal medical therapy (~10%–20%) or compliance issues (~5%–10%)
- Relatively narrow QRS width (~5%–10%) or non-LBBB RS morphology
- Severe valvular disease, particularly mitral regurgitation
- Primary RV dysfunction

Assessment and Troubleshooting

Step 1: Clinical Assessment for Reversible Causes

- Medical therapy optimization
- Volume overload: Increase diuretics
- AF: Pharmacologic rate control (or AVN ablation) or cardioversion
- Manage comorbidities
  - Cardiac obstructive pulmonary disease (COPD)
  - Anemia
  - Pre-renal azotemia
- Cardiac ischemia: Coronary angiography ± revascularization

Step 2: ECG: Assess for Fusion or Pseudo Fusion

- Lead I and V1
  - R/S ratio <1 in lead V1 or >1 in lead 1: Consider loss of left ventricular capture
- Lead II and V1 (compare baseline ECG at time of implant to present ECG)
  - ↑ R/↓ S in II and no change in morphology in V1: Loss of RV capture (PPV 93%; NPV 96%)
  - ↑ S in II and/or change in morphology in V1: Loss of LV capture (PPV 91%; NPV 71%)

Step 3: Device Interrogation

- Ensure the pacemaker is pacing the ventricle >95% of the time.
- Ensure an adequate and consistent LV and RV lead capture.

Step 4: Base Programming

- Rate response
  - Programmed in patients with chronotropic incompetence.
- Tracking rate
  - A maximum tracking/sensor rate of 140–150 bpm ensures pacing is delivered at higher rates.
- Mode switching
  - Consider a LRL during mode switching of 70 bpm.

Step 5: AV/AA/VV Delays

- AV delays
  - **Empiric**: 100–120 ms for sensed atrial signals (add 0–30 ms paced offset)
  - Echo-based mitral inflow (Ritter Method):
    - Program a non-physiologically short AV delay (SAVD).
      - The MVC_{SAVD} (interval between the V spike and the end of the MV A wave) designates the electromechanical delay between the pacing stimulation and the beginning of LV systole (i.e., mitral valve closure: MVC).
    - Program a long AV interval (LAVD: Slightly shorter than the intrinsic AV interval).
      - MVC_{LAVD}: Interval between the V spike and the end of the A wave designates the duration of the undisturbed maximal diastolic LV filling.
    - Optimal AV delay = SAVD + [(LAVD + MVC_{LAVD}) – (SAVD + MVC_{SAVD})] **or** LAVD – MVC_{SAVD} – MVC_{LAVD}
  - Iterative method
    - Program the LAVD.
    - Shorten the AVD by 20 ms until the mitral A wave is truncated (premature mitral valve [MA] closure).
    - Increase AVD by 10 ms until the mitral A-wave truncation is eliminated.
- VV delays *(LV-RV Offset)*
  - **Invasive hemodynamics**: Based on LV dP/dt or aortic pulse pressure.
  - **EGM-based**: This is a fusion between intrinsic and paced depolarization (QRS width).
  - **Automatic algorithms**: Found in newer devices, these are vendor-specific.
  - Note: No study has demonstrated an improvement in hard clinical endpoints from routine optimization of VV delays.

Step 6: Dyssynchrony Studies

- Evidence of dyssynchrony
  - Reevaluate the LV lead position (transvenous or epicardial).
    - An apical lead position is associated with a suboptimal response.
    - A targeted lead placement away from the scar with tissue doppler imaging may result in an improved response (NYHA Class and LVESV) as well as better survival.
    - Consider an epicardial or LV endocardial lead position.

- No evidence of dyssynchrony
  - Moderate to severe MR: Consider MV surgery.
  - No MR: Consider cardiac support devices.

CARDIAC IMPLANTABLE ELECTRONIC DEVICE (CIED) INFECTIONS

Incidence

- 1.9/1000 device-years (pacemakers) and 8.9/1000 device-years (ICDs)
- 1.37/1000 device-years (pocket) and 1.14/1000 device-years (blood stream or device infective endocarditis [IE])

Risk Factors

- Recent manipulation of the device (higher risk for generator changes)
- Early re-intervention
- Fever within 24 hours of implant
- Temporary pacing prior to permanent device
- Other:
  - Chronic kidney disease
  - Long-term glucocorticoids
  - >2 pacing leads
  - Operator inexperience
  - Diabetes mellitus
  - Underlying malignancy
  - Advanced patient age
  - Prior treatment with anticoagulants

Protective Factors

- Perioperative antibiotics: e.g., cefazolin (<1 hour pre) or vancomycin (<2 hours pre)
- Hematoma prevention
  - Pocket packing with antibiotic impregnated sponges
  - Topical thrombin
  - Pressure dressing for 24 hours

Causative Organisms

- ~70% *Staphylococcus* (40% coagulase negative *Staphylococcus* [Staph], 25% methicillin-sensitive *Staphylococcus aureus* [MSSA], 5% methicillin-resistant *Staphylococcus aureus*)
- ~10% gram negative
- ~10% culture negative

Types of CIED Infections

- Infection of the generator pocket
  - Involves a subcutaneous pocket containing the device and the subcutaneous segment of the lead

    - Etiology
        - Perioperative contamination of the pocket
        - Erosion of the device or leads through the overlying skin (with or without overt infection)
    - Presentation
        - Presents with local symptoms such as pain, swelling, tenderness, or overlying erythema.
        - Systemic signs of sepsis are relatively uncommon in pocket infection.
- Infection of pacing leads involves:
    - Transvenous portion of the lead
    - Associated with:
        - Bacteremia
        - Device-endocarditis (intracardiac lead vegetation)
        - Native valvular endocarditis
    - Etiology
        - Intravascular tracking from a pocket infection
        - Hematogenous seeding during a bout of bacteremia (Staph >> other)
    - Presentation
        - Endovascular infection with signs and symptoms similar to endocarditis
        - May present as a fever of unknown origin with vague symptoms (malaise, fatigue, anorexia).

Investigations

- Blood cultures (multiple cultures, from multiple sites, separated in time)
    - Usually these are positive with deep infection.
    - Usually these are negative with isolated pocket infection.
- Leukocyte count and erythrocyte sedimentation
    - They may be abnormal with a deep infection.
    - Usually these are normal with isolated pocket infection.
- The echocardiogram may demonstrate vegetation on the intracardiac lead(s).
    - If the transthoracic echo (TTE) is negative, then a transesophageal echo (TEE) must be performed.
        - TTE have a relatively low sensitivity compared to TEE (30% vs. 95%).
- Other investigations
    - Ultrasound examination of the pocket may demonstrate fluid collection.
        - Note: Never perform a percutaneous aspirate of a suspected pocket infection.
    - Gallium or radiolabelled WBC scan may demonstrate an uptake along the lead(s) or pocket.
    - Consider investigating for metastatic infection.
        - Mycotic aneurysm(s), nephritis, septic pulmonary emboli, septic phlebitis, osteomyelitis

Management

- Superficial or incisional infection without CIED involvement
  - 7–10 days of PO antibiotics with activity against Staph ± topical antibiotic cream
- Established CIED infection
  - Complete device and lead removal
    - Indications
      - Pocket infection (class I)
      - Deep infection (class I)
      - Valvular endocarditis without definitive CIED Involvement (class I)
      - Occult bacteremia: *Staphylococcus* (class I); gram negative (class IIa)
    - Send:
      - Pocket tissue gram stain and culture
      - Lead-tip culture
- Antibiotics
  - Broad-spectrum IV antibiotics pending intraoperative pocket and blood cultures
  - Antibiotic duration
    - **Pocket erosion**: 7–10 days of antibiotics
    - **Pocket infection**: 10–14 days of antibiotics
    - **Deep infection** without endocarditis *or* uncomplicated lead endocarditis
      - *Non-staphylococcus:* 14 days of IV antibiotics
      - *Staphylococcus aureus:* 2–4 weeks of IV antibiotics
    - **Lead endocarditis** complicated by septic deep vein thrombosis (DVT), osteomyelitis, or bacteremia:
      - 4–6 weeks of IV antibiotics
    - **Valvular involvement** (associated native or prosthetic valve endocarditis)
      - Standard therapy for infectious endocarditis (IE)
  - **Re-implantation** (epicardial or contralateral)
    - **Device-dependent pocket infection**: Re-implant after 72 hours of negative blood cultures.
    - **Non-device–dependent pocket infection**: Re-implant after completion of antibiotic course.
      - Consider a longer delay to ensure eradication of the infectious organism.
    - Device-dependent deep infection:
      - **Blood culture positive (BC+) but transesophageal echocardiography negative, or lead IE only**: Re-implant after 72 hours of negative blood cultures.
      - **BC+ and valve IE**: Re-implant after 14 days of negative blood cultures.

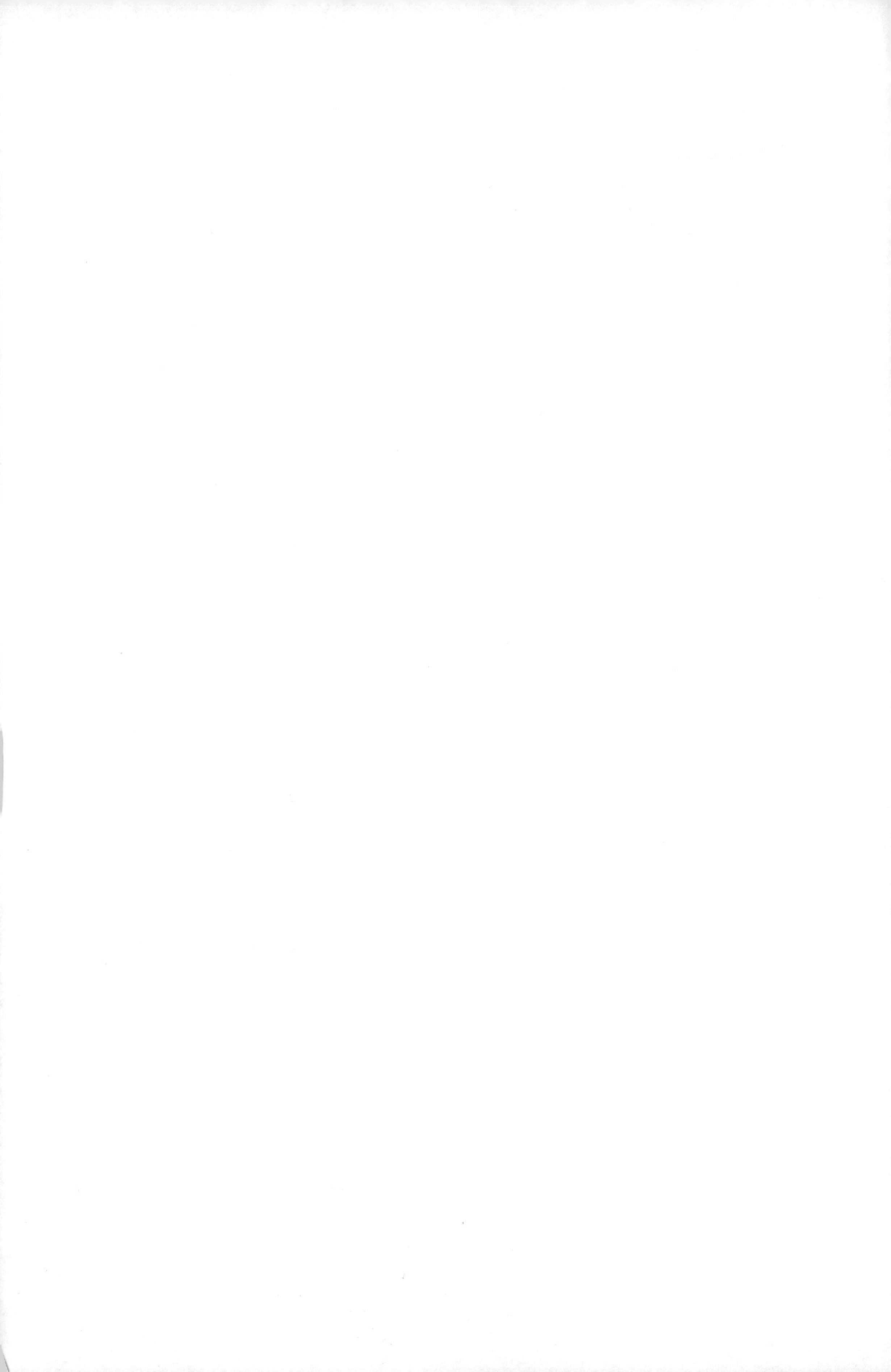

CHAPTER

14

Sudden Cardiac Death and Inherited Arrhythmias

SUDDEN CARDIAC DEATH (SCD)

SCD is defined as an unanticipated, non-traumatic death in a stable patient within 1 hour of symptom onset (witnessed) or within 24 hours of being observed alive and symptom-free (unwitnessed).

Anatomy and Physiology (Mechanism)

- **Malignant ventricular arrhythmias** (e.g., ventricular fibrillation [VF]) cause 75% of SCDs.
  - Of these, 45% are ventricular tachycardia (VT) that degenerates to VF.
- **Bradyarrhythmia** (heart block, asystole) is the other 25%.
  - Note: Pulseless electrical arrest (PEA) is increasingly recognized during resuscitation as a causative or contributory rhythm.

Causes of SCD

- Coronary artery disease (CAD; dominant mechanism, ~70%–80%):
  - Ischemic heart disease or coronary atherosclerosis
  - Congenital abnormalities of coronary arteries: Anomalous origin, AV fistula
  - Coronary spasm
  - Coronary dissection
  - Coronary artery embolism
  - Coronary arteritis
  - Myocardial bridging
- Cardiomyopathies (10%–15%):
  - Ischemic cardiomyopathy
  - Hypertrophic cardiomyopathy
  - Dilated cardiomyopathy
  - Valvular cardiomyopathy

The Clinical Cardiac Electrophysiology Handbook © 2016 Jason Andrade.
Cardiotext Publishing, ISBN: 978-1-942909-00-2.

    - Alcoholic/toxic cardiomyopathy
    - Infiltrative (e.g., sarcoidosis, amyloidosis, hemochromatosis, Fabry)
    - Arrhythmogenic right ventricular cardiomyopathy
    - Takotsubo cardiomyopathy
    - Left ventricular non-compaction cardiomyopathy
    - Myocarditis (e.g., acute, giant cell, chronic lymphocytic)
    - Neuromuscular diseases (e.g., muscular dystrophy, Friedreich's ataxia, myotonic dystrophy)
    - Congenital cardiomyopathy (corrected or uncorrected)
    - Commotio cordis
- Primary arrhythmias:
    - Long QT syndromes
    - Short QT syndrome
    - Brugada syndrome
    - Early repolarization syndromes
    - Catecholaminergic polymorphic ventricular tachycardia
    - Idiopathic ventricular fibrillation
    - Wolff-Parkinson-White syndrome (WPW)
- Non-cardiac causes include:
    - Sudden death during extreme physical activity
    - Drug overdose
    - Toxic/metabolic imbalances (e.g., hyper- or hypokalemia, thyroid storm, adrenergic storm, acidosis)
    - Acute intracranial hemorrhage
    - Massive pulmonary embolus
    - Asthma (or other pulmonary condition)
    - Aortic dissection

Epidemiology and Clinical Features

- SCD affects 200,000–300,000 per year in the United States (≈0.1% population incidence/year).
    - It is the initial clinical presentation in up to 20% of patients with CAD.
    - SCD accounts for up to 50% of CAD deaths.
- The highest proportion of SCD events occurs in the highest-risk subgroups.
    - Thirty percent of all SCD events occur in the highest-risk subgroup; however, the absolute number of deaths is relatively small owing to the subgroup being very focused.
        - This limits the overall population impact of intervention.
    - Fifty percent of all SCD events occur among subgroups of patients thought to be at relatively low risk for SCD.
        - Given the high absolute number of events in this population, the population impact of intervention is potentially great, if these patients could be identified.

Prognosis

- Survival falls rapidly after the initial minutes from the onset of cardiac arrest.
- The likelihood of survival to discharge is 23% for witnessed cardiac arrest, vs. 4% for unwitnessed arrest.
- Recurrence is highest in the first 6–18 months post index event.

IDENTIFYING PATIENTS AT RISK OF SUDDEN CARDIAC DEATH (SCD)

General Risk Stratification

Table 14.1 Factors Affecting Risk of SCD

	Risk of SCD
LVSD/HF *or* previous MI	5%
Any two of LVSD/HF, previous MI, or complex ectopy*	10%
LVSD/HF + previous MI + complex ectopy	15%
Survivor of SCD, or syncopal VT	20%–40%

HF: heart failure; LVSD: LV systolic dysfunction (LV ejection fraction [LVEF] <30%–40%); MI: myocardial infarction; SAECG: signal-averaged electrocardiogram (ECG).
*Complex ectopy = >10 premature ventricular contraction (PVC)/h, couplets, triplets, non-sustained ventricular tachycardia (NSVT)

- Predictors of recurrent cardiac arrest in the "survivor" of SCD include:
  - High brain natriuretic peptide (BNP)
  - Extensive (multivessel) CAD
  - Prior MI (within 6 months)
  - Chronic heart failure (CHF)/LV dysfunction
  - Ventricular electrical instability (complex ventricular ectopy)
  - Abnormalities on signal-averaged ECG (SAECG)

Investigations

Table 14.2 Investigations to Determine Risk of SCD

Parameter	Marker of Risk	Target Group
Family history	SCD, syncope, or known high-risk cardiomyopathies	All patients
ECG	NSVT, MI, LQTS/SQTS, Brugada pattern, pre-excitation, possible early repolarization	CAD, LQT, Brugada, WPW HCM
TWA	Positive TWA	CAD
SAECG	Positive late potentials	ARVC
EPS	Short anterograde AP ERP Inducible VT	WPW Cardiomyopathy Bundle branch reentry Tetralogy of Fallot
Echocardiogram	Low EF Asymmetric LVH	DCM HCM
Genetic testing	Disease causing mutation Several emerging adverse genetic polymorphisms	LQTS, Brugada HCM ARVC

ARVC: arrhythmogenic RV cardiomyopathy; DCM: Dilated cardiomyopathy; EPS: electrophysiology study; HCM: hypertrophic cardiomyopathy; LQT: long QT; LQTS: long QT syndrome; LVH: left ventricle hypertrophy; TWA: T-wave alternans.

Signal-Averaged ECG (SAECG)

- SAECG improves the signal-to-noise ratio of a surface ECG, thus facilitating the identification of low-amplitude signals at the end of the QRS.
  - The late potentials indicate regions of abnormal myocardium, which serve as the substrate for reentrant tachyarrhythmia.
- Abnormal findings include:
  - Filtered QRS duration (fQRS) ≥114 ms
  - Root mean-square voltage of terminal 40 ms (RMS40) <20 mcV
  - Duration of low amplitude signals (<40 μV) in the terminal QRS ≥38 ms
- Interpretation
  - Presence of abnormal SAECG increases the risk of arrhythmic events 6- to 8-fold post myocardial infarction (MI).
    - May signal the need for further risk stratification (i.e., EPS).
  - High negative predictive value (NPV; 89%–99%).
    - Normal SAECG is associated with a <5% change of inducible VT at EPS.

T-Wave Alternans (TWA)

- TWA is a beat-to-beat fluctuation in the amplitude or morphology of the T wave.
- TWA is typically measured on ECG with exercise.
- Its presence identifies high-risk patients (post MI and those with ischemic or non-ischemic dilated cardiomyopathy [NIDCM]).
- Its absence offers good discriminative function (i.e., high NPV).

Heart Rate Variability (HRV)

- HRV is a beat-to-beat variation in cardiac cycle length (CL) due to the autonomic influence on the SN.
  - It reflects a continuous assessment of the basal sympathovagal influence.
- Derived from 24-hour Holter monitoring.
- HRV independently predicts the risk of SCD and total mortality post MI (with/without LV dysfunction).

Heart Rate Turbulence (HRT)

- HRT is short-term oscillation of cardiac CLs after spontaneous PVCs.
  - Normally, there is a brief, baroreflex-mediated HR acceleration followed by a gradual deceleration.
  - In high-risk patients, the typical HRT response is blunted or missing, reflecting reduced baroreflex sensitivity.
- HRT is derived from 24-hour Holter monitoring.
  - RR intervals surrounding spontaneous PVCs (that fulfill criteria with respect to prematurity and compensatory pause) are averaged to create a "local tachogram."
- HRT independently predicts the risk of SCD and total mortality post MI (with/without LV dysfunction).

Baroreflex Sensitivity

- Baroreflex sensitivity offers a quantitative assessment of the ability of the autonomic system to respond to acute stimulation.
  - Most commonly it is performed by analyzing bradycardic response to intravenous phenylephrine bolus.
  - HR slowing in response to increased blood pressure (BP) indicates the baroreflex tone; a reduced response indicates increased risk.
- Baroreflex sensitivity independently predicts risk of SCD and is additive to HRV and TWA.

Cardiac Meta-Iodobenzylguanidine (MIBG) Scintigraphy or Positron Emission Tomography (PET)

- MIBG indicates sympathetic innervation; PET shows myocardial metabolism.
- Both are possibly better than SAECG, HRV, and QT dispersion at predicting SCD in patients with chronic HF.

Cardiac Magnetic Resonance Imaging (MRI)

- MRI allows for scar quantification and characterization (dense vs. heterogeneous).
- MRI is also useful to identify patients at high risk for ventricular arrhythmias (dilated cardiomyopathy [DCM], HCM, ARVC, post-MI).

Electrophysiology Testing (EPS)

- In general, the positive predictive value (PPV) is about 10% with a NPV of about 95%; however, the overall utility depends on the underlying pathology.
  - EPS is most useful for ischemic heart disease as well as VT induction in the context of ablation.
  - EPS for dilated cardiomyopathy or inherited arrhythmia syndromes suffer from the following issues:
    - Low inducibility
    - Low reproducibility of EPS
    - Limited PPV of induced VT
  - EPS for syncope due to suspected bradyarrhythmia suffers from the following issues:
    - Limited sensitivity with episodic bradycardia and syncope
    - Common false positive (~25%) and false negative tests

Specific Conditions

CAD

- Epidemiology
  - CAD is present in 60%–75% of SCD deaths.
    - A high proportion of those experiencing SCD have multivessel disease.
    - Only 30%–40% of these will have acute infarction.
    - It is estimated that 20% of first MI present as SCD.
- Risk factors for SCD:
  - Risk factor with good sensitivity but poor specificity:
    - Reduced LVEF (<40%; particularly if the LVEF is <30%)
  - Risk factors with good specificity but poor sensitivity include:
    - Previous cardiac arrest or a history of aborted SCD
      - Transmural MI (STEMI): VT/VF <48 h post event does not imply a worse prognosis.
      - Non-transmural MI (NSTEMI): VT/VF <48 h post event confers increased long-term risk.
    - Syncope
    - Non-sustained VT (spontaneous)
    - Inducible VT at EPS
      - If LVEF <40%, there is a 35%–45% yearly risk of SCD with an inducible VT at EPS.
      - If no inducible VT is present at EPS the annual risk of SCD is <5%.
    - Other
      - Late potentials on SAECG
      - Decreased HRV, microvolt TWA, HRT
      - Increased QRS duration, QT dispersion, or TWA

Non-Ischemic Dilated Cardiomyopathy (NIDCM)

- Epidemiology
  - 5-year mortality of ~20%
  - 30% of all deaths are sudden: VT/VF > bradyarrhythmia
- Risk factors for SCD:
  - Previous cardiac arrest or a history of aborted SCD
  - History of syncope
  - EF <35%
  - Non-sustained VT
  - Induction of monomorphic VT at EPS (absence of VT does not confer lower risk)

SUDDENT CARDIAC DEATH (SCD) IN ATHLETES

Incidence

- Annually, 1–3 SCD per 100,000 (RR of 2 to 3 vs. non-athletic peers)

Causes

- HCM (30%–40%)
- Congenital coronary artery anomalies (15%–20%)
- ARVC (5%)
- Ion channel disorders (<5%)
- Autopsy negative (<5%)
- Other causes include:
  - Myocarditis
  - Trauma: Commotio cordis or trauma involving structural cardiac injury
  - Aortic: Ruptured aortic aneurysm, aortic valve stenosis
  - Atherosclerotic CAD
  - Asthma (or other pulmonary condition), heat stroke, drug abuse (i.e., cocaine)

Screening

- Annual clinical history (personal and family) and physical examination
- ECG
  - Common abnormalities in athletes (95%)
    - Sinus bradycardia, first-degree AV block
    - Notched QRS in V1 (incomplete RBBB), early repolarization, Isolated voltage criteria for left ventricular hypertrophy (LVH)
  - Uncommon abnormalities in athletes (<5%)
    - Chamber enlargement or hypertrophy: Left atrium, right ventricle
    - Bundle branch or fascicular block
    - Pathologic Q waves, ST segment depression, T-wave inversion
    - Brugada-like early repolarization
    - Long or short QT interval
    - Ventricular arrhythmias
- If the history or ECG is positive, then proceed to further investigations:
  - ECG, stress test, 24-hour Holter monitor, cardiac MRI, angiogram, EPS

Exercise Restriction

- HCM
  - Restrict the patient to low-intensity/recreational sports (particularly with obstructive variant).
- Gene carriers without a phenotype (HCM, ARVC, DCM, channelopathies)
  - Restrict to low-intensity/recreational sports (European Society of Cardiology); no restriction (Bethesda 36).
- Ion channelopathies (QTc >440 ms in men and >460 ms in women):
  - Restrict to low-intensity/recreational sports.
  - A recent trend is to favor less restriction, especially if adequately β-blocked.
- Brugada syndrome, catecholamine-induced polymorphic VT
  - Restrict to low-dynamic/low-static sport.
  - Recent trend to less restriction
- Marfan syndrome
  - Restrict to low-intensity/recreational sports unless the aortic root <40 mm.
  - If < moderate-severe MR and no family history of aortic dissection or SCD, restrict to moderate-intensity competitive sports.
- WPW syndrome
  - No restriction if asymptomatic (use care in dangerous environments)
  - Post-ablation may resume competitive sports after 1–3 months
- PVCs or NSVT (<10 beats; <150 bpm; suppresses with exercise)
  - No restriction if asymptomatic or structurally normal heart
  - If CV disease, only allowed to participate in low-intensity/non-competitive sports
- ICDs
  - Restrict to low-intensity/recreational sports without risk of device trauma.

CHANNELOPATHIES

Channelopathies are rare, heritable syndromes.

Long QT Syndrome (LQTS)

General Information

- The incidence of LQTS is 1 in 2500.
- LQTS accounts for 3000–4000 annual sudden deaths in childhood in the United States.
- Mutations are more frequent than the clinical phenotype:
  - The average QTc penetrance is 25%–60%.
  - Only 35%-40% of gene carriers are identified by clinical diagnostic criteria.
  - Exercise testing improves detection and genetic prediction.

Classification

Table 14.3 Classification of LQTS Types

	LQT1	LQT2	LQT3	LQT4	LQT5	LQT6
Epidemiology	40%–55%	35%–45%	8%–10%		3%	2%
Gene/ protein	KvLQ1 or KCNQ1	KCNH2 or HERG	SCN5A	Ankyrin-B	KCNE1 (minK)	KCNE2 (miRP1)
Channel	Slow delayed rectifier	Rapid delayed rectifier	Sodium channel	Ion channel anchor	Coassembles with KvLQT1	Coassembles with HERG
Current	I_{Ks} (α)	I_{Kr} (α)	I_{Na} (α)	I_{Na}, I_{K}, I_{NCX}	I_{Ks} (β)	I_{Kr}
Channel function	↓	↓	↑	↓	↓	↓
Action potential	Delayed phase 3	Delayed phase 3	Prolonged phase 2	—	Delayed phase 3	Delayed phase 3
Triggers	Exercise Swimming	Emotion Auditory	Rest Sleep			
T wave	Broad T Late onset	Bifid T Low amplitude	Asymmetric, late and peaked			
Epinephrine or isoproterenol	↑ QT	↓ QT	↓ QT			
Mexilitine	—	—	↓ QT			
Events <10y	40%	16%	2%			

- LQT7 – Andersen-Tawil syndrome
  - *KCNJ2* mutation leads to loss of function alters inward rectifier K current through the Kir2.1 channel.
  - Clinical
    - Potassium-sensitive periodic paralysis
    - Dysmorphic features: Short stature, hypertelorism, palate defect, broad nasal root
  - ECG: Pseudo long QT with prominent U wave
  - Ventricular arrhythmias: Very large PVC burden (up to 50% ectopy), bidirectional VT
  - Prognosis: Benign

Epidemiology and Clinical Features

- LQTS is mostly asymptomatic.
- Common symptoms include syncope, seizures, and cardiac arrest.

- Associated symptoms may include:
  - Sensorineural deafness (Jervell & Lange-Nielsen: Autosomal recessive)
  - Periodic paralysis (Andersen-Tawil: Autosomal dominant heterozygote)
- Family history
  - Positive for LQT or SCD

12-Lead ECG

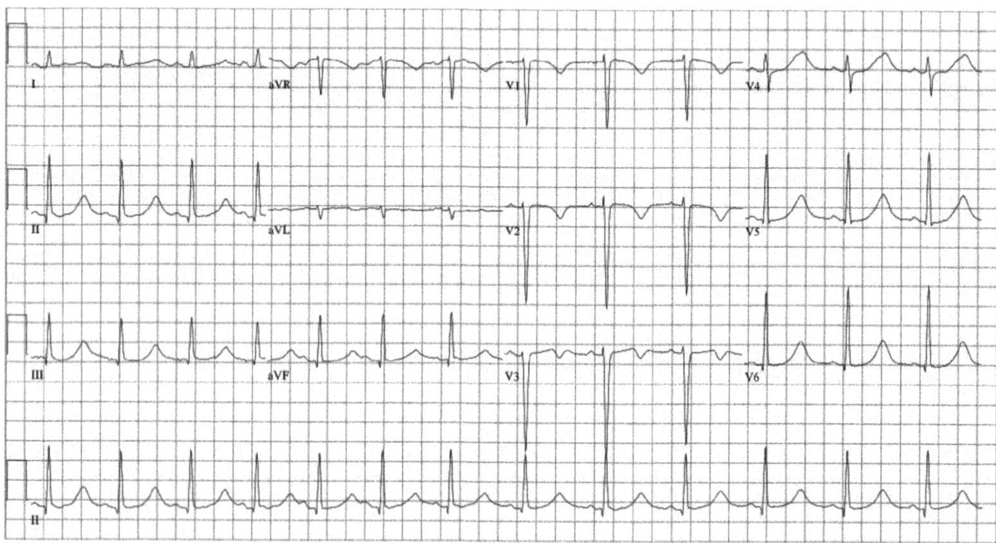

- Measuring the QT interval
  - Average QT and RR interval over ≥3 QRS complexes in ≥3 ECG leads.
  - Measure from the onset of the QRS complex to the end of the T wave (the point where the tangential line from the steepest terminal portion of the T wave crosses the isoelectric line).
  - **Corrected QT** (QTc)
    - **Bazett's formula:** $QTc = QT/\sqrt{(RR \text{ in seconds})}$
    - **Normal**: 390–450 ms (men) or 390–460 ms (women)
    - Most borderline prolonged intervals are normal when repeated.

Diagnosis: Schwartz Score

- The Schwartz score combines ECG and clinical parameters to estimate the probability of inherited LQTS with high specificity (80%–100%) but low sensitivity (70% for score ≥4; >30% for <4).
  - **ECG parameters** include:
    - QTc: ≥480 ms: 3 points; 460–470 ms: 2 points; >450–460 ms (males): 1 point
    - Torsade de pointes: 2 points
    - T-wave alternans: 1 point
    - Notched T wave in three leads: 1 point
    - Resting HR below second percentile for age (children): 0.5 point

- **Syncope** (points for torsade and syncope are mutually exclusive)
  - With stress: 2 points
  - Without stress: 1 point
- **Family history** (cannot use same family member for both points)
  - Family members with LQTS: 1 point
  - Sudden death in family member <30 years without a defined cause: 0.5 point

- Interpretation
  - Probability of having LQTS: Low <1, intermediate 2–3, or high ≥4

Other Investigations

Exercise Testing

- Normal response: QT interval shortens with exercise and increased heart rate.
- Abnormal response (LQTS); see Table 14.4

Table 14.4 Exercise Testing in LQTS

	QT Interval with Exercise	Peak Exercise and Early Recovery QTc	QTc Interval 4–6 Minutes Post Exercise
LQT1	Decreased shortening	Prolonged	Exaggerated lengthening with HR decline
LQT2	Shortening	Normal	Exaggerated lengthening with HR decline
LQT3	Marked shortening	Normal	

- Burst exercise protocol may improve diagnostic yield.
  - Maximal exertion against a fixed workload (200 W) is undertaken for 1 minute to provoke rapid HR acceleration (simulates sudden adrenergic surge).

Pharmacologic (Epinephrine) Challenge

- Infusion of IV epinephrine at escalating doses (0.025 to 0.3 mcg/kg/min)
- **Paradoxical response**: An increase in uncorrected QT by ≥30 ms occurs during an epinephrine infusion.
  - This is observed in 92% with LQT1 but only 13% in LQT2 and none in LQT3.
  - It should shorten in normal subjects (false positive rate is 20%).
  - Marked T- and U-wave emergence changes.

Genetic Testing

Genetic testing is useful with:

- Established diagnosis of LQT on clinical grounds
  - Identification of a specific genotype may influence prognosis and modify treatment.
    - High risk or known pathologic mutations can be used for cascade screening if they are identified.
    - But variants of unknown significance (VUS) are found in 10% of cases.
      - These are typically unhelpful in establishing a diagnosis and prognosis.

- Borderline clinical criteria for LQTS
  - Identification of a mutation may confirm the diagnosis.
  - Note: Failure to identify a known mutation does not exclude the diagnosis, as genetic testing identifies mutations in only ~75% of affected individuals.
- Asymptomatic family members of patients with an identified disease causing LQTS mutation
  - Genetic testing can confirm or exclude the diagnosis.

Management

Chronic Management

- Non-pharmacologic therapy
  - Avoid drugs that prolong the QT interval or reduce serum K^+ or Mg^{2+} concentration (www.qtdrugs.org).
  - Exercise restriction: This is a contentious area with a trend to favor less restriction, especially if β-blocked.
    - Conventional advice is restriction to low-intensity/recreational sports.
      - LQT1: Limit swimming or perform only under supervision.
      - LQT2: Avoid exposure to acoustic stimuli especially during sleep.
    - However, recent evidence indicates that the risks are lower than previously assumed.
  - Genetic counseling
- Pharmacologic therapy
  - β-blockers
    - Mainstay of treatment
      - β-blockers prevent the adrenergically-mediated increases in plateau inward Ca^{2+} current that cause excess action potential duration (APD)/QT prolongation that occur in situations of sympathetic stimulation, particularly in the absence of I_{Ks} (LQT1), an outward current that is enhanced by adrenergic stimulation and normally offsets the inward Ca^{2+} current increase.
      - Improves QT adaptation with more gradual changes in sinus rates
    - Indications
      - LQTS clinical diagnosis (class I)
      - LQTS molecular diagnosis but normal/borderline QTc (class IIa)
    - Outcome
      - Highly effective at preventing SCD in LQT1
      - Less effective for LQT2 and relatively ineffective in LQT3
    - Possible adjunctive therapies
      - Nicorandil (LQT1), spironolactone (LQT2), mexiletine (LQT3)
- Invasive therapy
  - Implantable cardioverter-defibrillator may be used in the following classes of patients:
    - Survivors of aborted cardiac arrest (Class I)
    - Syncope and/or VT while receiving β-blockers (Class IIa)
    - High-risk patients (>50% event rate, Class IIb)
      - QTc ≥500 and LQT1 or LQT2
      - LQT3 and male gender

- Sensorineural hearing loss (JLN)
- Poor compliance with or intolerance of β-blockers
  - Intermediate (30%–50%): QTc >500 ms LQT3 (F); QTc <500 ms LQT2 (F) and LQT3
  - Low risk (<30%): QTc <500 ms LQT1 and LQT2 (M)

- Dual-chamber pacemaker for overdrive pacing.
  - Most helpful for LQT3.
- Cardiac sympathetic denervation:
  - Preganglionic denervation interrupts the major source of norepinephrine in the heart.
    - Conceptually it is appealing because it addresses the pathophysiology, in contrast to ICD, which responds to the disease and (rarely) may perpetuate the arrhythmia by a shock/pain-induced hyperadrenergic state.
  - Indications are similar to an ICD (e.g., syncope, torsade de pointes, or cardiac arrest on β-blockers), but in situations where an ICD is not preferred.
  - Techniques used include:
    - Left cervicothoracic sympathectomy: Resection of the left stellate ganglion and the first four or five thoracic ganglia (often results in Horner's syndrome).
    - High thoracic left sympathectomy (HTLS): Resection of the lower part of stellate ganglion along with the first four thoracic ganglia (usually does not result in Horner's syndrome).

Complications

Bradyarrhythmia

- An AV block occurs in <5% of patients.
- Bradycardia occurs in 20%–30% of patients.
  - More frequent with LQT3 (abnormal sodium current → SA node dysfunction)

Tachyarrhythmia

- PVCs
  - Multiform (5%)
  - Uniform (4%)
- Torsade de pointes
  - Initiation (short-long-short sequence).
    - PVC results in a slight pause, in which the RR interval lengthens for one beat (the "long" RR in the sequence).
    - This pause causes the following QT interval to prolong.
    - If, during this lengthened QT interval, a second PVC occurs during the vulnerable period of repolarization, torsade de pointes can result
  - During torsade de pointes:
    - Ventricular rate of 160–250 bpm, irregular RR intervals
    - Cycling of the QRS axis through 180 degrees every 5–20 beats
  - Episodes are usually short-lived and terminate spontaneously.
    - Repeated or prolonged episodes may induce syncope or progress to VF.

CATECHOLAMINERGIC POLYMORPHIC VENTRICULAR TACHYCARDIA (VT)

General Information

- VT develops during exertion or with acute emotion.
- The estimated prevalence is 1:10,000.
- The mean age of onset is 7–12 years, but it may manifest later in life.
- It is caused by abnormal leak of Ca^{2+} from subcellular stores (sarcoplasmic reticulum) via RyR2 during diastole, causing triggered activity.
  - RyR2 opening is sensitive to intracellular Ca^{2+} concentration, so abnormal opening can occur due to excess intracellular Ca^{2+} load, excess sensitivity of RyR2 to Ca^{2+} (RyR2 mutations) or insufficient intracellular buffering of Ca^{2+} by the Ca^{2+} binding protein calsequestrin.

Classification

- Catecholaminergic polymorphic ventricular tachycardia (CPVT) 1 (autosomal dominant [AD]): Mutation in ryanodine receptor (RYR2), which is involved in intracardiac Ca^{2+} handling.
- CPVT 2 (autosomal recessive [AR]): Mutation in calsequestrin (CASQ2), which is a calcium-buffering protein of the sarcoplasmic reticulum.

12-Lead ECG

- Usually normal
- May have sinus bradycardia, pulse rate (PR) shortening, or prominent U waves

Exercise Testing

- Ventricular arrhythmias (typically onset at a HR threshold of 110–130 bpm) due to Ca^{2+} loading are caused by increased adrenergic drive (increases intracellular Ca^{2+} entry via $I_{Ca,L}$) and increased HR (Ca^{2+} enters cell with each heart beat).
  - Generally starts as PVCs followed by NSVT then sustained VT.
  - VT is polymorphic or "bidirectional": beat-to-beat 180° change in QRS axis

EP Testing

- EP testing is not useful.

Management

- Medical therapy
  - **β-blockers** are generally effective (nadolol or propranolol preferred).
    - Spontaneous or exercise-induced VT (class I)
    - Asymptomatic genetic diagnosis (class IIa: childhood; IIb: adulthood)
  - **Flecainide** is an adjunct in those with incomplete protection.
- Implantable cardioverter-defibrillator
  - Survivors of cardiac arrest (class I)
  - Syncope and/or documented sustained VT on β-blockers (class IIa)

- Left cardiac sympathetic denervation (LCSD)
  - Consider for those refractory to or intolerant of β-blockers.
- Prognosis
  - CPVT is the most malignant of the inherited causes of sudden death.
    - Eighty percent of affected individuals experience a syncopal episode.
    - Thirty percent of affected individuals experience a cardiac arrest.

BRUGADA SYNDROME

Epidemiology

- Found in 1–5/10,000; more common in SE Asians
- Family history in 21%; 80% men
- Average age at presentation is 30–50 years (2 months to 77 years)

Classification

- B1 (20%): *SCN5A* gene; α-subunit of Na^+ channel (I_{Na})
- Six other genes identified, relatively rare causes

12-Lead ECG

- rSR′ (incomplete or complete RBBB)
  - ≥ 2 mm of ST elevation in two of V1–V3 (rapid descent off R′ on RV side)
    - Inceased with vagal, bradycardia, exercise, fever, tricyclic antidepressant (TCA), cocaine, alcohol, propranolol, class 1a, 1c, or III
    - Decreased with exercise, adrenergic, tachycardia, isoproterenol
  - Coved morphology
    - Begins at the top of where the R′ is down sloping and ends in an inverted T wave
- **Clinical Subtypes**: Type 1 is diagnostic; types 2–3 are suggestive
  - **Type 1**: Coved ST segment elevation ≥2 mm followed by a negative T wave

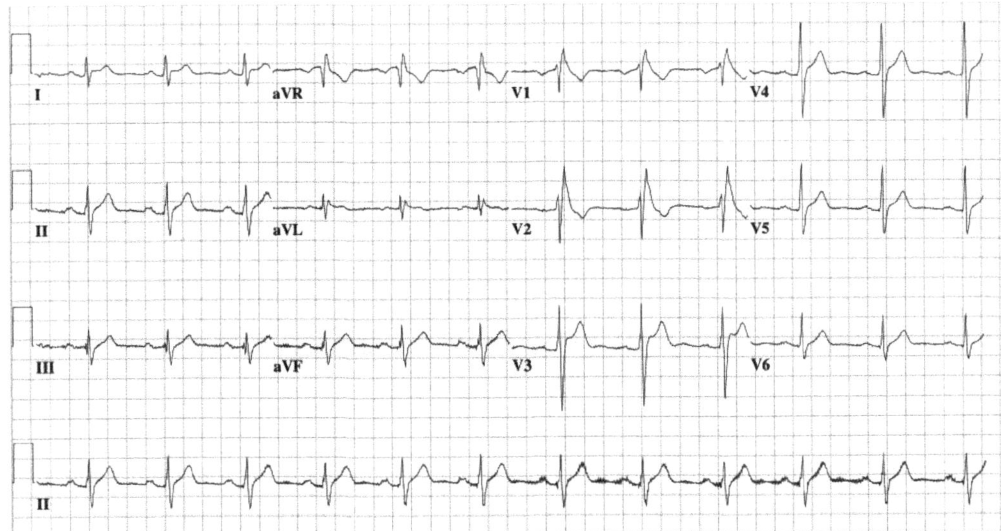

- **Type 2**: Saddleback high takeoff ST elevation ≥0.2 mV followed by positive or biphasic T wave
- **Type 3**: Saddleback or coved ST segment with <0.1 mV ST elevation

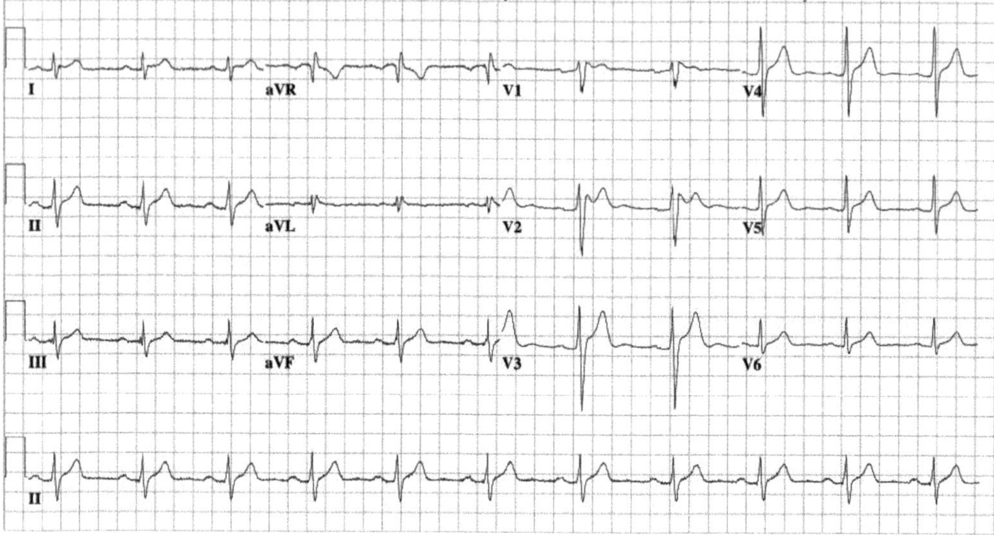

Diagnosis

- Type 1 morphology in the right precordial leads V1, V2, positioned in the second, third, or fourth intercostal space occurring either spontaneously or after provocative drug test with IV administration of class I antiarrhythmic drugs
- Type 2 or 3 pattern on baseline ECG that converts to the type 1 pattern with a Na-channel blocker

Investigations

- Sodium challenge
  - Drugs
    - Ajmaline 1 mg/kg IV over 10 mg/min
    - Flecainide 2 mg/kg IV over 10 min IV (max 150 mg) or 400 mg PO
    - Procainamide 10–15 mg/kg IV over 10–30 min (max 50 mg/min, 1 g total)
  - Monitoring
    - 12-lead ECG q10 minutes during infusion and q30 minutes post infusion for 1–2 hours
    - Place the right precordial leads in second interspace (improves sensitivity)
  - Terminate the sodium challenge when:
    - Diagnostic type 1 ST-segment elevation or Brugada ECG develops
    - ST segment in type 2 increases by ≥1–2 mm
    - Premature ventricular beats or other arrhythmias develop
    - QRS widens to ≥130% of baseline

- EP testing
  - Low PPV (23%) but high NPV (93% over 3 years of follow-up)
  - Recent guidelines do not support routine use.
    - May be helpful when contemplating a primary prevention ICD

Management

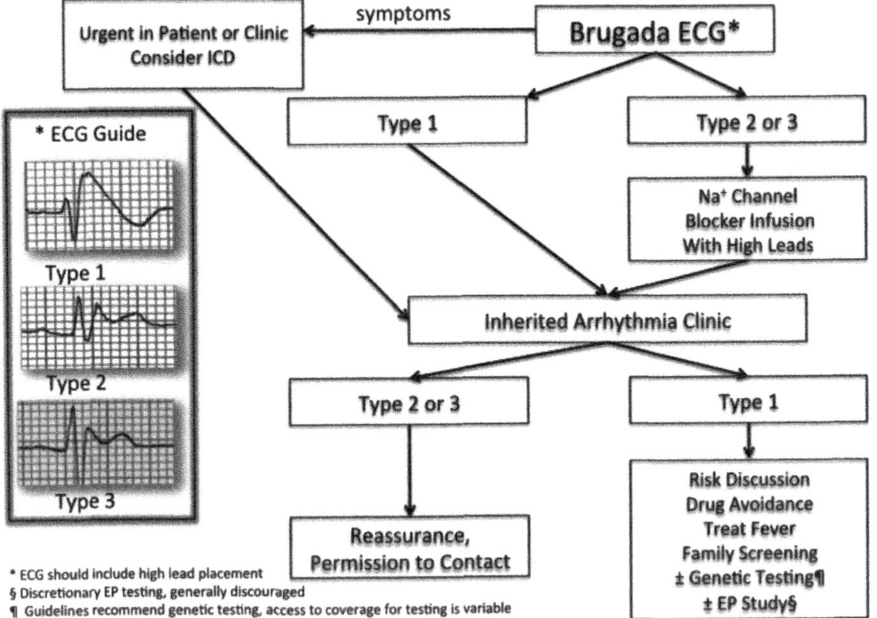

- Non-pharmacologic therapy
  - Avoid drugs that prolong the affect sodium channels (www.brugadadrugs.org).
  - Aggressively treat fever.
  - Restrict exercise: Restricted to a low-dynamic/low-static sport.
    - A recent trend is for less restriction.
  - Genetic counseling
- Pharmacologic therapy
  - β-blockers may increase mortality.
  - Quinidine has been shown to prevent shocks in patients with VT storm.
- ICD
  - Survivors of sudden death (class I: 17%–62% recurrence over 4–8 y)
  - Syncope + spontaneous type 1 pattern (class IIa: 6%–19% recurrence at 2–3 y)
  - Documented VT (no sudden cardiac arrest [SCA]): Class IIa

Prognosis

- Asymptomatic patients at increased risk can be identified by:
  - Presence of spontaneous type 1 ST-segment elevation
  - Presence of late potentials, QRS fragmentation or early repolarization
  - Inducibility of VT/VF using programmed stimulation

Complications

- VT storm occurs in 18%.
  - Isoproterenol augments the cardiac L-type channel
  - Quinidine blocks the I_{to} current
- Spontaneous VF may be treated with:
  - Quinidine or bepridil, which block the I_{to} current
  - Cilostazol, a phosphodiesterase III inhibitor that increases inward L-type calcium channel current

ARRYTHMOGENIC CARDIOMYOPATHY

Epidemiology

- Incidence is 1 per 1000–5000; accounts for 11% SCD in Northern Italy, but has lower incidence in other geographies.
- Mean age at diagnosis is 31 y (more common between 20 and 50 years of age; rarely diagnosed before 10 y).

Etiology

- Disease of the desmosome: Mutations are in genes encoding for desmosomal proteins in an autosomal-dominant fashion with variable penetrance and expressivity.
- A rare variant is Naxos disease (familial palmoplantar keratosis; 117q21).
  - Cardiac: RV structural (100%), ECG abnormalities (92%), LV involvement (27%)

Pathology

- RV free wall myocardium is replaced by fibrous ± fatty tissue with scattered myocardial cells.
- **Fibrolipomatous**: Myocardial atrophy/thinning with fibrous-fatty replacement ± patchy inflammation
  - RV aneurysms and LV involvement in the minority
- **Lipomatous**: Normal/↑ myocardial thickness with fatty replacement and infrequent inflammation
  - Minimal RV aneurysms and LV involvement

Classification

- "Classic" arrhythmogenic right ventricular cardiomyopathy (ARVC)
  - Early and predominant RV involvement [RV inflow → apex → infundibulum (right ventricular outflow tract [RVOT]) → LV]
- Left-dominant arrhythmogenic cardiomyopathy (LDAC)
  - Early and predominant LV involvement [circumferential band in outer 1/3 of LV and right septum]
- "Biventricular" variant

Clinical Features

- Palpitations (67%), syncope (32%), atypical chest pain (27%), dyspnea (11%), RV failure (6%)
- Symptomatic ventricular arrhythmia (50%): Varies with the severity of disease.
  - Sustained/non-sustained monomorphic ventricular tachycardia from RVOT
- Events may be precipitated by exercise and resolve with rest.
- RV is more thin-walled than left, so it is more susceptible to mechanical forces.

12-Lead ECG

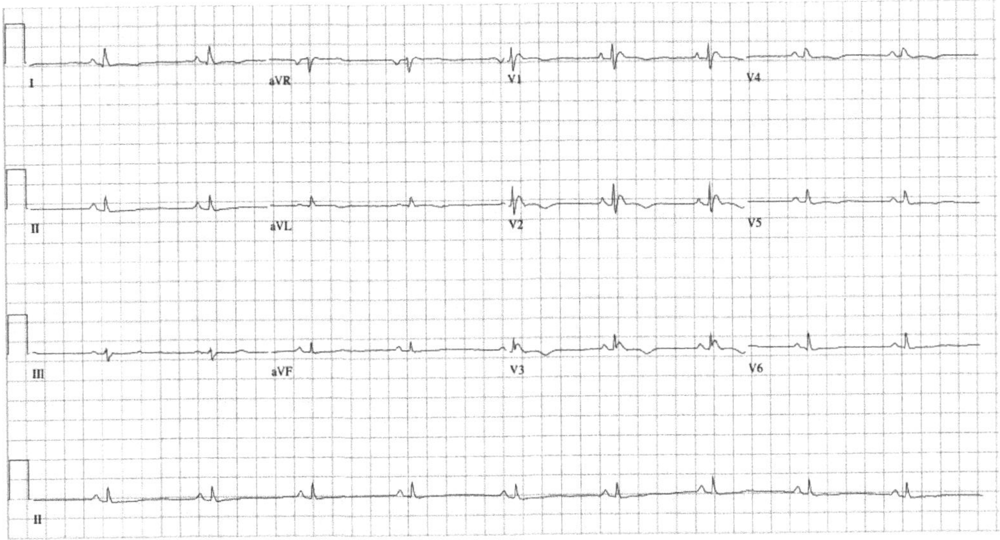

- About 40%–50% have a normal ECG at presentation, but they may develop progressive changes over time.
  - Major diagnostic finding is a T-wave inversion in the precordial leads beyond V1
  - Prolonged QRS duration (>110 ms) in the right precordial leads (V1–V3)
  - Prolonged S upstroke (interval from S nadir to isoelectric baseline 55 ms)
  - Incomplete RBBB with an Epsilon wave (V1 > I or V6); Epsilon wave is rare

Other Investigations

- Chest x-ray may identify globular cardiac enlargement.
- Echocardiogram
  - Suggestive features:
    - RV dilatation or isolated dilatation of RVOT or apical dyskinesia
    - Localized bulging and dyskinesia of inferobasal wall, trabecular disarrangement
    - Highly reflective irregularly shaped moderator band

- **Radionucleotide angiography** has an 80% sensitivity and specificity and PPV 100%.
  - Abnormal RV contraction, low right ventricular ejection fraction (RVEF)
- MRI
  - RV enlargement
  - RVOT ectasia
  - RV free wall end-diastolic crinkling (accordion sign)
  - Reduced RVEF or RV wall motion abnormalities
  - RV myocardial fatty infiltration (nonspecific finding)
- Other:
  - SAECG shows late potentials in 50%.
    - One third of the criteria is sufficient to be positive for Task Force Criteria.
    - Extent of abnormalities is proportional to the degree of RV enlargement/ fibrosis.
  - Exercise testing
    - Unmasks RV conduction delay including epsilon waves
    - May provoke PVCs or VT for the RV
  - Isoproterenol infusion
    - 8–30 mg for 3 min → VT/sustained arrhythmia (LBBB pattern)
  - Myocardial biopsy (ideally should be imaging ± voltage guided)
    - Lacks sensititivity because ARVC may not be found in the RV septum.
    - Fifty percent of those meeting criteria for ARVC may have focal RV myocarditis
  - Electrophysiology testing
    - Not useful at risk stratification

Diagnostic Criteria

- Revised Task Force Criteria
  - **Definite diagnosis** requires that patient have 2 major criteria, *or* 1 major and 2 minor criteria, *or* 4 minor criteria from different categories.
  - **Borderline**: Patient has 1 major and 1 minor *or* 3 minor criteria from different categories.
  - **Possible**: Patient has 1 major criterion or 2 minor criteria from different categories.
- Major criteria include:
  - Global and/or regional dysfunction and structural alterations:
    - By 2D echo: Regional RV akinesia, dyskinesia, or aneurysm and 1 of:
      - Parasternal long axis (PLAX) RVOT ≥32 mm (end diastole, indexed for body size [PLAX/body surface area {BSA}] ≥19 mm/m^2)
      - Parasternal short-axis (PSAX) RVOT ≥36 mm (end diastole, indexed for body size [PSAX/BSA] ≥21 mm/m^2)
      - Fractional area change ≤33%

- By MRI: Regional RV akinesia, dyskinesia or dyssynchronous contraction and 1 of:
  - Ratio of RV end diastolic volume (EDV) to BSA ≥110 mL/m^2 (male) or ≥100 mL/m^2 (female)
  - RVEF ≤40%
- By RV angiography: Regional RV akinesia, dyskinesia, or aneurysm
- Endocardial biopsy findings:
  - Residual myocytes <60% by morphometric analysis (or <50% if estimated), with fibrous replacement of the RV free wall myocardium in ≥1 sample, with or without fatty replacement of tissue on endomyocardial biopsy
- Repolarization abnormalities
  - Inverted T waves in right precordial leads (V1, V2, and V3) or beyond in individuals >14 years of age (in the absence of complete RBBB QRS ≥120 ms)
- Depolarization/conduction abnormalities
  - Epsilon wave (reproducible low-amplitude signals between end of QRS complex to onset of the T wave) in the right precordial leads (V1–V3)
- Arrhythmias
  - Non-sustained or sustained VT of LBBB morphology with superior axis (negative or indeterminate QRS in leads II, III, and aVF and positive in lead aVL)
- Family history:
  - ARVC/D confirmed in a first-degree relative who meets current Task Force Criteria
  - AVRC/dysplasia (AVRC/D) confirmed pathologically at autopsy or surgery in a first-degree relative
  - Identification of a pathogenic mutation associated or probably associated with ARVC/D

- Minor criteria consist of:
  - Global and/or regional dysfunction and structural alterations include:
    - By 2D echo: Regional RV akinesia or dyskinesia and 1 of the following (end diastole):
      - PLAX RVOT ≥29 to <32 mm (indexed for body size [PLAX/BSA] ≥16 to <19 mm/m^2)
      - PSAX RVOT ≥32 to <36 mm (indexed for body size [PSAX/BSA] ≥18 to <21 mm/m^2)
      - Fractional area change >33% to ≤40%
    - By MRI: Regional RV akinesia/dyskinesia or dyssynchronous RV contraction and 1 of the following:
      - Ratio of RV EDV to BSA ≥100 to <110 mL/m2 (male) or ≥90 to <100 mL/m^2 (female)
      - RVEF >40%– ≤45%
  - Endocardial biopsy shows residual myocytes 60%–75% by morphometric analysis (or 50%–65% if estimated), with fibrous replacement of the RV free wall myocardium in ≥1 sample, with or without fatty replacement of tissue.
  - Repolarization abnormalities, including:
    - Inverted T waves in leads V1 and V2 in individuals >14 years of age (in the absence of complete RBBB) or in V4, V5, or V6
    - Inverted T waves in leads V1, V2, V3, and V4 in individuals >14 years of age in the presence of complete RBBB

- Depolarization/conduction abnormalities, including:
  - Late potentials by SAECG in ≥1 of the following 3 parameters in the absence of a QRS duration of ≥110 ms on the standard ECG
    - Filtered QRS duration (fQRS) ≥114 ms
    - Duration of low amplitude signals (<40 μV) in the terminal QRS ≥38 ms
    - Root mean-square voltage of terminal 40 ms (RMS40) <20 mcV
  - Terminal activation duration of QRS ≥55 ms measured from the nadir of the S wave to the end of the QRS, including R′, in V1, V2, or V3, in the absence of complete RBBB
- Arrhythmias
  - Non-sustained or sustained VT of RV outflow configuration, LBBB morphology with inferior axis (positive QRS in leads II, III, and aVF and negative in lead aVL) or of unknown axis
  - >500 ventricular extrasystoles per 24 hours (Holter)
- Family history
  - History of ARVC/D in a first-degree relative in whom it is not possible or practical to determine whether the family member meets current Task Force criteria.
  - Premature sudden death (<35 years of age) due to suspected ARVC/D in a first-degree relative.
  - ARVC/D confirmed pathologically or by current Task Force Criteria in second-degree relative.

Management

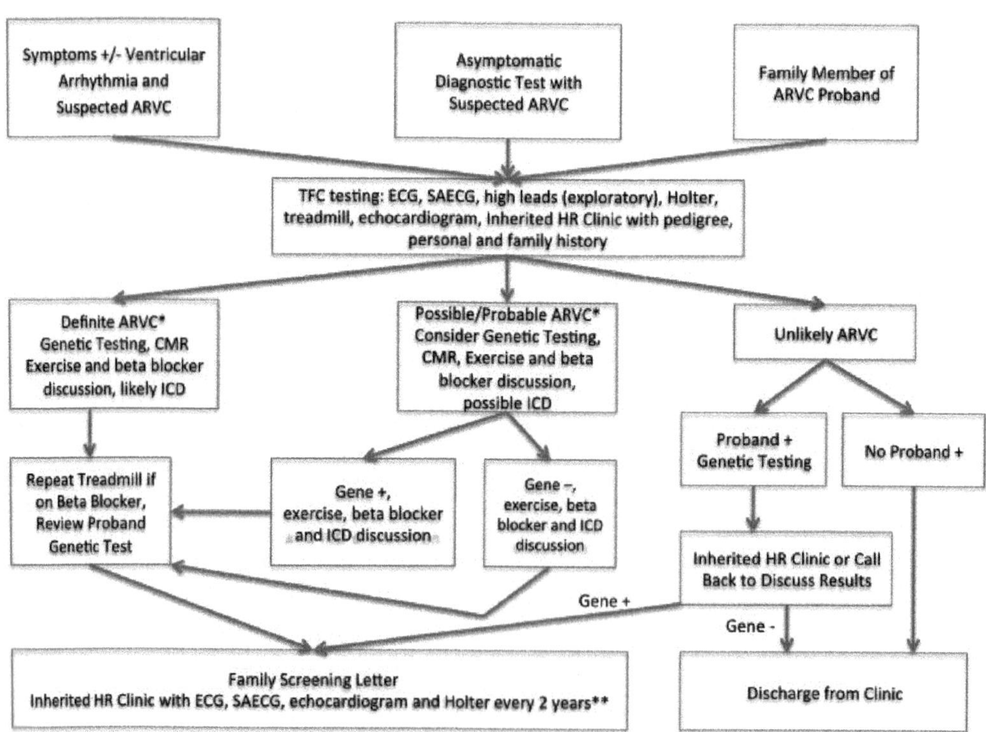

- Non-pharmacologic therapy
  - Exercise restriction: Restricted to modest intensity, non-endurance sports
    - Desmosomes hold cells together; when they are abnormal, the heart has difficulty maintaining structural integrity under mechanical stress.
    - Strong inferential evidence that endurance exercise accelerates disease progression and can exaggerate the phenotype; malignant arrhythmias tend to occur during exercise.
  - Screen family members
  - Genetic counseling
- Pharmacologic therapy
  - Empiric β-blockade
  - AADs are often used as an adjunct to ICD therapy
    - Sotalol (~70% efficacy)
    - Amiodarone (~15% efficacy)
- Invasive therapies
  - Catheter ablation
    - For patients intolerant of AADs
    - Often requires epicardial ablation
  - Implantable cardioverter-defibrillator
    - Secondary prevention (resuscitated cardiac arrest)
    - Primary prevention
      - ARVC with extensive disease (including LV involvement)
      - ≥1 family member with SCD
      - Undiagnosed syncope (VT/VF cannot be excluded as the cause)

Prognosis

- High-risk groups for SCD:
  - Younger patients (odds ratio ~0.8 per 5–year interval)
  - Present with syncope or have recurrent syncope
  - Previous history of cardiac arrest or a history of VT with hemodynamic compromise
  - Clinical signs of RV failure or LV involvement
  - ARVC type 5 (ARVC5): Uncommon outside of Newfoundland, Canada, but malignant course.
- Course in asymptomatic patient is highly variable (incomplete natural history).
  - Over ~9 years:
    - 10% eventually develop changes on echo
    - 50% develop symptomatic VT
    - 5% progress from mild to moderate
    - 8% progress from moderate to severe
  - Life expectancy of 40–60 years
- Course in patients with VT: There is a relatively low risk of death with AAD treatment.

LEFT DOMINANT ARRHYTHMOGENIC CARDIOMYOPATHY (LDAC)

- **Pathogenesis**: LV fibrofatty tissue replacement
  - Circumferential band in the outer 1/3 of the myocardium and on the right side of the IV septum
- **Clinical features**
  - Similar to ARVC: Palpitations to overt syncope secondary to malignant ventricular arrhythmias
- **Diagnostic criteria**
  - ECG
    - Inferior-lateral T-wave inversion (V5–V6 ± V4, I and aVL)
  - Arrhythmia
    - Sustained or non-sustained RBBB-type VT (ECG, Holter or exercise-resting)
    - Frequent PVCs (RBBB morphology)
  - Imaging
    - LV aneurysms
    - Mild LV dilatation and/or systolic impairment (with arrhythmia presentation)
  - Biopsy/cardiovascular magnetic resonance (CMR)
    - Myocyte loss with fibrofatty replacement on histology
    - Extensive LGE (late gadolinium enhancement) of LV myocardium (subepicardial/midmyopcardial)

HYPERTROPHIC CARDIOMYOPATHY (HCM)

Epidemiology

- HCM is diagnosed when the patient has LV hypertrophy (septal thickness >14 mm) in the absence of abnormal loading conditions.
- The prevalence of 0.2% (i.e., 1:500) does not vary worldwide ("global disease").

Classification and Differential Diagnosis

- HCM with (or without) sarcomeric protein mutations
  - Usually Alzheimer's disease (AD); 50% overall; >16 genes; >430 mutations
    - β-myosin heavy chain (45%), myosin-binding protein C (25%), troponin T (15%)
    - Other: α-myosin heavy chain, troponin I, troponin C, α-tropomyosin
- Non-HCM syndrome with LVH
  - Acquired hypertrophy
    - Athletic heart
    - Obesity
    - Amyloid
    - Outflow tract obstruction with secondary hypertrophy
  - Inherited:
    - Storage disorder
      - Glycogen: Pompe, PRKAG2, Forbes, Danon
      - Lysosomal: Fabry, Hurler's
    - Disorders of fatty acid metabolism, carnitine or phosphorylase B kinase deficiency
    - Syndromic (Noonan's, LEOPARD, Friedreich's, Beckwith–Wiedermann)

Clinical Features

- Angina secondary to subendocardial ischemia (↑ myocardial O_2 demand, reduced myocardial blood flow)
- Dyspnea (90%, secondary to diastolic dysfunction, ↓ LV emptying due to obstruction) and HF (10%–15%)
- Presyncope/syncope due to arrhythmia (ventricular/atrial), LV outflow obstruction, or reflex syncope
  - Post exercise, there is a decrease in ventricular volume (↓ cardiac output [CO] and HR) and catecholamine drive.
- Hallmark signs of HCM with obstruction are:
  - Pulse: rapid carotid upstroke; bifid or bisferins pulse ("spike and dome")
  - Jugular venous pressure (JVP): Prominent A-wave
  - Precordial palpation: Double apical impulse, "triple ripple" (palpable S_4)
  - Precordial auscultation
    - Normal or paradoxical S_2 (more commonly associated with HCM than AS), $S_4 > S_3$
    - Harsh systolic ejection murmurs (SEM) at the left lower sternal border (LLSB) or apex that does not radiate to carotids ± murmur of mitral regurgitation
      - ↓ with maneuvers that ↑ preload and systemic vascular resistance (↓ obstruction), e.g., passive leg raise, stand → squat, isometric handgrip, amyl nitrate; also, negative inotropes, vasoconstrictors, volume expansion, bradycardia
      - ↑ with maneuvers that ↓ preload and systemic vascular resistance (↑ obstruction), e.g., Valsalva maneuver, squat → stand; also, inotropes, vasodilators, diuretics/hypovolemia, tachycardia

12-Lead ECG

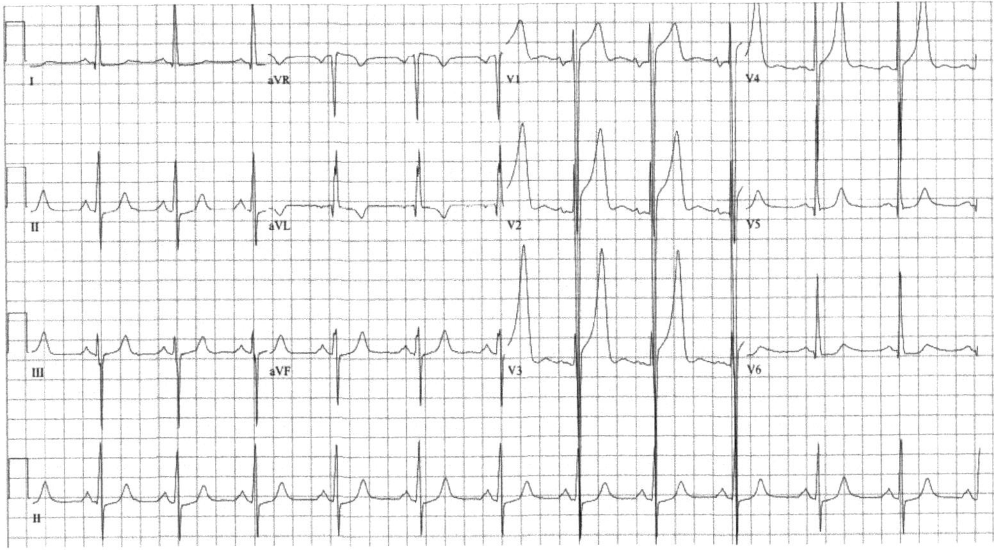

- >75% have an abnormal ECG; abnormalities may precede echo abnormalities.
  - LVH
  - LA enlargement
  - Pseudoinfarction: Deep, narrow Q waves in aVL and V6

Investigations

- Echocardiography
  - LVH: Disproportionate hypertrophy (>14 mm) ± normal or ↓ LV volume
    - Asymmetric septal hypertrophy (ASH; 60%): Septum 1.5 LV ± RV free wall
    - Also: Concentric (30%), apical (10%)
  - Left atrial enlargement
  - Mid-systolic aortic valve closure and fluttering
  - Systolic anterior motion (SAM) of anterior mitral valve leaflet (AMVL) with or without mitral regurgitation
    - Venturi effect (suction of AMVL into LVOT) vs. Forward "pushing" pressure of flow vs. AMVL
  - LVOT obstruction (mid-cavitary or outflow tract): 1/3 none, 1/3 at rest, 1/3 are provokable
    - **Resting**: Resting gradient >30 mm Hg
    - **Latent**: No obstruction at rest but gradient ↑ to >30 mm Hg after maneuvers.
    - **Provokable**: Mild obstruction at rest but gradient ↑ to >30 mm Hg post Valsalva, PVC, exercise, nitrate, or calcium-channel blocker
      - Note: Dobutamine is not preferred because it can provoke obstruction in normal individuals, leading to a "false positive."
  - Diastolic dysfunction (due to LVH)
- Exercise testing
  - 4 categories of blood pressure response:
    - Normal
    - Flat BP response: BP rise <20% from baseline
    - Hypotensive response: Initial rise then a >20 mm Hg fall from peak
    - Hypotensive response: Continuous decline
- Cardiac catheterization
  - Angiography findings include:
    - Diastolic vessel obliteration
    - May have a large septal perforator.
  - ↑ LV end-diastolic pressure with variable systolic gradient across LVOT
    - "Spike and dome" on pressure tracing
  - Brockenbrough
    - PVC → ↑ diastole → ↑ filling → ↑ wall stress → ↑ LV inotropy and contractility
    - Increased SAM and outflow obstruction with a decrease in aortic systolic and pulse pressure
- Cardiac biopsy findings include:
  - Myofibrillary disarray (pathognomonic)
  - Myocyte hypertrophy
  - Interstitial fibrosis

- Cardiac MRI
  - Evolving into an accepted risk factor for SCD, but quantitative estimates of scar burden have yet to determine clear risk cutoffs.
  - Indications
    - Suspect HCM when the echo is inconclusive.
    - Known HCM when additional information may impact management.
  - The degree of delayed enhancement is associated with a higher prevalence of:
    - Ventricular arrhythmia (NSVT and ventricular ectopy)
    - Exercise-induced arrhythmias
    - Cardiac death and possibly SCD and ICD discharge
- Genetic testing
  - The yield is 50%–70%, depending on strength of phenotype.
  - A large archive of culprit mutations is available; however, genetic information is not known to influence prognosis.
  - A major utility is screening family members to determine surveillance or discharge from follow-up.
- Electrophysiology study
  - Inducible VT: Sen 82%, Sp 68%, PPV 17%, NPV 98% for SCD
- Look for characteristics differentiating HCM from athlete's heart (see Table 14.5).

Table 14.5 Characteristics that Distinguish HCM from an Athlete's Heart

	Hypertrophic Cardiomyopathy	Athlete's/heart
Clinical	Female sex Family history of HCM	
ECG	Bizarre ECG pattern	
Echo	Unusual pattern of LVH IVSd >17 mm LV cavity < 45 mm Marked LA enlargement Abnormal LV filling (diastolic dysfunction)	Thickness decreases with deconditioning IVSd 14–17 mm LV cavity > 55 mm
Other		Max VO_2 > 45 mL/kg/min Max VO_2 >110% predicted

Management

- Screen first-degree relatives of patients with HCM.
  - Ideally, genetic screening enables discharge of 50% of at-risk family members.
  - Confirmed gene carriers should receive physical examination, ECG, and echo q2y until the age of 22 years, then q5y thereafter.
  - If no genetic test available, then first-degree relatives should receive physical examination, ECG, and echo q3–5y between the ages of 25 and 60.
- Exercise restriction:
  - **Gene carriers without phenotype**: No restriction (Bethesda 36); restricted as below (ESC)

- **Clinical phenotype**: Restricted to low-intensity/recreational sports
  - **Avoid recreational sports in which:**
    - Participation is intense and simulates competitive organized athletics.
    - Burst exertion, in which an abrupt increase in heart rate is triggered, is common.

- Relieve the obstruction (hypertrophic obstructive cardiomyopathy).
  - Avoid factors that ↑ obstruction.
  - Verapamil or β-blockers (first-line) or diltiazem or disopyramide (second-line) if symptoms persist
    - Negative inotropes with bradycardic effects
  - Dual-chamber dyssynchronous pacing
    - Theoretically ↓ obstruction by activating the RV and then the LV sequentially
    - However, no difference in symptoms, SAM or LVOT gradient (RCTs negative)
  - Alcohol septal ablation vs. surgical myomectomy:
    - Indications
      - Symptoms (class I)
        - NYHA Class 3–4 refractory to medical therapy
        - NYHA Class 2 but objective limitation (e.g., VO_2 max)
        - Exercise induced syncope
        - Gradient ≥30 mm Hg at rest or ≥60 mm Hg with exercise
      - Outcomes (class IIa)
        - Long-term mortality data only available for surgical myomectomy
        - Possibly decreases the ICD discharge rate
    - Complications
      - Perioperative mortality (0%–3% for surgery and alcohol)
      - VF (2.2%)
      - AV block (1%–2% for surgery; 10% [5%–30%] for alcohol septal ablation)
      - MI, coronary dissection (1.8%), or spasm (1.4% alcohol septal ablation)
- Sudden death risk assessment
  - Should be performed in all patients with HCM at initial evaluation (class I).
  - Should be repeated every 12 to 24 months (class IIa).
- Atrial fibrillation management:
  - Can result in sudden deterioration due to high ventricular rates and loss of atrial contraction.
    - AF in HCM is associated with increased risk of embolism, HF, and death.
  - Rate control (class I)
    - Can require high doses of β-blockers or non-dihydropyridine calcium-channel blocker (NC-CCB).
  - Rhythm control
    - Amiodarone and disopyramide are the preferred AADs (class IIa)
    - Sotalol, dofetilide, and dronedarone are second line (class IIb)
    - Radiofrequency (RF) ablation for AF (class IIa): Refractory symptoms or unable to take AADs
    - Surgical MAZE procedure with LA appendage closure (class IIa)
  - Anticoagulation is recommended for all patients (class I indication).

Complications

- Yearly mortality is ~2%–3%.
- HF occurs in 5%–10% of cases with an associated 0.5% per year mortality.
    - Initial diastolic dysfunction progresses to a
    - "Burnt-out phase" of systolic dysfunction resembling dilated cardiomyopathy
- Arrhythmia: VT, atrial arrhythmia (AF, AFL)
    - Myocyte disarray and fibrosis: Abnormal conduction with reentry
    - Hypertrophy: Heterogeneous repolarization
    - Gene mutation: Abnormal calcium handling
- Infective endocarditis (<10%)

Sudden Death and HCM

- **Epidemiology**: Overall annual mortality due to sudden death: 1%.
    - Initial peak: 1.5% per year for those <15 years
    - Quiescent period: <1% per year for those 16–65 years
    - Late peak: 2% per year for those 66–75 years
- **Etiology**
    - Fibrosis and disarray produce abnormal impulse propagation ± block, resulting in reentry.
    - Hypertrophy leads to heterogeneous repolarization, leading to abnormal impulse propagation.
    - Gene mutation causes abnormal calcium handling, which leads to abnormal impulse propagation
- **Risk stratification**
    - Secondary prevention (~10%/year appropriate ICD discharge):
        - Prior cardiac arrest or sustained VT (class I)
    - Primary prevention (~4-5%/year appropriate ICD discharge):
        - Start with "more-established" risk factors. If any are present, there is an indication for ICD therapy (class IIa).
            - Family history of premature SCD in a first-degree relative
                - Particularly ominous if multiple relatives, or when it occurs at a young age
            - Unexplained or suspected arrhythmic syncope
                - Especially if recent (within 6 months), or if it occurs at a young age (<18 years).
            - LV wall thickness ≥30 mm
                - Mortality is low for wall thickness <20 mm (2/1000 vs. 18/1000 for a septal thickness of >30 mm)
                - Particularly ominous if it occurs at a young age (<30 years).
        - Look at the "less-established" risk factors:
            - Documented non-sustained VT on Holter (definition: ≥3 beats at ≥120 bpm)
                - Particularly ominous if it occurs at young age <30 y; or with exercise
            - Abnormal BP response to exercise (class IIa)
                - Flat (increases <20 mm Hg) or hypotensive response (drops 20 mm Hg)
            - Interpretation
                - If all are absent, no ICD is required.
                - If any are present, further risk stratification is required.

- Potential risk factors
  - Late gadolinium enhancement on cardiac MRI (class IIb)
  - "High-risk", double, or compound mutations (class IIb)
  - Marked LVOT obstruction (≥30 mm Hg: class IIb)
  - Interpretation
    - If all are absent, no ICD is required (class IIb).
    - If any are present, ICD therapy is advisable (class IIa).
  - Emerging risk factors
    - **HCM morphology**: Apical aneurysm, catenoid septal morphology
    - **Multiple risk factors**: 1 RF (OR 2), 2 RF (OR 3), 3 RF (OR 6.5), 4 RF (OR 10)

- Device selection
  - Single-chamber devices are reasonable in younger patients without a need for pacing.
    - Dual-chamber devices are not associated with a reduction in inappropriate shock but are associated with more implant-related complications.
  - Dual-chamber devices are reasonable for patients with:
    - Sinus bradycardia
    - Paroxysmal AF
    - Elevated resting outflow gradients >50 mm Hg and significant heart failure symptoms who may benefit from RV pacing (most commonly, but not limited to, patients >65 years of age).
  - Subcutaneous ICD may have a role because of lead durability issues, but T-wave sensing and defibrillation threshold (DFT) concerns should lead to caution.

Key References for Further Reading

- Corrado D, Basso C, Schiavon M, Pelliccia A, Thiene G. Pre-participation screening of young competitive athletes for prevention of sudden cardiac death. *J Am Coll Cardiol.* 2008;52(24):1981–1989.
- Elliott PM, Anastasakis A, Borger MA, Borggrefe M, Cecchi F, Charron P, et al. 2014 ESC Guidelines on diagnosis and management of hypertrophic cardiomyopathy: The Task Force for the Diagnosis and Management of Hypertrophic Cardiomyopathy of the European Society of Cardiology (ESC). *Eur Heart J.* 2014;35(39):2733–2779.
- Priori SG1, Wilde AA, Horie M, Cho Y, Behr ER, Berul C, et al. HRS/EHRA/APHRS expert consensus statement on the diagnosis and management of patients with inherited primary arrhythmia syndromes: document endorsed by HRS, EHRA, and APHRS in May 2013 and by ACCF, AHA, PACES, and AEPC in June 2013. *Heart Rhythm.* 2013;(12):1932-1963.

CHAPTER

15

Syncope

UNDERSTANDING AND MANAGING SYNCOPE

Syncope is defined as a sudden, transient loss of consciousness and postural tone with spontaneous recovery.

- Incidence of syncope is 6.2/1000 person years with a 30% recurrence.
- Syncope accounts for 3% of emergency room (ER) visits and 1%–6% of hospital admissions.
- If the cause of syncope is cardiac, there is a 20% 1-year mortality rate.

Etiology

- Cardiac causes (20%)
  - Arrhythmia
    - Tachyarrhythmia: Supraventricular tachycardia (SVT), atrial fibrillation (AF)/atrial flutter (AFL), ventricular tachycardia (VT)
    - Bradyarrhythmia: Bradycardia, AV block, or bundle branch block (BBB)
  - Mechanical obstruction
    - Valvular: Aortic stenosis, pulmonary stenosis, mitral stenosis
    - Hypertrophic obstructive cardiomyopathy
    - Pump failure: MI, tamponade
    - Other: Atrial myxoma, pulmonary embolism
- Neurocardiogenic causes (60%)
  - Pathophysiology (Bezold-Jarisch reflex)
    - Peripheral venous pooling results in a drop in preload triggering a hypercontractile state. This results in mechanoreceptor stimulation (posterior-inferior LV) triggering a medullary vasodepressor brain stem reflex. This results in decreased sympathetic and increased vagal tone, leading to lower heart rate (HR), blood pressure (BP), and blood vessel tone.
  - Subtypes:
    - Carotid sinus hypersensitivity (lower BP, lower HR, or both)
    - Vasovagal syncope: "Common faint," cardioinhibitory, and vasodepressor variants
    - Situational syncope: Micturition, defecation, deglutition, cough, swallow, pain

Cardiotext Publishing, ISBN: 978-1-942909-00-2.

- Neurologic
  - Vertebrobasilar insufficiency, usually associated with dysarthria and dysphagia
  - Subarachnoid haemorrhage
  - Seizure (bicortical failure): Sudden loss of postural tone followed by tonic-clonic movements. Incontinence and post-event confusion are common.
  - Atypical migraine
- Orthostatic hypotension
  - Pathophysiology: Postural hypotension resulting in symptoms of cerebral hypoperfusion, leading to decreased effective circulating volume
  - Potential causes include:
    - Volume depletion due to hemorrhage, diuresis, diarrhea, sepsis, salt wasting, and supine hypertension
    - Hyperthyroid, diabetes (hyperglycemia), pheochromocytoma, adrenal insufficiency, diabetes insipidus (DI)
    - Venous pooling: Postural, morning, postprandial, pregnancy
- Drugs
  - Antihypertensive (sympatholytic, vasodilator, diuretic), nitrates, alcohol
  - Antidepressant (tricyclic antidepressant [TCA]), antipsychotic, anti-Parkinsonian drugs, benzodiazepines, narcotics
  - Autonomic neuropathy (diabetes mellitus, alcohol, B_{12}, amyloid, Bradbury-Eggleston, Shy-Drager)
  - Neurologic (stroke, posterior fossa tumours, upper cervical cord lesions)
- Other
  - Psychiatric: Somatization, pain, anxiety
  - Metabolic: Hypoglycemia, dumping syndrome, hypoxia, hypocapnea

Clinical

- History/physical examination is diagnostic in 40%–50% (50% of cases are undiagnosed).
- Structured history may help improve the diagnostic yield, and is evidence-based:
  - Calgary syncope score (*Eur Heart J.* 2006;3:344–350); vasovagal syncope if score ≥ –2; see Table 15.1

Table 15.1 Calgary Syncope Score

Component	Score
1. History of bifascicular block, asystole, SVT, diabetes	–5
2. History of bystanders noting a bluish skin tone during the episode	–4
3. Syncope beginning after the age of 35 years	–3
4. Do you remember anything about being unconscious	–2
5. Lightheaded spells or fainting with prolonged sitting or standing	1
6. Do you sweat or feel warm before a faint?	2
7. Do you have lightheaded spells or faint with pain or in medical settings?	3

- Age of onset
  - Young
    - Predominantly these cases are vasovagal.
    - Uncommon causes such as idiopathic VT, prolonged QT, and HCM should be considered with an atypical history.
  - Older
    - Strongly consider an arrhythmic cause.
- Number of episodes
  - Single/multiple over long period (~benign)
  - Multiple over short period (~malignant)

Table 15.2 Characteristics of Syncope Episodes that Point to Neurocardiogenic vs. Arrhythmia

	Neurocardiogenic	Arrhythmia
Triggers	Prolonged standing Pain, emotional upset, fear/anxiety CSH: Turning head, seat belt, shaving Situation: Defecation, coughing, eating, drinking	Seated or supine
Prodrome	Nausea, diaphoresis, presyncope Pallor, palpitations, visual changes	Sudden LOC without warning
Onset – Offset	Abrupt – Slow	Abrupt – Abrupt
Resolution	Immediately after lying down	
Residual symptoms	Fatigue/weakness (usually severe), nausea Diaphoresis, headache	

CSH: carotid sinus hypersensitivity; LOC: loss of consciousness.

- Medical history
  - Diabetes
  - Psychiatric disorders
  - Coronary arterial disease (CAD) (if present, then 26% chance cardiac syncope; if absent, then 24% vasovagal syncope)
- Medications/drugs (especially changes):
  - Antiarrhythmic
  - Antihypertensive
  - Recreational drugs, alcohol

Table 15.3 Differentiating Postural Orthostatic Tachycardia Syndrome (POTS) from Neurocardiogenic Syncope

POTS	Neurocardiogenic Syncope
0.2% prevalence; 80% female	37% prevalence; 55% female
15 to 50 years old, otherwise healthy	
Profoundly symptomatic • Sympathetic symptoms • Tremulousness, GI upset, fatigue, poor sleep	Usually asymptomatic • Vasodilation symptoms: Warm, flushed prodrome
Frequent lightheadedness/presyncope; rare syncope	Intermittent syncope

GI: gastrointestinal.

- Examination
  - Orthostatic vitals after the patient has been supine 2 minutes, and stands 1 minute
    - Abnormal responses:
      - Symptomatic
      - Hypotensive (BP decreases by >20/10 mm Hg)
      - Tachycardic (HR increases by <10 bpm or >30 bpm)
  - Fundoscopy, carotid bruits, carotid upstroke
  - Carotid sinus massage
    - Abnormal: >3 second pause, BP decrease >50 mm Hg or >30 mm Hg + symptoms
    - Yield improved by performing upright
  - General cardiac exam: Aortic stenosis (AS)/HCM, pulmonary stenosis (PS), mitral valve prolapse (MVP), atrial myxoma, pulmonary hypertension (HTN)

Investigations

- Investigations are directed by the findings from the history and physical examination.
- For all patients, perform the following tests:
  - **Blood**: Complete blood count (CBC), electrolytes, urea/creatinine (Cr), Mg/Ca, ABG, troponin, glucose/HbA1c, B_{12}, thyroid stimulating hormone (TSH), serum protein electrophoresis (SPEP)
    - This is a standard approach, but the yield is very low unless the history is suggestive.
  - **12-lead ECG**: Look for signs of ischemia/infarct, left ventricular hypertrophy (LVH), BBB, arterioventricular (AV) block, WPW, arrhythmogenic right ventricular cardiomyopathy (ARVC), long QT syndrome (LQTS), Brugada
  - Ambulatory monitoring
    - **24- to 48-hour Holter monitor**: For those with frequent symptoms
    - **Emerging intermediate-duration monitors**: Adhesive patch-based systems
    - **Implantable loop recorder**: For those with infrequent symptoms and negative non-invasive tests
      - Offers 3× ↑ yield over event recorder, tilt table, and electrophysiology study
  - **Echo**: LV dysfunction, atrial stenosis, HCM, cardiomyopathy (dilated cardiomyopathy [DCM], ARVC)
- Other tests to be performed as indicated:
  - **Stress test**: Ischemia, LQTS, exercise-induced arrhythmias
  - **Tilt-table testing** is most useful in patients with intermediate pre-test probability of disease.
  - **Signal averaged ECG** may identify late potentials or arrhythmic substrate (VT).
  - **EPS** is rarely indicated; may have a role in pauses, ventricular/supraventricular arrhythmias, coronary arterial disease (CAD), LV dysfunction (<40%).
  - **Adenosine** (triphosphate) 20 mg IV: pause >6 seconds or AVB >10 seconds is positive (predicts recurrent symptoms) and may predict utility of pacemakers but has limited uptake.
  - **Tests of autonomic function** (rarely used)
    - Standing time (normal >10 minutes), handgrip, (normal BP ↑ >10 mm Hg)
    - Mental arithmetic (normal BP ↑ >5 mm Hg)
    - Drug responses (atropine: heart rate [HR] ↑ >25 bpm)

Management

- ER-based risk prediction tools (San Francisco rule, Rose rules, OESIL score) are often used to determine prognosis and guide decision to admit.
  - The findings predominantly reflect comorbidity burden and the presence of heart disease.
  - No evidence shows that their use influences outcome, or that there is a preferred tool.
- Syncope units are advocated by syncope experts that reflect multidisciplinary expertise combined with rapid access to expert consultation and appropriate investigations.
  - These likely help reduce admission rates but have not been shown to influence outcome.
- Driving restrictions
  - Influenced by local jurisdictional policy
  - Consider discretionary vs. mandatory reporting environment, as well as national guidelines.
- Hospitalization
  - Underlying heart disease and risk if VT/sudden cardiac death (SCD), old age, presence of serious injury, frequent/recurrent symptoms
  - Diagnosis of a serious cardiovascular or neurologic aetiology
- Treat the underlying cause

Neurocardiogsyncope, Orthostatic Hypotension, and POTS

- Non-pharmacologic approaches include:
  - Avoid high-risk activities
  - Increase salt and water intake and avoid volume depletion.
    - Liberalize/supplement NaCl (150 mEq qam if no chronic heart failure [CHF]).
  - Avoid triggers:
    - Generally person-specific
    - May include: Heat, alcohol, prolonged standing/sitting, pain, large meals
  - Recognize prodromal symptoms
    - If present, strongly consider sitting and/or lying down.
    - Counterpressure maneuvers using isometric exercises (e.g., link arms, compress calves) may avert a syncopal episode.
- Pharmacologic agents include:
  - Volume-increasing agents:
    - Florinef (mineralocorticoid) 0.1 mg daily or bid (can increase to 1 mg/24h) ± nonsteroidal anti-inflammatory drugs (NSAIDs)
    - Side effects: Fluid retention (CHF/supine HTN), ↓ K (50%), ↓ Mg (5%)
    - Monitor: Potassium (weekly × 1 month then q2–3 months if stable), Mg
  - Sympathomimetics
    - Midodrine 2.5–10 mg tid (alpha agonist)
    - The only agent with strong evidence to support use, limited by frequent dosing
    - Side effects include supine HTN, piloerection, pruritus, paresthesia.
- **Disorder-specific approaches**:
  - Neurocardiogenic syncope
    - Reassure the patient:
      - The disorder is generally benign.
      - Rare episodes with a specific trigger do not require treatment.

- Non-pharmacologic and pharmacologic as above
    - β-blockers may be beneficial after age 42 (POST trial).
    - Selective serotonin reuptake inhibitor (SSRI) decreases serotonin release with medullary stimulation.
    - Theophylline blocks the peripheral vasodilator effects of adenosine.
- Pacemaker:
    - Generally not helpful
    - May have some benefit in patients with patients with predominantly bradycardia (see below)

- **POTS**
    - Search for other causes of tachycardia.
    - Remove stimulants, e.g., caffeine, alcohol, drugs, etc.
    - Reassurance: Benign; watchful waiting often resolves POTS.
    - Well-tolerated measures: Recumbent exercise, support hose, liberal salt/fluid, and florinef are helpful.
    - Poorly tolerated measures: These include β-blockers, calcium-channel blockers (CCBs), digoxin, midodrine, clonidine, pyridostigmine.
- **Orthostatic hypotension**
    - Address reversible causes, e.g., hypovolemia
        - Note: 500 cc of fluid will generally increase the BP 30 mm Hg for 3 hours.
    - Non-pharmacologic interventions:
        - Postural training with rising slowly from supine
        - Consider high graduated pressure stockings: Major muscle compression
    - Pharmacologic approaches:
        - Volume-increasing agents (salt, fludrocortisone) and sympathomimetics (midodrine)
        - Dopamine receptor antagonists: Domperidone, metoclopramide
        - Miscellaneous: Non-selective β-blockers, night-time vasodilation

- Pacemaker indications include:
    - Recurrent syncope
        - Secondary to spontaneous carotid sinus hypersensitivity + carotid sinus massage (CSM) causes asystole ≥3 seconds (class I)
        - Without a clear provocative event and CSM causes asystole ≥3 seconds (class IIa)
    - Recurrent neurocardiogenic syncope associated with bradycardia
        - Ideally with demonstration of spontaneous pauses ≥6 seconds or persistent bradycardia during the syncopal events (ISSUE3 trial).
        - Observations at time of tilt testing are not good predictors of spontaneous events, limiting prediction of benefit from pacemakers.
    - Undiagnosed syncope when other causes (esp. VT) have been excluded or major SN abnormalities are discovered/provoked at EPS (class IIa).

TILT TABLE TESTING

Indications

- Tilt-table testing is indicated for
  - Recurrent episodes of syncope of undetermined etiology
    - In the absence of organic heart disease
    - In the presence of organic heart disease after cardiac causes of syncope have been excluded.
  - Unexplained single syncopal episode in high-risk settings.
    - Occurrence or potential risk for physical injury or occupational hazard.
  - When deemed of clinical value to demonstrate neurocardiogenic syncope to the patient.
    - May be useful for teaching counterpressure maneuvers.

Procedure

- Patient preparation: NPO with IV fluids running at 75 mL/hour, 3-lead ECG monitor, continuous BP monitoring
- Supine equilibrium (pre-tilt phase)
  - Begin at least 5 minutes before venous cannulation is performed.
  - Connect the blood pressure (BP) and ECG prior to venous cannulation, because cannulation may induce vagal events.
  - It takes a minimum of 10 minutes after venous cannulation to come to equilibrium.
- Baseline tilt to 60°–80° (increasing angle increases sensitivity but also reduces specificity)
  - The passive phase lasts a minimum of 20 minutes and a maximum of 45 minutes.
- The drug challenge phase duration is 15 to 20 minutes if the passive phase has been negative.
  - Intravenous isoproterenol at 1–3 mcg/min
    - Aim to increase the heart rate by 20%–30% over baseline.
    - Administered with or without returning the patient to the supine position.
  - Sublingual nitro-glycerine 400 mcg spray in the upright position
- The end-point of the test is defined as:
  - Induction of syncope (positive test).
  - Completion of the planned duration of tilt, including drug provocation (negative test).

Types of Responses

- Type 1: **Mixed**
  - HR falls at the time of syncope, but not to <40 bpm, or falls to <40 bpm for <10 seconds with or without asystole of <3 seconds.
  - BP falls before the heart rate falls.
- Type 2A: **Cardioinhibition without asystole**
  - HR falls to <40 bpm for more than 10 seconds, but asystole of more than 3 seconds does not occur.
  - BP falls before the heart rate falls.
- Type 2B: **Cardioinhibition with asystole**
  - Asystole occurs for more than 3 seconds.
  - BP falls coincides with or occurs before the HR falls.

- Type 3: **Vasodepressor**
  - The HR does not fall more than 10% of its peak at the time of syncope.
  - Exception 1: Chronotropic incompetence
    - There is no HR rise during the tilt testing (i.e., <10% from the pretilt rate).
  - Exception 2: There is an excessive HR rise (POTS)
    - An excessive HR rise (i.e., >130 bpm) both at the onset of the upright position and throughout its duration before syncope.

Interpretation of Tilt Table Testing

- Interpretation varies depending upon the clinical setting.
  - Patients without structural heart disease:
    - Tilt testing can be considered diagnostic (particularly if positive).
    - No further tests need to be performed when spontaneous syncope is reproduced.
  - Patients with structural heart disease
    - Arrhythmias and other cardiac causes of syncope should be excluded before considering the response to positive tilt test as evidence of neurocardiogenic syncope.

Caveats

- The upright tilt table test has limited specificity, sensitivity, and reproducibility.
  - Structured histories are considered better tools than tilt testing by most syncope experts.
- The hemodynamic response to upright tilt testing may differ from the hemodynamic mechanism of spontaneous syncopal episodes.

INDEX